Russia's Torn Safety Nets

Health and Social Welfare during the Transition

Edited by

Mark G. Field and Judyth L. Twigg

St. Martin's Press
New York

ISBN 0-312-22916-X

Library of Congress Cataloging-in-Publication Data

Russia's torn safety nets : heath and social welfare during the transition /
Mark G. Field
and Judyth L. Twigg, editors.
    p. cm.
  Includes bibliographical references and index.
  ISBN 0-312-22916-X
  1. Russia (Federation)—Social conditions—1991–   2. Quality of
life—Russia (Federation)
3. Medical care—Russia (Federation).   I. Field, Mark G. (Mark George)
II. Twigg, Judyth L.
HN530.2.A8 R869   2000
306'.0947—dc21 99–055563

Designed by Letra Libre, Inc.

First published: April 2000
10 9 8 7 6 5 4 3 2 1

CONTENTS

PART II. SOCIAL ISSUES

PART III. REPLACING THE SAFETY NET?

LIST OF TABLES AND FIGURES

This volume is dedicated to the memory of Stephen P. Dunn, a person of great courage who, in spite of formidable personal obstacles, devoted his life to understanding the Russians as people rather than as abstractions.

CHAPTER 1

Introduction

Mark G. Field and
Judyth L. Twigg

MORE THAN 40 YEARS AGO, IN A PAPER ENTITLED "Ten Theories in Search of Soviet Reality: The Prediction of Soviet Behavior in the Social Sciences," Daniel Bell wrote:

> Surely, more has been written about the Russian Revolution and the ensuing forty years of Soviet rule than about any comparable episode in human history. The bibliography of items on the French Revolution occupies, it is said, one wall of the Bibliotheque Nationale. A complete bibliography on the Soviet Union—which is yet to be compiled and may never be because of the geometric rate at which it multiplies—would make that earlier cenotaph to scholarship shrink the way in which the earlier tombs diminished before the great complex at Karnak.

He continues by exclaiming: "And yet how little of this awesome output has stood the test of so short a span of time!"[1] Bell penned these lines when the West, and particularly the United States, was obsessed with what made the Soviets (or the Russians, since in those days the terms were synonymous) "tick" and how to predict what they would do next.

One shudders to contemplate how much more has been written about the USSR in the 40 years that have elapsed since Bell wrote these lines, and again how little has stood the test of time. For example, in the billions of words that have poured out of Sovietologists and Kremlinologists, how many predicted, or even hinted, at the collapse of the Soviet Union in December 1991? There is no doubt that a great number of accurate studies were made about the nature of the Soviet system, its economy, and its political structure. And yet, how much did we understand the texture of Soviet life: the grittiness of apartment houses that were decaying even before tenants moved in; the crowding of communal housing, where several families had to share facilities; the constant shortages and the ubiquitous lines at the stores that dispensed the basics; the contrast between the bombast of the propaganda and the shabbiness of existence; and thus the everyday experiences of its millions of citizens, particularly the fate of those who lived on the margins: the weak, sick, crippled, homeless, or discriminated against because of their gender, religion, or nationality. Indeed, Sergei Khrushchev, emphasizing that his father wanted to improve housing, has left us a graphic description of living conditions:

> In Russia, several generations . . . grandparents, their children and grandchildren, ten or more people, might be cooped up in one room of 150 square feet. They slept on the floor. In the morning long lines formed for the only toilet at the end of a hall with doors to a dozen similarly overpopulated rooms. It is hard to describe in words what it's like to stand in such a line; it has to be experienced.[2]

The collapse of the Soviet Union was indeed a revolution, but fortunately a bloodless one. It generated extraordinary hopes among the population: the new regime, an "antimodel" of socialism, would solve the many problems that had plagued the previous system by introducing several features of capitalism, including a market system and privatization, and a decentralization of governmental activities and responsibilities that amounted to a devolution of political power toward the regions. This would be followed by the creation of a new infrastructure and new institutions that would reinforce the foundation of democracy, and the creation of a civil society that would replace the many functions performed earlier by the Communist Party.

It did not quite work out this way. The transition from socialism to a protocapitalistic system produced a series of "unintended consequences," exacerbated many of the problems that existed in the prior era, and created new ones that constitute the core of the crisis of Russian society at the end of the 1990s. The major purpose of this collection of essays is to shed some light on the human costs of this transition, and particularly to illuminate the shredding of the safety nets that existed under the Soviet regime, safety nets that depended on the workings of the state. This phenomenon was well illustrated by Janine Wedel when she wrote that under the Soviets private enterprise had been virtually eliminated and that "entire communities of workers had been created around state-run enterprises. These 'company towns,' guaranteeing not only lifetime employment but also housing, social security, and health and day care, exemplified a slice of socialist life." She goes on to note that in "transforming these 'white elephants' [state-owned enterprises] . . . [the aim was] to drive a silver stake through the heart of socialism."[3] The "silver stake" has indeed slain socialism, and at the same time, it has also destroyed or severely affected the vast array of social services that socialism offered, and for which privatization and the market have failed to provide functional substitutes, at least until now. Thus the social contract that was struck between the state and the people under the communist regime has been to a large extent abrogated, leading to what some have called "state desertion," and leaving millions of people stranded in despair, poverty, and destitution. It has been estimated that the top 10 percent of the population possess half of the nation's wealth, and the bottom 40 percent less than 20 percent of that wealth. Somewhere around 40 or more million people live below the poverty line, currently defined at about $30 per month. Privatization has also led to a flight of capital abroad estimated at $200–500 billion, paralleling a stark decrease in production, both industrial and agricultural, and thus a decline of the gross domestic product.[4] The famous, and now notorious, "shock therapy" became more shock than therapy, leading to political instability, corruption, and criminalization at the highest levels of government.

It is perhaps the realization that the market cannot do it all, as was believed in the early phase of the transition, that is one of the more intriguing aspects of the postcommunist period. Certainly in many instances, the market is more efficient than the command economy. Frederick von Hayek, for example, argued that the price system is an efficient means to send signals throughout the economy, adding that "the marvel is that in a case like that of a scarcity of one raw material, without an order being issued . . . tens of thousands of people whose identity could not be ascertained by months of investigation are made to use the material . . . more sparingly, that is, they move in the right direction."[5] And it is certainly true that the adjustment of supply and demand in a market situation is much more efficient than the command economy, as is illustrated by the parable of the potatoes and the sack. Briefly, the task is to fit as many potatoes as possible into a sack, or, conversely, to reduce waste space to a minimum. The command economy solution would be to assign each potato an ordinal number, then measure and make a profile of each one, and with a team of specialists and computers match each potato to a mate so that the waste space is at its irreducible minimum. The other solution would be to toss the potatoes into the sack and shake vigorously. The difference in waste space would be around 5–10 percent, but the procedure immensely cheaper than the command economy solution—a solution adopted by Soviet central planners at enormous cost in terms of lost efficiency and productivity, squandering of scarce resources, and almost complete inattention to product quality and assortment and consumer demand.

And yet the market also needs, in most instances, a strong government and regulatory system in order to operate effectively, backed by respect for property rights and a legal structure and enforcement mechanisms that are beyond corruption. These elements are mostly lacking in today's Russia. But perhaps of even greater moment is the fact that the market is not equipped to handle many aspects of private and public life. This is the case before us in Russia: its major safety nets have been torn by privatization and the market, as well as by the downsizing and crippling of the public sector and the of role of government in providing services that the private sector is unable, unwilling, or not geared to give, for example, public health services. As a result, it is not surprising that there is in Russia a certain nostalgia for some aspects of the Soviet system, with its support (however meager it might have been) for many of these safety nets and for the predictability of life under the Soviet type of socialism, a nostalgia that has political implications. In other words, with all of its fatal flaws, the Soviet system did institutionalize among the population certain expectations about the legitimate role of the state, expectations that are now being frustrated on a large scale. This tension will remain as long as those who grew up under the Soviet regime constitute the majority of the population.

The contributors to this volume detail the consequences of the collapse of the Soviet mechanisms of state support on which so many millions had come to rely. In the first section on health issues, the authors examine the varied aspects of health and demographic dilemmas so severe that Russian commentators and government officials have designated them a matter of national security. Mark G. Field begins with an assessment of the broad dimensions of the health and demographic situation, arguing that although the crisis finds its roots as far back at the 1960s, matters have been sharply exacerbated by the Soviet collapse. The term *katastroika,* as Field points out, was coined originally by A. Zinoviev during *perestroika* to capture the essence of increased mortality rates and declining birth rates, the former due not only to a crescendo of infectious and degenerative diseases but also, and in some instances even primarily, to increased rates of homicides, suicides, traffic and industrial accidents, and the like.[6] The immediate and longer-term consequences of these trends include declining economic productivity and therefore, among other things, a reduced capacity of society to support the increasing numbers of those in need. Judyth Twigg's chapter observes that a lack of funds, as in many other sectors of the Russian economy, hinders the state's ability to tackle even the most pressing health concerns. She argues that, although a new system of national compulsory medical insurance has channeled some new resources toward hospitals, clinics, and public health services, the legacy of the inefficient, gross output–oriented Soviet health care system continues to prevent the deep structural reorganizations and reforms that would be necessary to put the still meager resources at hand to effective use. In other words, money is a necessary but not sufficient condition for repair of Russian health care.

Julie Brown and Nina Rusinova examine one major set of participants in any health care system, the patients. Drawing on extensive survey research performed in St. Petersburg throughout the 1990s, Brown and Rusinova paint a bleak picture, identifying who has fallen through the torn medical safety nets, and how this has taken place. Their surveys reveal that more and more people are being required routinely to pay for their supposedly "free" medical care; that those in the poorest health are also frequently those suffering the most from low and declining living standards; and that, in sum, many or most Russians would list "getting sick" as one of their greatest fears, largely due to their limited understanding of the evolving Russian medical marketplace and their limited resources for navigating it. Kate Schecter focuses on another aspect of Russia's decaying health care system—the medical profession itself. She observes that Russian physicians suffer from an inability, rooted in Soviet tradition, to unite against the many hardships that have been imposed upon them by the socialist-to-capitalist transition. In particular, the fact that the vast majority of Russian physicians are women, coupled with the post-Soviet degradation of women's status in society, have made the burdens of the transition particularly deeply felt by Russia's physicians.

The large and growing numbers of Russian drug addicts and abusers are discussed in John Kramer's essay. He demonstrates that the collapse of the Soviet state greatly diminished the capacity of state authorities to combat the problems of illicit drug use, trafficking, and indigenous production. The irony, he points out, is that it is the positive elements of the decline and fall of the Soviet Union— the opening of borders and freeing of the population from police-state control—that have paved the way for the drug problem to accelerate. David Powell addresses a related problem, the rise in Russia of HIV and AIDS, which of course has spread in tandem with intravenous drug use among Russian citizens. Today, it is primarily the behavior of IV drug users and their sexual partners that is responsible for a looming AIDS crisis, although a substantial proportion of the spread of the disease is also due to heterosexual and homosexual activity among non–drug users, particularly prostitutes. Efforts to quell the emerging tidal wave of HIV in Russia have suffered from a lack of funds for treatment and prevention, and from continuing societal taboos against discussing many aspects of the disease. According to Powell, if this situation is not addressed promptly and effectively, Russia will find AIDS to constitute a form of "self-induced genocide." Finally, Ethel Dunn, in her chapter on the disabled in Russia, describes how popular misunderstanding and shunning of people with disabilities continues to plague this unfortunate segment of the population. Government funding to address their wide array of problems is limited, and education and training programs still suffer from stereotypes and misdiagnoses that result in potentially effective contributors to society being left isolated and ignored. Dunn also details the degree to which some groups of disabled Russians, particularly veterans of the Soviet conflict with Afghanistan, have achieved limited success in calling attention and resources toward their plight through political mobilization, but suggests that most efforts in this regard have been ineffective.

The second section of the book expands beyond health to a wider array of social issues, all of which have similarly suffered from the collapse of the Soviet safety net infrastructure. Valerie Sperling begins with a discussion of what she terms an "explosion of overt sexism" in post-Soviet Russia. The Soviet image of women as full and equal citizens has vanished, she argues, having been displaced by a political system in which women participants are routinely denigrated, an economic situation in which women have been disproportionately affected by rising unemployment and overt on-the-job sexual harassment, and a new media culture that thrives on a portrayal of women as little but objects of sexual desire and gratification. Walter Connor turns to issues of work and labor, demonstrating that the Soviet legacy of "false" full employment has now resulted in both hidden unemployment (in the form of enterprises that continue to pay, or pretend to pay, workers who have no productive work to do) and hidden employment (in the form of people and firms who do not report performed work, income, and profit, primarily for reasons of tax evasion). Connor also discusses the ineffective nature of strikes, mostly symbolic gestures with no real power, as a tool of organized labor in the post-Soviet period, and the equally ineffective status of post-Soviet labor and trade unions.

Justin Burke's chapter describes the large number of ethnic and national groups affected, most adversely, by forced and reluctant migration and repatriation since the Soviet collapse. He points out that in many cases it is the newly dire socio-economic conditions in the more remote regions of Russia—regions that were heavily subsidized and supported in Soviet times—that have prompted many people to leave their homes. Burke also outlines the plight of the pockets of ethnic Russians who now find themselves a disenfranchised minority in many parts of the former Soviet Union. Victoria Velkoff and Kevin Kinsella turn to the social implications of the aging of Russia, echoing and expanding on many of the themes earlier composed by Mark Field. They detail regional patterns of demographic shifts, gender differentials (including high rates of widowhood), and living arrangements among the elderly. Their ultimate argument rests on the immediate and future need for restored safety nets in order to service the demands of this growing part of the population. Cynthia Buckley and Dennis Donahue continue with a discussion of perhaps the most basic and important of these demands: pensions. They observe that the Soviet pension system was one of the more iron-clad parts of the social safety net, one that is now in trouble as Russia can find neither the money to match the guarantees provided by the old system, nor the political where-withal to implement the structural reforms necessary to render the system more efficient and effective. This section concludes with Deborah Ball's assessment of the Russian military as a microcosm of the social ills affecting society as a whole. While the Soviet military included as one of its basic tasks the appropriate socialization of the country's younger generation, the Russian armed forces—having suffered from over a decade of institutional decay and ne-glect—lack the capacity to continue this mission. Instead, the ranks of the armed forces suffer from a declining quality of the draft co-hort, rampant drug abuse and sexually transmitted disease, and in-creases in violent crime, including systematic and severe "hazing"-type abuse of young conscripts. Ball observes that it is un-likely, despite grandiose intentions, that the military will in the foreseeable future be able to resume its previous function of educa-tion and indoctrination.

Finally, the last section of the volume deals with attempts to re-store the most urgent and desirable elements of the old Soviet safety net, attempts that have largely involved foreign aid of various kinds. Edward J. Burger's essay on health-related assistance from the West, and particularly the United States, dismisses these attempts as largely ineffective. Drawing on examples of more successful postwar aid programs to Latin America and Greece, Burger argues that for-eign aid to specific social sectors in Russia cannot succeed outside of a larger, more coherent and consistent foreign aid and foreign policy strategy toward Russia. This strategy has been sorely lacking. He points out that many Western aid programs have failed because they have treated Russia as a tabula rasa on which existing Western mod-els can be imposed, without sufficient consideration of the crucially important Soviet experience and context within which the "reform-ers" are working.

Collectively, these chapters make the case that, while nobody would want to return to the Soviet Union of personal restrictions, closed media, labor camps, and uniformly shoddy industrial output, it is important to recognize that Soviet socialism provided important social benefits which protected the vast majority of the population from abject misery and poverty. Now those benefits have either diminished or disappeared, and people are left to fend for themselves to a degree seldom required even in the most "free" market economies in the world. The irony, which is a key theme running throughout many of these chapters, is that it is the very legacy of that Soviet system that now hinders the building of effective post-Soviet institutions that might ease these social burdens. Despite its inherent difficulties, the task now standing before Russia is to create a humane capitalism, a task that will centrally involve the repair and restoration of those key safety nets, in order to give even society's weakest and most disadvantaged the opportunity and tools to compete in and contribute to the new market economy and society.

NOTES

1. Daniel Bell, "Ten Theories in Search of Soviet Reality," *World Politics* 10 (April 1958): 327–356.
2. Sergei Khrushchev, "The Cold War through the Looking Glass," *American Heritage,* October 1999, 40.
3. Janine Wedel, *Collision and Collusion: The Strange Case of Western Aid to Eastern Europe* (New York: St. Martin's Press, 1998), 49 and 50–51.
4. Some of these statistics on income distribution, poverty, and capital flight were taken from John Lloyd, "The Russian Devolution," *The New York Times Magazine,* 15 August 1999, 34–62.
5. Frederick von Hayek, *The Road to Serfdom,* cited in James K. Glassman, "How Nations Prosper: Markets, Government, and the Culture of Capitalism," *Harvard Magazine,* July-August 1998, 23.
6. Michael Ellman, "The Increase in Death and Disease under 'Katastroika'," *Cambridge Journal of Economics* 18 (1994): 329–355.

PART I

Health Issues

CHAPTER 2

The Health and Demographic
Crisis in Post-Soviet Russia:
A Two-Phase Development

Mark G. Field

AMONG THE MANY SCOURGES THAT ARE HAUNTING post-Soviet Russia
is a health and demographic crisis of major proportions, with ominous implications reaching into the third millennium. Indeed, the
health of the population has been one of the major casualties of the
collapse of the Soviet regime, and of the transition to a new political and economic system, although the crisis had its origins considerably earlier, in the 1960s. The major aspects of that crisis consist
of a yearly decrease in the size of the population, stagnant or decreased life expectancy, increased premature mortality, the return of
infectious diseases, rising morbidity, a degradation of the environment, and practically every other index related to the well-being of
the population, including a length of life differential between the
sexes in favor of women unprecedented in peace time and unique in
the world in its magnitude. Since 1994 there have been some improvements as the population adjusts to the new conditions, although it is too early to determine whether this trend will continue,

given the renewed shocks caused by the economic crash of August 1998.

The major purpose of this paper is to relate the nature and the dimensions of the health and demographic crisis to the turmoil that is gripping Russia today, but that began in the mid-1960s and was exacerbated by the collapse of the Soviet regime at the end of 1991. In essence, as pointed out by Meslé and Shkolnikov,[1] this was a two-phase crisis (1960s to 1991, and 1992 to the present). Although references will be made to the statistical and quantitative evidence that must necessarily undergird any such enterprise, the major approach of this chapter is qualitative. It is an attempt to understand an extraordinarily complex phenomenon that some have dubbed *katastroika,*[2] that is, both a reflection of past events and a harbinger of future problems. It stands to reason, for instance, that a significant decrease in the birth rate at a certain point in time will have a reverberating impact in the years to follow, as that cohort ages. It will mean a decrease in the number of students in the schools and universities, later on in the availability of the work and armed forces, in the number of children born when that cohort reaches adulthood, in the dependency ratio, i.e., the number of those working and producing the wealth of the society, and those (children, students, the unemployed, the handicapped, and the retired and elderly) who to some degree must be supported by the "active" population. A high mortality rate among the adult population or a segment of that population will affect the socialization and support of children and adolescents, may increase the number of orphans or single-parent families, and creates special dependency burdens for society and nation. Thus the nature of a population as a mirror of both past events and present conditions will produce "echoes" in the future.

Population Dynamics

A population is in a constant state of metabolism or change as newborns join it and those who die leave it. It is the balance between these two events that determine the "natural" growth, the steady state, or the decline of a population. But they are not the only factors in population dynamics. A population is also affected by immigration and emigration of people (the functional equivalents of births and deaths). And finally, one should also consider the acquisition or loss of territory and its population. Migration and territorial changes lead to a shifting of already living populations. Most fundamental, of course, is the production or reproduction of people through births, and their loss through deaths.

Russian Population Dynamics

One of the major aspects of the Russian health and demographic crisis is that since 1992, the year Russia started as an independent country after the collapse of the Soviet Union, the population has been in a state of decline as deaths surpass births. The natural population decline is of the order of 0.4–0.6 percent annually. In numerical terms, in 1980 the annual increase in population was about one million; by 1989 that figure was cut by half; in 1991 it was only 224,600; and in 1993 the number of deaths exceeded births by 750,400, making Russia the first industrial nation to experience such a sharp decrease in its population for reasons other than war, famine, or disease.[3] In 1995, the excess of deaths was 840,000. At the end of July 1999, the Russian government reported that during the first five months of that year, the population dropped by 346,700 persons, whereas in the corresponding time period for 1998, the decrease was 191,600, perhaps a reflection of the meltdown in the economy in August 1998.[4] It is therefore not surprising that projections into the future are bleak and raise the specter of depopulation. The situation, logically, resembles that of withdrawing more money from a bank account than depositing. Eventually there would not be any left, particularly since this process would accelerate in time as the result of compound interest (as a population [capital] decreases so does the number of potential parents and of children [interest] born to them).

The decrease was the result of two simultaneous phenomena, each of about the same magnitude: a decline in births, an increase in deaths. Births went down by *two-thirds* between 1988 and 1994. "Women are afraid nowadays to give birth," said Tamara Gorbunova, chief physician of Moscow's Maternity Hospital No. 25. "It's enough to walk down the street to understand why . . . we are dealing with an economic problem."[5] And add to this that women die in childbirth from five to ten times as often as their counterparts in the West. In the years between 1985 and 1996, the crude birth rate dropped from 16.7 per 1,000 population to 14.6 in 1989, 9.4

in 1993,[6] and 8.8 in 1996.[7] Between 1990 and 1995, 9,522,000 infants were born, whereas 9,985,000 would have been born if the birth rate obtaining in 1989 had remained constant.[8] This represents a shortfall of 463,000 births (13.6 percent). In the Soviet period, the use of contraceptives was limited, and women resorted to abortions as the major birth control measure. In 1988, the proportion of women 15–49 who used oral contraceptives was insignificant, 1.2 percent, and intrauterine devices 12.4 percent. Since then these proportions have steadily increased: in 1994 they were 3.7 percent and 19.8 percent, respectively.[9] These figures may well be conservative. Nonetheless abortions continue to play an important role in birth control now, as they did in the past. Since 1970 (with the exception of 1985) the number of officially registered abortions exceeded the number of births by a factor of more than two. In 1993, for instance, there were 234.9 abortions per 100 live births; in 1994 the figure was 217.02. But these were only the registered procedures. If to these we add those unregistered terminations, the estimate is well over three abortions per live birth, perhaps as many as four. It may be expected, however, that as means of birth control beside abortion become more available, the number of abortions will decline, and there are some preliminary indications to that effect.[10]

In order to assess the significance of these figures on the population and its reproduction, one can use the fertility index, which is the average number of children women bring into the world per lifetime. This then yields the net reproduction index, i.e., the degree to which each death is replaced by one birth. In order to have a reproduction index of 1, or zero population growth, it is necessary for women to bear slightly over two children per lifetime. A survey of Russian men and women about their ideas of the "ideal, wished for, and expected number of children" for the years 1991–1995 showed that the "expected" number was well below 2, i.e., below reproduction (see table 2.1).

Furthermore, the increased proportion of births that are illegitimate, and particularly those births to women in their teens, has led to an increase of low-weight births, and to the problems that these newborns and infants will face in their early years. In 1970, 10.6 percent of births were illegitimate (9.6 percent for the urban population, 13.4 percent for the rural population). Since then that percentage has steadily increased and stood at double the 1970 figure

Table 2.1 Ideal, Wished-For, and Expected Number of Children, for Men and Women, Russia, 1991–1995

| | Number of Children | | | | | | | | | | | |
| | Ideal | | | | Wished-For | | | | Expected | | | |
Sex	1991	1992	1994	1995	1991	1992	1994	1995	1991	1992	1994	1995
Men	2.02	1.59	2.04	2.01	2.22	1.94	1.63	1.89	1.68	1.41	1.09	1.60
Women	2.21	1.45	2.00	2.16	2.29	1.93	1.68	2.01	1.94	1.30	1.08	1.56
Both sexes	2.10	1.53	2.02	2.12	2.25	1.96	1.65	1.95	1.77	1.33	1.08	1.58

Source: Naselenie Rossii 1996: 86.

in 1995, or 21.1 percent (21.0 percent for the urban population, 21.3 percent for the rural one.)[11] Single mothers (and many of them are teenagers) are usually at a disadvantage emotionally, psychologically, and financially to provide a healthy environment for their children. Motherhood also often prevents them from pursuing a career or even holding a job. The child, often unwanted, runs the risk of abandonment, institutionalization, poverty, and psychological problems, and the temptation to engage in antisocial and criminal behavior.[12] There is increased evidence of homeless children and the inability of the state to provide for them.

Projections into the future confirm the bleak picture of a population in decline. These are essentially guesses based on a series of assumptions: they are usually expressed in "optimistic," "middle," and "pessimistic" terms and, of course, the more distant into the future the projection, the less the degree of accuracy. On January 1, 1996, the Russian population was 147,976,000. An optimistic 1996 projection by the State Committee on Statistics of the Russian Federation forecast for the year 2000 a figure of 146,500,000; the pessimistic estimate was 144,300,000. For the year 2010 the projections are 147,600,000 and 133,600,000 respectively, in every case lower than the figure for 1996.[13] Without immigration from other parts of the former Soviet empire the figures would be even bleaker. Moving to the middle of the twenty-first century, the State Statistical Committee predicted in December 1998 that by that time the population would shrink by one-half.[14]

The decrease in births has been accompanied by a steep increase in deaths. For example, the crude mortality rose from 11.3 per 1,000 population in 1985 to 11.4 in 1991, 14.5 in 1993, and 15.4 in 1994. After that it declined slightly, to 14.3 in 1996.[15] In the first nine months of 1993 Moscow saw two-and-a-half times as many deaths as births; in St. Petersburg the ratio was nearly three deaths to one birth.[16] Such discrepancies were last seen during the German invasion of Russia in World War II, and the siege of Leningrad.[17] As a matter of fact, in the next century the city could simply die out, and according to Vladimir Yesipov, "only migration from other regions can save St. Petersburg."[18] What is significant is that mortality has risen particularly among the younger male population.

One of the aspects of the increase in mortality, especially adult mortality, has been a dramatic decrease in life expectancy (at birth and other ages), and again particularly for men. Life expectancy at birth for males was 64 years in 1989; it declined to 63.5 in 1991, and by an incredible three years between 1992 (62 years) and 1993 when it reached a low of 59 years. The decline continued until 1994 when male life expectancy went down to 57.5 years, so that Russian men lived shorter lives than their counterparts in Indonesia, the Philippines, and certain parts of Africa. Higher death rates for men could be found only in very poor underdeveloped third world countries. Although female life expectancy has also decreased, the decline has been much smaller and the amplitudes of the changes much smoother. As a matter of fact, female life expectancy has been stagnant compared to the declining male life expectancy, as we shall see below.

It is also noteworthy that infant mortality, a proxy index of well-being and of medical care, increased during the first phase of the health crisis. But during the second phase, while adult male mortality increased and life expectancy decreased, infant mortality tended, as we shall see below, to decline. For instance, it went from 22.1 per 1,000 population in 1989, to 18.6 in 1994, and 17.0 in 1997 (preliminary figures). This should alert us to the different nature of the health crisis after 1991, and to the impact on health and mortality of the transition crisis and of what has been generally termed "shock therapy."

It is therefore not surprising that this "negative increase" with all its implications for the future has caused anxiety, and has been seized as a political issue by conservatives as an indictment of the policies of the Yeltsin government and what has been called the neo-liberal policy pursued by Russia since 1992.[19] What Russia may be dealing with, as suggested by Aleksander Prokhanov, is homicide on a large scale, adding, "I don't think when you are killing off a half million men every year [that] it is unfair to call it genocide."[20] Though to some extent hyperbolic and meant to be provocative if not alarming, Prokhanov captures the essence of the crisis, particularly in the light of the continued inertia by the Duma and the Russian government about the health of the population.[21] That perennial prophet of doom Aleksandr Solzhenitsyn weighed in when he wrote in 1993 that "Russia lies utterly ravaged and poisoned . . . its people are on the brink of perishing physically . . . perhaps even biologically."[22] But what these commentators conveniently forget is that there also was an excess of deaths before the collapse of the Soviet Union. Excess deaths or premature mortality means deaths that under "normal circumstances" would not have occurred,[23] as is the case, for instance, of male deaths during a war. Thus between 1975 and 1985, there were among men aged 20–50 an excess of deaths of about 1.6 million, the equivalent of the combined losses among the military and civilian populations during World War II of Great Britain, the United States, and France. This is "1.6 million Russians," as Vishnevskii put it, "sons, husbands many of whom could have been alive today because preserving their lives did not enter into the priority of their time."[24]

Nineteen ninety-two was a critical year, since it marked not only the beginning of the Russian Federation as an independent state, but also the time when the population began to decline, as we noted earlier. For the first time since World War II, the parallel curves of higher births than deaths intersected and assumed a "scissors" configuration.

It might then be tempting to trace the beginning of the health and demographic crisis to that moment, and to the momentous upheavals caused by the transition from a command economy to a pre- or protocapitalistic, market and democratic system. But the crisis had its origins in the mid-1960s, for reasons we will examine in some detail below. The first inkling the West had of a problem was the unexpected rise in mortality, and particularly, at first, infant mortality, at the end of the 1960s.

Phase 1 (mid-1960s–1991)

Writing in 1983, eight years before the collapse of the regime, Roland Pressat, a French demographer, remarked that "one has never seen, in peace time, a regression of health conditions (as can be measured by mortality) on such a scale."[25] A few years later, a Russian sociologist, commenting on the social and economic polarization taking place in postcommunist Russia, observed that about 90 percent of the population lived below the poverty line (the subsistence minimum) and added, "History has never seen such a decline in living standards during peacetime."[26] In 1994, Lee Hockstader wrote that "Russia is facing . . . demographic and public health crises virtually unprecedented in peace time."[27] What these comments have in common, and they are far from unique, is a sense of astonishment at demographic indices characteristic of a wartime situation, and thus not only unprecedented but unexpected in peacetime. But was it really peacetime?

It was in fact *wartime,* although only a Cold War, which the Soviet Union eventually lost, and which helps to account not only for the deterioration of health and demographic indices after the mid-1960s but also for an impoverishment and demoralization of the population after 1991 of the type usually associated with a lost conflict, a search for scapegoats, and a sense of national humiliation as in the Weimar Republic. Slobodan Vitanovic has argued most cogently about the existence of such a war:

> It would be a great error to think that the Third World War has been avoided. It took place and it was long. The particularity of that war consists in the fact that it was political, ideological and first of all, economic. Fortunately there were no combats, but if the weapons were not for this time utilized, they were being constantly produced, and military expenditures have surpassed those of all preceding wars. . . . If the Third World War has been political, ideological, and particularly economic, victory, or seen from the other side, capitulation was of the same type.[28]

One may surmise that the beginning of the crisis was the Cuban episode of the early 1960s, which the Soviets apparently considered a defeat and loss of national prestige, the result of one of Khrushchev's "hare-brained" schemes. After his removal in 1964, the succeeding (Brezhnev) regime apparently decided to engage in a national defense buildup to establish and maintain military and nuclear parity (if not superiority) to the United States, and this with a gross national product several times smaller than its adversary. From 1952 to 1959, according to CIA estimates, the annual percentage increase in Soviet defense spending was 0.4. From 1960 to 1969 that figure jumped to 5.7 (more than 14 times). In 1970 to 1974, it was 3.3, then tapering down to 1.3 from 1975 to 1984, rebounding to 4.3 in 1985 to 1987, then decreasing drastically in the latter part of the Gorbachev regime to -0.4 (1988–1900).[29] Khrushchev's son, Sergei, has written that "the leaders who replaced Father hurried to 'correct his mistakes' by giving a new impetus to the arms race and producing tens of thousands of tactical nuclear weapons. By 1989 the Soviet army had seven thousand nuclear cannon. The Cold War was prolonged by twenty years."[30] The expenditures for the Soviet military-industrial complex, including the very expensive space and moon race[31] (with its military aspects and prestige overtones) must have strained the already meager resources available for the civilian sector in the classical conflict between guns and butter, the latter including, in particular, the support of the major safety nets bearing on the health and the well-being of the population, including such items as medical care and public health, housing, child care, and the environment. And, except for the military-industrial complex, the Brezhnev years have also been characterized as the years of stagnation and of a decaying economy.

When Gorbachev came to power in 1985 he was surprised at the proportion of national resources devoted to defense. In his *Memoirs* he wrote:

> We ... were aware of how heavily our exorbitant military expenditures weighed on the economy, but I did not realize the true scale of militarization of the country until I became General Secretary.... Although the leaders of the military-industrial complex opposed it, we published those data.... Military expenditure was not 16% of the state budget ... but rather 40%.... It was not 6% but 20% of the Gross National Product. Of 25 billion rubles in total expenditures on science, 20 billion went to the military for technical research and development.[32]

And at the prestigious Academy of Sciences basic science research institutes, 60 percent of efforts were devoted to developing innovations geared toward military projects.[33] Expenditures of human and material resources on armaments provide, it is assumed, a sense of security against potential attacks by an aggressor, and yet, paradoxically, they also deprive the very population they "protect" of the means that otherwise could be used for their welfare, health, and general well-being. This has been called, metaphorically, "buying death with taxes."[34] The "costs" of national defense have never been better articulated than by President Eisenhower early in his presidency:

> Every gun that is made, every warship launched, every rocket fired, signifies, in the final sense, a theft from those who hunger and are not fed, those who are cold and are not clothed. The world in arms is not spending money alone. It is spending the sweat of its laborers, the genius of its scientists, the hopes of its children.... We pay for a single destroyer with new homes that

could have housed more than 8,000 people. . . . Under the cloud of threatening war, it is humanity hanging from a cross of iron.[35]

What this meant for the Soviet Union, in terms of daily life, is illustrated from 1981 secret police documents describing how the population felt about food shortages. Otto Latsis reports:

> . . . and how could the people understand why we worked and sweated for a pittance, and for a pittance we could not buy any-thing . . . this for decades after the end of the war. . . . It is possi-ble to subsist without a market for a few years during a war as resorted to by many countries. But only we managed in the course of a half century . . . to preserve a command system that devoted a proportion of its resources to war: almost two-thirds of the ma-chine building industry worked for defense . . . [first we had coupons for produce], then coupons without produce, then the disappearance of all goods.[36]

An evaluation of the impact of these conditions on the gradual impoverishment and health of the population is difficult, particu-larly because, a few years after the indices began their downward slide, the Soviet regime imposed an embargo on the publication of many vital statistics in the fear that they might expose its demo-graphic "weaknesses" to the world. According to demographer Leonid Rybakovsky, in 1976 the Party Central Committee created a "Commission on the Non-Publication of Data." At one meeting of the commission, a general stated that "we must not reveal the num-ber of boys born in the Soviet Union. Our enemies could use this in-formation. We must make it a state secret."[37]

This statement was made in 1976. But the first inkling the West had that something was amiss was the unexpected rise in infant mor-tality in the early 1970s.[38] Infant mortality, as mentioned earlier, is also usually seen as a proxy index of the well-being of a population and of the effectiveness of medical care. Infant mortality is defined as the deaths of infants born alive within the first year of life. It is usu-ally expressed as a rate of deaths per 1,000 live births. In 1971, the infant mortality was reported in official statistics as 22.9, less than one-tenth the figure for pre-Revolutionary Russia (1913), and about one-quarter what it was in 1950. Such decline was attributed to the superiority of the Soviet system. But the figure rose to 24.7 for 1972,

26.4 for 1973, and 27.4 for 1974.[39] An embargo was then imposed on the publication of such data, for reasons noted earlier. General mortality also rose, as we have seen, again to levels unprecedented in peace time. As a result, life expectancy also began to decline for men and women, but at a faster rate for men. The only upturn was noted in 1987 and a few years thereafter, primarily the result of the anti-alcohol policy imposed by the Gorbachev regime after 1985 but soon discontinued for financial and political reasons (see table 2.2).

The rise in mortality in the mid- and late 1960s came as a surprise because it diverged from trends in the West. In general, mortality in Russia and in the West declined steadily after the end of World War II, due primarily to the introduction of antibiotics and the control of the major infectious diseases. This meant that the

Table 2.2 Life Expectancy at Birth, Men and Women in Russia, 1979–1997

Year	Men	Women	Differential (in years, female by male)
1979–80	61.5	73.0	11.5
1980–81	61.5	73.1	11.6
1981–82	62.0	73.5	11.5
1982–83	62.3	73.6	11.3
1983–84	62.0	73.3	11.3
1984–85	62.3	73.3	11.0
1985–86	63.8	74.0	10.2
1986–87	64.9	74.6	9.7
1988	64.8	74.4	9.6
1989	64.2	74.5	10.3
1990	63.8	74.3	10.5
1991	63.5	74.3	10.8
1992	62.0	73.8	11.8
1993	58.9	71.9	13.0
1994	57.6	71.2	13.6
1995	58.3	71.7	13.4
1996	59.8	72.5	12.7
1997	60.8	72.9	12.1

Source: *Demograficheskii ezhegodnik 1998* (Moscow: Goskomstat, 1999).

major noninfectious diseases began to assume a much more important role in the mortality and morbidity picture, as people lived longer and became candidates for such conditions as heart and cerebro-vascular diseases, cancer, and diabetes. This has been called the epidemiological transition. This transition necessitated a different, more nuanced, more complicated, and eventually more expensive approach than that used to cope with infections. Preventive medicine, in the Soviet context, consisted primarily of screening checkups rather than population-based health promotion measures.[40] At the same time, the Soviet health care system lacked the flexibility administratively and structurally to adjust to the morbidity and mortality conditions that could no longer be handled by the relatively simple and inexpensive massive measures that had controlled the spread of infectious diseases and indeed had cast Soviet socialized medicine as such a model. Moreover, the paternalistic approach of the Soviet health philosophy precluded giving a significant role to the individual in adopting a life-style that would permit him/her to cope with the newly emerging health conditions such as a reduction of alcohol abuse, smoking, sedentary behavior, and high-fat diet.[41]

Finally, given the strains imposed by defense expenditures and a stagnating economy, the funding of the health services declined from the mid-1960s, when about 6 to 6.5 percent of GNP went to health (a respectable figure in line with what most Western countries spent at that time), to 2–3 percent or less when the Soviet Union collapsed. This may, however, be an underestimation, since it does not include the "under-the-table" payments to medical personnel that had become increasingly common and almost customary, given the miserly salaries of most health personnel. It is quite possible that, at present, about half of all expenditures on health come from individual payments rather than from public funds.

In 1988, Dr. Evgenii Chazov, a highly respected physician and cardiologist and former head of the elite Kremlin Medical Service, who had been appointed minister of health by Gorbachev, resigned his position. He did so in protest against what he defined as the "residual principle" in the financing of health services. This meant that the funding of these services came last, or about last, after all the other line budget items had been taken care of. The result was that too little was available. In all other developed countries, the percentage devoted to health care increased. In the Soviet Union it went down.

The health crisis that unfolded after the mid-1960s was one of gradual evolution: it affected the entire population, from infants to the elderly, and in general reflected a slide toward impoverishment and its consequences for the well-being of the population and the demographics of the nation. As we have argued, that crisis was the result of a multiplicity of factors, among which were the rise of defense expenditures in a generally decaying and corrupt economy, the inability of the Soviet Union to deal with the new conditions of morbidity that required a different approach from the one that had previously served it well, and the generally paternalistic attitude of the regime, which encouraged a passive attitude and the lack of a sense of responsibility for one's own health.

Phase 2 (1992–1999)

Phase 1 of the Russian health and demographic crisis came to an end with the collapse of the Soviet system at the end of 1991. The second phase began in 1992 at the time Russia became an independent nation. This transition not only exacerbated the trends visible in Phase 1, but introduced an element of shock, uncertainty, and unpredictability particularly in the economy, with the freeing of prices early in 1992 and a high level of inflation that wiped out the savings of the majority of the population.

It was, using the metaphor of the Cold War, indeed a "postwar situation," accompanied by a sharp and highly visible polarization of the population between an ever larger and ever poorer and disaffected group, and a smaller, more affluent, and more powerful contingent of "New Russians." The vaunted "shock therapy" advocated by Western consultants resulted in more trauma than healing. To this one should add the demoralization at the loss of the Soviet empire and prestige of Russia, reducing it from superpower to international beggar. Many years ago, one of the founders of sociology, Emile Durkheim, in his classic study *Le Suicide,* observed that "whenever serious readjustments take place in the social order, whether or not due to a sudden growth or to an unexpected catastrophe, men are more inclined to self destruction."[42] As noted earlier, it was in 1992 that the birth rate became smaller than the death rate, and the population began to decline; it was after 1992 that mortality due to external or violent causes began to increase, for example in homicides, suicides, traffic accidents (often related to alcohol), poisonings, and increases in heart diseases often exacerbated by alcohol intake. It can be estimated that in 1992, the excess or premature mortality of men before the age of 70 was 282 per 1,000 deaths of all ages, and in 1995 the figure was 385. In other words, according to Vishnevskii, in 1992 more than a quarter, and in 1995 more than a third, of male Russian deaths were "premature," in the sense that they died "before their time," mostly from violence or from cardiovascular diseases. Cancer did not increase appreciably. Deaths due to violence (trauma), particularly in the age range 20–60, constituted almost 40 percent of premature deaths, and cardio-vascular diseases accounted for 31 percent of such deaths. Among women premature mortality was not as high as among men, but their concentration among a small group of conditions was even larger than among men. The important causes of female deaths were heart disease and strokes, accounting for more than 42 percent of all deaths of women between the ages of 55 and 70.[43]

The temptation would be to attribute the phenomena in that second phase to impoverishment and the degradation of health services. And yet, if this were the case, then the infant and elderly mortality, which are particularly sensitive to these factors, and which indeed were characteristic of the first phase and suggested that there was something going on that affected the population as a whole, should also have increased. Yet these were not particularly affected. In fact, in some years after 1992, infant mortality declined. In 1990, the infant mortality was 17.4; it increased to 18.6 in 1994, but declined afterward to 17.4 in 1996, 17.0 in 1997, and (according to preliminary data) 16.6 in 1998.[44] That second phase thus tended to affect primarily the adult population. This suggests that factors other than pauperization, the food supply, or a further breakdown of health care were the major culprits. It was more likely the result of a shock due to the sudden change of macroeconomic and social conditions. And in fact, that transition was traumatic and, we might as well call it, murderous at least for some, more specifically adult males, and psychologically difficult for many others. Nicholas Eberstadt has noted that "these [deaths] are suggestive of extreme social stress," adding that in the modern world, significant and general increases in mortality "always betoken either social instability, or regime fragility, or both."[45] Again, Durkheim emphasized the negative effects of abrupt change and stressed that it is *change* rather than any related impoverishment that is critical, further specifying

that "change results in a temporary disruption of the normal mechanisms through which society imposes limits on behaviour, which in
turn results in increased rates of suicides."[46] According to the
deputy director of Moscow's Serbsky Center for Social and Forensic
Psychiatry, there is a "booming population of depressives. . . . Suicide has soared since 1991, accompanied by skyrocketing rates of
alcohol abuse. . . . The whole country is suffering from the shocks of
economic decline, unemployment and uncontrollable life events.
These are known to trigger borderline mental illness, like depression, post-traumatic stress disorder, and aggression."[47] But by the
same token, and following Durkheim's suggestion that changes for
the *better* as well as for the *worse* are traumatic, there are reports
from Russia that some of the New Russians who became very rich
suddenly are not able to handle their new situation and are seeking
psychiatric help to cope with their new wealth.[48] Although, as Walberg and his colleagues emphasize, there are many other causes of
death in Russia besides suicide, the Durkheimian hypothesis of the
role of rapid and unexpected change that leads to increased personal
pathology and mortality seems to apply to Russia in the second
phase of the health and demographic crisis. Man is a creature of
habit, and social life is based on a probabilistic model that is severely strained during periods of sudden and unexpected events.
This accounts, among other factors, for the nostalgia of many Russians for the meager but predictable certainty of life under the Soviet system. There is also not only a polarization between the poor
and the affluent, but a new one between the old and the young.
Thus, as Aavramova has pointed out, a totally new phenomenon
has appeared in the Russian family as a result of the new economic
circumstances: "children learning to operate in a market environment before the other members of the family, and thus becoming the
family's principal breadwinners. . . . These children begin to 'lay
down the law' as they redefine their relations with their parents."[49]

   And finally, Walberg and his colleagues point out that trends
since 1995 also suggest that Durkheim was prescient when he wrote
that "once some sort of social equilibrium is re-established and individuals are able to reposition themselves in the new social order,
self-destructive behaviours should decline."[50] As the following figures indicate, both male and female life expectancy began to increase after 1994. By the beginning of 1998, according to
preliminary data, male life expectancy rose by 3.6 years, and female

life expectancy by 2.1 years. According to Vishnevskii, of the years of male life expectancy lost between 1991 and 1994, more than half were regained by early 1998, and for women the gain was two-thirds. The improvement was most marked for age groups from 30 to 60, and most particularly for those 30 to 45. This was due primarily to a decrease in mortality caused by accidents, poisonings, trauma, and violence among the younger groups, and cardio-vascular diseases among the older, a mirror image of what happened between 1992 and 1994.[51] It may be too early at this writing (1999) to estimate the impact of the economic meltdown of August 1998, but it is hardly likely to be positive if the past is any indication.

Meanwhile, male life expectancy (61 years) still remains exceedingly low, indeed below the figure for the years between 1970 and 1980, and for women it remains at the level of these years,[52] among the lowest of industrial nations. And has the general economic or political condition radically improved after 1994? Not quite: according to Shkolnikov and his colleagues, the mortality decrease is not associated with the improvement of socio-economic standards, *which simply never occurred,* but with a gradual adaptation of the population to the new realities of life.[53]

Sex Differentials in Life Expectancy

There remains one other intriguing issue, visible in both phases of the Russian health crisis: Why is the life expectancy of Russian women so much greater than that of men? Indeed, the gap is the greatest in the world today, unprecedented in peacetime, although we argued earlier that the period between the mid-1960s and 1991 was "wartime," but war of a special type, and that the events after 1991 were the equivalent of a postwar situation, with all the implications of such a situation.

But this is not enough to explain the life expectancy differential between Russian men and women.[54] The question is: How is it that men and women, subject to the same macroscopic and often traumatic events, living in the same area under the same climatic conditions, reacted so differently? How is it that the difference is twice or more than that of developed, industrial countries? To some degree it may be advanced that there is a genetic and physiological factor, in that women are "better built" because of their reproductive functions. "Women," according to Donald K. Grayson, "are designed to have children, and what enables them to have kids, enables them to deal better with privations."[55] Recent research suggests that there are prenatal factors at work that will affect the health and longevity of both sexes, but that women are better protected. This is particularly true of the role played by hormones. During their reproductive years women have much less heart disease than men of the same age, estrogen being responsible for part of the difference.[56] But there are, of course, a host of other factors that affect longevity, some of which we will explore below. In general, the difference (in the absence of events such as wars that would affect selectively the mortality of men and women) is around six years. In 1998 in the United States, the difference was 5.5 years for the white population, and 7.4 for African Americans. In earlier years the difference was even smaller or insignificant. For example, in 1920 the average life span of American men and women was about the same. In Russia's postcommunist years the gap has been around 12–14 years (see figure 2.1, constructed from the data in table 2.2). This gap is not only unprecedented but also the largest recorded in the world today.[57] The gap during and shortly after the Cold War was also of the same general order of magnitude. It should be noted that the difference is larger in the rural areas, presumably because of the use of agricultural machinery and alcohol consumption. It is thus particularly marked for the adult years. As figure 2.2 shows, in 1993 the rural mortality for ages 20–25 was five times greater for males than for females, and in the urban areas it was over four times greater. It is therefore not surprising that concern has been expressed in the Russian media that the nation is on its way to becoming a country of widows[58] and, we might add, of fatherless children.[59]

It seems clear that it is not in physiological, or economic, or climatic factors alone that we can seek answers to the Russian gender gap in life expectancy. It is more likely that it lies in the cultural and sociological arenas. In a paper published in 1960, Vera S. Dunham explored what she called the "strong woman motif" in Russian and Soviet literature.[60] She identified that "motif" as an integral part of Russian culture with a tradition going back to the nineteenth century. She found a depiction of women as pillars of strength, stability, and continuity. They were "heroines," depicted in contrast to weak-willed, confused, ineffectual men, who enjoyed boasting and posturing but who lacked steadfastness, determination, and courage in the face of adversity. And Dunham adds that the multifaceted

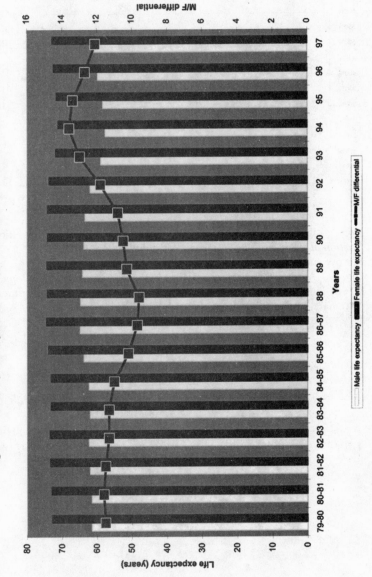

Figure 2.1: Life Expectancy at Birth, Men and Women in Russia, 1979-1997

**Figure 2.2   Male Mortality Rates in Russia in 1993 (Relationship be-
tween Male and Female Mortality Rates in Percentage Terms)**

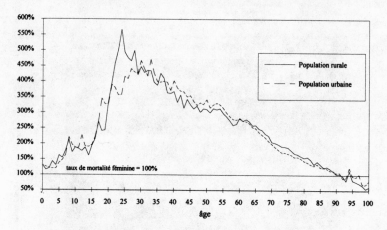

Note: Right hand box indicates Rural Population and Urban Population
Caption at the bottom left: Female Mortality Rate = 100%
Bottom middle: age is age
Source: Alexandre Avdeev and Alain Monnier, *Mouvement de la Popula-
tion de la Russie 1959–1994: Tableaux Démographiques* (Paris: Institut
National d'Études Démographiques, 1996), 32.

character of women encompasses "positive qualities such as self-lessness, endurance, and the ability to adjust to stress." If women appear to be strong, men on the other hand appear to be much more at risk than women. Thus, the cultural tradition of drinking vodka as a male prerogative may contribute, to a large extent, to the higher male mortality. Alcohol drinking is thus seen as a culturally determined way, among others, for men to deal with stress and other problematic areas. As Avdeev and Monnier put it, excess male mortality [may] reside in certain male behavioral patterns, alcoholism in particular.[61] But there may be other factors that, within the context of the Soviet system, have exacerbated the culturally determined problematics of life under the socialist system and, interestingly enough, in the postsocialist system. As Peter Makara, a Hungarian sociologist concerned with health, has pointed out, the increased mortality cannot simply and directly be linked to a deteriorating health care system and other conventional factors, such as impoverishment. Rather the health crisis, as a reflection of a more general societal unrest, includes such elements as a low value placed on human life and health and intensive tensions between a depressed standard of living and aspirations and their gratification. To further compound that problem there is a chronic lack of genuine communities, human relationships, and social support systems.[62] If we accept the hypothesis that socialism, according to Makara, imposed heavy burdens on the population, we must also accept the idea that these burdens fell on both men and women. Then what accounts for the fact that women fared much better than men and lived considerably longer? We may advance the hypothesis that in socialist society, and to a large degree in the postsocialist society after 1991, the sense of frustration, the discontinuity between aspirations and achievements, the feeling of helplessness, the lack of relationship between efforts and rewards, whether in the political or more particularly in the occupational sphere, affected men much more than women: they affected everyone but to a different degree.[63] Men often used the West as a point of reference and comparison to judge their own fate, and thus felt alienated, helpless, frustrated, and angry. Women, by contrast, although they also were involved in the occupational sphere (because of economic necessity in most instances), found the center of their concerns and preoccupations in the family and household, and in the care of family members, be they children, spouse, or elderly parents. In one sense the family, and the responsibilities it entailed, provided meaning for their lives and a sense of "coherence," as Antonovsky used the term.[64] Thus it is at the sociological level, in terms of social roles, as pointed out by Peggy Watson,[65] that a better understanding may be reached. She writes, "in a state-controlled public sphere . . . the opportunities for realising traditional masculinity are strictly limited. . . . For men under state socialism . . . there is a specific 'incongruity' between gender expectation and outcome. State socialism thus fosters a pattern of fixed coping strategies which is (within limits) adaptive for women, but . . . maladaptive for men as men."

It seems that different gender roles place men more at risk than women both in Soviet and post-Soviet society, and that indeed women do play an important role in keeping society going. To do this requires strength and determination and a sense of purpose that seems to be lacking, in general, in men. But another question remains: is this a Russian phenomenon, as Dunham seems to claim, or is it the product of the nature of life under a Soviet-type regime, or more probably a combination of both? Thus, in 1998, the life expectancy in many of the former Soviet republics also showed a sex differential of great magnitude, though smaller than in Russia: in Latvia, Lithuania, Estonia,[66] and Belarus it was between 12.5 and 12.3. In the Ukraine and Kazakstan it was 11.8 and 11.2 respectively.[67]

In addition to the biological, psychological, and sociological elements mentioned, there is a cultural factor that might provide supplemental explanation. This factor has been most noticeable among the Russian population, but it undoubtedly affects other populations subjected to a Soviet-type regime. Russian sociologists puzzled by the low life expectancy of adult men report that there is simply no feeling among the majority of people that it is worthwhile worrying about the future. As Antonov of the Moscow State University put it, "The Soviets demanded that men sacrifice their lives for Communism. . . . Nobody put the cost of life before the cost of building . . . society. . . . We were taught to suffer . . . and that we will probably die in the next war. . . . Why worry about how you are going to survive to an old age?"[68]

In addition to the idea that human life is cheap, there seems to be a kind of indifference or fatalism about one's own life that translates, as we have already mentioned, into the pervasiveness of alcoholism. It may be remembered that the anti-alcohol campaign led to a sharp decrease in mortality, particularly male of course, and that its abandonment led to a resumption of the negative trends in life expectancy and mortality. Another manifestation of that indifference is the rise in suicides and homicides affecting primarily the men. Gennady Gerasimov, a former spokesman for Gorbachev, some time ago wrote that "a death wish is haunting Russia," pointing out that in the two years before 1994, 100,000 Russians had committed suicide, and the rate had climbed to 38 per 100,000 as against 26.5 in 1991. He related this trend to the disorientation that accompanied the transition from a command to a market economy. He quoted the former minister of social security to the effect that fathers committed suicide because they could not provide for their children.[69]

Not only fathers contemplate suicide. A reporter visiting Novosibirsk in 1997 went to a youth club for males. When the discussion turned to alcohol's effect on their future, "Sergei, 22, blurted out: 'I tried to commit suicide,' pulling up his sleeve to reveal the scars of slit wrists. 'Me too,' Alex said, displaying a similar set of scars. Quickly, all five of the young men rolled up their sleeves . . . excitedly comparing suicide methods and scarred reminders."[70]

In addition to alcoholism, suicide, and homicide (and alcohol-related traffic accidents), male mortality is also related to the more "traditional" causes of death. Specter reported (in 1997) that there are few more shocking trips one can take in Russia than to the general wards of a major hospital. What is striking is almost always the age of the patients and their condition. "Lung disease, heart attack, cancer, alcohol poisoning, high blood pressure . . . a nurse . . . reeled off the afflictions of five men, *none of them yet 50:* 'The usual stuff. They are all going to die'" (emphasis added).[71]

Although this disregard for life, which some profess to see as a kind of "Russian disease of the soul," may go back a hundred years or so (Dostoyevski wrote about it in the late nineteenth century),[72] it seems to have been reinforced by the very nature of the Soviet system. Shkolnikov and Malkov, for instance, attribute it to the regime's paternalism, "the development and the spread of a psychology of passivity and irresponsibility in Russia,"[73] to which we have already alluded in reference to the inability of the Soviet system to deal with noninfectious diseases by encouraging the individual to take charge of his own health through a change of life-style. The Soviet regime paid workers very little but provided in return a series of modest but predictable services such as free health care.

And the low pay, the lack of a significant relationship between efforts and reward, the futility of performing well (or better than one's peers) led, again according to Shkolnikov and Malkov, to mass demoralization and apathy. These conditions "permit us to better understand the causes of this special inertia and indifference which kept Russians from an active concern to their own health, that strange case which our society has maintained for decades about the losses caused by the elevated mortality."[74]

And thus, whether one accepts Russian culture, or the nature of the Soviet system, or both as a major contributor to the health crisis, it seems to be well established that this crisis affected men to a much larger degree than women in the area of mortality, and that the present situation exacerbates trends already visible in the mid-1960s. Furthermore,

> Women . . . pay greater attention to their health, more frequently see a doctor and take medical advice, and spend more money on drugs. As for men, they are not eager to take medical advice, tend to ignore their illnesses, more frequently indulge in binge drinking and smoking and, as a result, die suddenly "on their feet," at a relatively younger age.[75]

This is not to argue, in any way, that women are immune to the larger macrosocial phenomena that have affected and are affecting Russia. When life expectancy falls or mortality increases, this affects both sexes, but it affects men to a much larger degree than women. Thus between 1990 and 1994, both sexes experienced a loss of life expectancy, but the male loss was twice that of women (6.6 years as against 3.2, respectively). The amplitudes of the changes, whether positive or negative, have been much more moderate for women. Finally, it should be noted that these changes have affected, particularly in the second phase of the health crisis, primarily adult males and females, and cannot thus be traced directly to the conventional explanations of the failings of the health care system or the general degradation of the standard of living, since they did not have the same impact on either infant, child, or geriatric mortality, as noted earlier. And the recent improvement in vital statistics after 1994 argues, as we have already noted, for a gradual adaptation of the population to the situation. But this adaptation has been reflected in a decrease in mortality due primarily to the stresses of rapidly changing circumstances, i.e., a reduction in deaths due to suicides, accidents, traumas, violence, and so on. On the other hand, this is not to dismiss grave health problems that have surfaced or resurfaced as a result of the deterioration of public health and a return of the infectious diseases that had been controlled earlier.

The Return of Infectious Diseases

Among the infectious diseases that have staged an ominous comeback, tuberculosis has reached epidemic proportions in Russian communities and among the prison population,[76] where incarceration almost amounts to a death sentence.[77] In particular, an alarmingly large and rising number of cases are resistant to available drugs.[78] According to a memorandum prepared by the ministry of the interior, "By the year 2000 the incidence of tuberculosis will increase 50 times compared with now; mortality will increase seventyfold; and deaths in children are expected to rise ninety-fold."[79] Tuberculosis is only one of many diseases that are plaguing Russia as a result of the dislocations, the impoverishment, and the difficult life conditions under which a majority of the Russian population must live. In addition to tuberculosis, a whole series of other conditions also controlled earlier during the Soviet regime have now reappeared. Cholera, diphtheria, plague, polio, typhoid fever, and the scourge of typhus[80] have staged ominous comebacks. Sexually transmitted diseases, including syphilis and AIDS, are on the rise. A former health minister, Tatiana Dmitrieva, forecast that by the year 2000, one million Russians will be infected with HIV.[81]

In addition to these conditions, cardiovascular problems constitute another serious threat to the population. In 1997 it was reported that the mortality rate from cardiovascular diseases was from five to six times higher in Russia than in the developed countries of the West. Deaths from cardiovascular diseases per 100,000 men aged 40–45 were 102 in France, 127 in Italy, 170 in Greece, and 549 in Russia. For men aged 45 to 74, the rates were (for men per 100,000) the following: 330 in France, 399 in Spain, 453 in Italy and 1,343 in Russia. Among women, the rates are lower but the differences of the same order. For women age 45–54, the death rate is 30 for Frenchwomen and 166 for their Russian counterparts. According to Rafael Oganov, director of the Russian Federation Research Institute for

Preventive Medicine, cardiovascular diseases are the number-one killer throughout the world, but this colossal disparity in death rates stems from Russia's social and economic conditions and its people's life-style. The deteriorating financial situation of the majority of the population, an inadequate and unbalanced diet, stress-inducing uncertainty about the future, and an ever greater predilection for harmful habits (drinking, smoking, drug use)—these are the reasons for the high death rates from cardiovascular disease in Russia.[82]

Even the slight improvements noted earlier (such as an increase in life expectancy between 1994 and 1997) are being threatened by the meltdown of August 1998. Thus the increase in the availability of contraceptives noted earlier had led to a modest decrease in abortions and abortion-related maternal deaths, which were, as mentioned earlier, five to ten times higher than in the West. But the financial crisis has also led to the increased inability of Russian women to afford contraceptives, most of which are imported from abroad.[83] At every step, the crisis of Russian society is reflected in the state of its health.

Conclusions

Russia is facing a multidimensional health and demographic crisis. In this paper, we have been able to deal with only part of the problem. This is a two-phase crisis, the first one beginning in the mid-1960s and dominated by the consequences, among others, of the strains imposed by the Cold War and a faltering economy. The second phase, which might be called the postwar period, was marked by the dismantling of the Soviet system, the transition from a command to a market economy, and the problems caused by shock therapy that had their dismal impact upon the health, the morale, and the morbidity and mortality of the population. This impact has been particularly severe on the male adult population, whose life expectancy dropped to the level of a third-world country. Recent data suggest a slow and gradual improvement as the population apparently is getting used to the changes, but is at the same time threatened by resurfacing epidemics of infectious diseases. The prospects for the future remain bleak, and the projections are guarded for at least the next half-century. Predictions are notoriously difficult and risky. As has been said, autopsies are easier than prophecies or fortune-telling. The vicissitudes of the health crisis in Soviet Russia and in postcommunist Russia are reflections of larger macroscopic events in the political, the economic and the social spheres. These events, this *katastroika* to which we already referred, will have profound repercussions in the near and distant future. They will place strict limits and impose heavy burdens on development, on the size of the labor force, on the dependency ratio, on the place and power of Russia on the international scene, and on Russia as the focus of epidemics that may affect the security and the health of populations inside and outside its borders. This is a largely silent crisis that has not received the attention nor the priority it deserves.[84] As in the past, people will continue to pay with their lives and their health for the instability and the folly of those who govern them.

NOTES

Figure 2.2 is reprinted with the generous permission of the Institut National d'Études Démographiques, Paris.

1. France Meslé and Vladimir Shkolnikov, "La Mortalité en Russie: une crise sanitaire en deux temps," *Revue d'Etudes Comparatives Est-Ouest* 26, no. 4: 25–34.

2. The expression was coined by A. Zinoviev. See Michael Ellman, "The Increase in Death and Disease Under 'Katastroika,'" *Cambridge Journal of Economics* 18 (1994): 329–355, ref. 1.

3. Michael Specter, "Climb in Russia's Death Rate Sets Off Population Implosion," *The New York Times*, 6 March 1994.

4. "Russian Population Sees Larger Decline," *The Boston Globe*, 31 July 1999, A18.

5. Lee Hockstader, "Death and Disease Rates Soar in Russia," *Guardian Weekly*, 13 March 1994, 18.

6. UNICEF, *Public Policy and Social Conditions: Central and Eastern Europe in Transition*, Regional Monitoring Report, no. 1 (November 1993), 89 pp.

7. *Demograficheskii Ezhegodnik 1997* (Moscow: Goskomstat Rossii, 1998)

8. *Naselenie Rossii 1996* (Moscow: Institut narodnokhoziastvennogo prognozirovaniia RAN, 1997), 77.

9. *Naselenie Rossii 1996*, Figure 6.6, 91.

10. Celestine Bohlen, "Russian Women Turning to Abortion Less Often," *The New York Times*, 29 March 1999, A3.

11. *Naselenie Rossii 1996*, 87.

12. Mark G. Field, "The Health Crisis in the Former Soviet Union: A Report from the 'Post-War' Zone," *Social Science and Medicine* 41, no. 11 (1995): 1469–1478.
13. *Naselenie Rossii 1996, 6.*
14. *Kommersant,* 3 December 1998.
15. *Goskomstat Rossii* 1997, 7.
16. *Estestvennii dvizhenie naselenia Rossiiskoi Federatsii za 9 mesiatsev 1993 goda* (Moscow: Goskomstat, 1993).
17. Nicholas Eberstadt, "Marx and Mortality: A Mystery," *The New York Times,* 6 April 1994, A21.
18. Vladimir Yesipov, "St. Petersburg Will Die a Natural Death," *Kommersant-Daily,* 25 August 1998, 4, translated in *Current Digest of the Post-Soviet Press (CDPSP)* 50, no. 34 (1998): 20.
19. See, for example, Mark G. Field, David M. Kotz, and Gene Bukhman, "Neoliberal Economic Policy, 'State Desertion,' and the Russian Health Crisis," in Jim Y. Kim, Joyce V. Millen, Alec Irwin, and John Gershman, eds., *Dying for Growth: Global Inequality and the Health of the Poor* (Cambridge, MA: Courage Press, 2000), 155–173.
20. Cited by Michael Specter, *The New York Times,* 8 June 1997.
21. Commenting on the seeming disinterest of the government in health matters, Anatolii Vishnevskii asks rhetorically, "Has not the time arrived to change priorities?" See "Russkii krest," *Novie izvestiia,* 24 February 1998.
22. Aleksandr Solzhenitsyn, "The Relentless Cult of Novelty and How It Wrecked the Century," *The New York Times Book Review,* 7 February 1993, 3.
23. See, for instance, José Luis Bobadilla, Christine A. Costello, and Faith Mitchell, eds., *Premature Death in the New Independent States* (Washington, D.C.: National Academy Press, 1997).
24. Vishnevskii, "Russkii krest."
25. Roland Pressat, "Une évolution anachronique: la hausse de la mortalité en Union soviétique," *Le Concours Médical* 105, no. 21 (21 May 1983): 2431–2434.
26. M. N. Rutkevich, "Social Polarization," *Sociological Research: A Journal of Translations from Russia* (September-October 1993): 58.
27. Hockstader, "Death and Disease Rates."
28. Slobodan Vitanovic, "La politique de culture et les transformations dans le monde actuel" (paper presented at the General Assembly of the Société Européenne de Culture, Venice, Italy, 1993).
29. Noel E. Firth and James H. Noreen, *Soviet Defense Spending: A History of CIA Estimates, 1950–1990* (College Station: Texas A&M University Press, 1998), Figure 5.2, p. 102.

30. Sergei Khrushchev, "The Cold War through the Looking Glass," *American Heritage,* October 1999, 35–50.
31. See, for example, Bill Keller, "Eclipsed: Thirty Years Ago, the Soviets Lost the Race to the Moon, They Might Have Won—If Only They Had Acted Like Good Communists," *The New York Times Magazine,* 27 June 1999, 30–37, 52, 55, 61, 63.
32. Mikhail Gorbachev, *Memoirs* (London: Bantam Books, 1995), 277.
33. Cited in Judyth L. Twigg, "Russia's Space Program: Continued Turmoil," *Space Policy* 15 (1999): 69–77.
34. Victor W. Sidel, "Buying Death With Taxes: Impact of Arms Race on Health Care," in *The Final Epidemic,* eds. R. Adams and S. Cullen (Chicago: University of Chicago press, 1981), 40, 43–44.
35. Dwight D. Eisenhower, "The Chances for Peace" address delivered before the American Society of Newspaper Editors, April 16, 1953, in Public Papers of the Presidents, Dwight D. Eisenhower, Washington, D.C., 1953, 179–188.
36. Otto Latsis, "Conversations Overheard in Voronezh," *Izvestiia,* 14 May 1996, 5. Latsis refers to the introduction of ration cards in many areas of the Soviet Union at that time, another measure reminiscent of a wartime situation.
37. Laurie Garrett, "Crumbled Empire, Shattered Health," *Newsday,* 26 October 1997, A42.
38. Christopher Davis and Murray Feshbach, *Rising Infant Mortality in the USSR in the 1970s* (Washington, D.C.: U.S. Department of Commerce, June 1980).
39. These figures are usually considered underestimates for purposes of international comparisons, because of the manner in which the Soviets defined infant mortality. What is important is that, in Soviet terms, the infant mortality went up. For details, see Mark G. Field, "Soviet Infant Mortality: A Mystery Story," in *Advances in International Maternal and Child Health,* eds. D. B. Jelliffe and E. F. P. Jelliffe (Oxford: Clarendon Press, 1986), 25–65.
40. "Health in Russia Is Broke, But Who Is Going To Fix It?" *The Lancet* 353, no. 9150 (30 January 1999): 337.
41. See, for example, Michael Wines, "Lean Times at the Russian Dinner Table," *The New York Times,* 6 December 1998, section 4.
42. Cited in Peter Walberg, Martin McKee, Vladimir Shkolnikov, Laurent Chenet, and David Leon, "Economic Change, Crime, and Mortality Crisis in Russia: Regional Analysis," *British Medical Journal* 317 (1 August 1998): 312–318.
43. Vishnevskii, "Russkii krest."
44. Bohlen, "Russian Women."

45. Nicholas Eberstadt, "The Demographic Disaster: The Dark Soviet Legacy," *The National Interest* (Summer 1994): 53–54.

46. Nicholas Eberstadt, "The Demographic Disaster."

47. "Depression: Spirit of the Age," *The Economist,* 19 December 1998, 113–117.

48. David Filipov, "Cure-All Gives Russian Mafia A Lease on Life," *The Boston Globe,* 28 June 1999, A2.

49. E. Aavramova, *Social and Demographic Dimensions of the Economic Transition: Impact on Families with Children* (New York: UNICEF, 1994).

50. Walberg, et al., "Economic Change."

51. Vishnevskii, "Russkii krest."

52. Vishnevskii, "Russkii krest."

53. Vladimir Shkolnikov, Andrea G. Cornia, David A. Leon, France Meslé, "Causes of the Russian Mortality Crisis: Evidence and Interpretations," 1998, unpublished draft.

54. For a more detailed discussion, see Vladimir Shkolnikov, Mark G. Field, and Evgenii M. Andreev, "Gender Gap in Russian Mortality in Time and Socio-Demographic Dimensions," in *Challenging Inequities in Health: From Global to Local,* eds. Margaret Whitehead, Finn Diderichsen, Timothy Evans, and Abbas Bhuiya (Oxford University Press, in press).

55. Jane E. Brody, "Sex and the Survival of the Fittest: Calamities Are a Disaster for Men," *The New York Times,* 24 April 1996, C5.

56. *Harvard Men's Health Watch* 3, no. 7 (February 1999): 4–5.

57. Meslé and Shkolnikov, "La Mortalité en Russie."

58. "Russia May Become a Country of Widows," *Segodnia,* 19 July 1995, 12.

59. For a general examination of the relationship between demographics and the family, see Valerii V. Elizarov, "The Demographic Situation and Problems of Family Policy," *Sociological Research* 38, no. 1 (January-February 1999): 79–90.

60. Vera Sandomirski Dunham, "The Strong Woman Motif," in *The Transformation of Russian Society: Aspects of Change Since 1861,* ed. Cyril E. Black (Cambridge: Harvard University Press, 1960), 459–483.

61. Alexander Avdeev and Alain Monnier, *Mouvement de la population de la Russie 1959–1994: Tableaux Demographiques* (Paris: Institut National d'Etudes Demographiques, 1996), no. 1, graphique 17, 32.

62. Peter Makara, "Policy Implications of Differential Health Status in East and West Europe: The Case of Hungary" (paper prepared for the XIIIth International Conference on the Social Sciences and Medicine, 1994). A slightly different version of this paper has been published as

"Dilemmas of Health Promotion and Political Changes in Eastern Europe," *Health Promotion International* 6, no. 1 (1991): 41–47.

63. It should be noted that in state-controlled economies, economic frustrations become political frustrations because the public perceives the political sphere as the basic mechanism for distribution of all economic goods and as the source of prosperity, but also because the experience of economic problems has been infused with a sense of political injustice and moral outrage. See Peggy Watson, "Explaining Rising Mortality Among Men in Eastern Europe," *Social Science and Medicine* 47, no. 7 (1995): 923–934.

64. Aron Antonovsky, *Health, Stress, and Coping: New Perspectives on Mental and Physical Well-Being* (San Francisco: Jossey Bass, 1979).

65. Watson, "Explaining Rising Mortality."

66. France Meslé and Véronique Hertrich, "Sex Mortality Differences in the Baltic Countries" (paper presented at the International Conference of Vilnius, 8–9 October 1998, on Regularities and Inconsistencies of Demographic Development: Preconditions for the Replacement of Generations, Paris, INED, 1998).

67. See, for example, the contribution to this volume by Victoria A. Velkoff and Kevin Kinsella.

68. Specter, "Climb in Russia's Death Rate."

69. Gennadi I. Gerasimov, "A Death Wish Is Haunting Russia," *The New York Times,* 17 December 1994, 23.

70. Garrett, "Crumbled Empire."

71. Michael Specter, "Deep in the Russian Soul, A Lethal Darkness," *The New York Times,* 8 June 1997, 1.

72. Specter, "Deep in the Russian Soul."

73. V. M. Shkolnikov and L. P. Malkov, *Prodolzhitelnost' zhizni v Rossii* (Moscow: Tsentr demografii i ekologii cheloveka), in progress.

74. Shkolnikov and Malkov, *Prodolzhitelnost' zhizni.*

75. N. Rimashevskaia, "The Individual Health Potential in Russia," The Institute of Socio-Economic Studies of the Population, Russian Academy of Sciences (Moscow and Amsterdam: September-October 1992), unpublished.

76. M. Franchetti, "Thousands of Russians Die in TB Gulag," *Sunday Times,* 28 September 1997.

77. Garrett, "Crumbled Empire."

78. M. E. Kimmerling, "Inadequacy of the Current WHO Re-Treatment Regimen in Russia: MDRTB [multi-drug-resistant tuberculosis] in a Central Siberian Prison," *International Journal of Tuberculosis and Lung Disease* (1999), in press.

79. Laurie Garrett of Newsday, cited in Murray Feshbach, "Dead Souls," *The Atlantic Monthly,* January 1999, 26–28.

80. Hermann Feldmeier, "Die Rückkehr des Fleckfieber in Russland: Wiederaufleben alter Seuchen in Osteuropa," *Neue Zürcher Zeitung, Internationale Ausgabe,* 8 March 1999, 5.

81. Feshbach, "Dead Souls."

82. "Russians Have the Weakest Hearts," *Segodnia,* 11 September 1997, 2, in *CDPSP* XLIX, no. 37 (1997): 17.

83. Bohlen, "Russian Women."

84. A recent and very useful exception is William C. Cockerham, *Health and Social Change in Russia and Eastern Europe* (New York: Routledge, 1999).

CHAPTER 3

Unfulfilled Hopes: The Struggle to Reform Russian Health Care and Its Financing

Judyth L. Twigg

ONE OF THE SOVIET UNION'S MOST NOTABLE accomplishments was the development of its system of health care. Soviet citizens enjoyed universal access to free medical care, through either the workplace or neighborhood clinics, with an emphasis on preventive health maintenance. Although the quality of secondary and tertiary care was not up to Western standards, and access to some specialists and treatments frequently required patients to contribute gifts and other "side payments," the extension of basic primary care services to even the most sparsely populated rural areas of Soviet territory was a remarkable achievement.

It is an achievement rendered even more notable by the consistently low level of resources the Soviet government devoted to health care. Health and medicine were financed according to a "residual principle," meaning that, along with education and other social programs, they made do with the budgetary scraps remaining after more high-priority items like defense and heavy industry had their fill. After reaching a peak in 1955, with health-related articles comprising 20.8 percent of the total government budget, health care spending plummeted to a steady state of between five and six percent of the Soviet budget from the early 1960s through the early 1980s.[1] Even so, the Soviet people came to rely on the safety net provided by the government health care network.

As the Soviet Union collapsed, so too did that health care safety net. This chapter will outline Russia's efforts to replace Soviet socialized medicine with a more market-oriented system of universal health insurance. It will argue that these efforts have left health care even more woefully underfunded than in the past, and that the Russian people have suffered from the collapse of universal access and free provision of basic health services. It will also detail several strategies for intensive growth recently proposed by health reformers in response to the budget difficulties, ending with some remarks on the continuing impact of the August 1998 financial crisis.

Russia Adopts Medical Insurance

It became clear to Russian leaders even before the Soviet Union's final demise that something had to be done to rescue health care. The economic instability and growing state budget deficits of the 1980s had resulted in dramatic shortages of basic medicines and medical equipment, increasingly lengthy queues for surgeries and other procedures, and an exodus of skilled health professionals to more stable and lucrative professions.

The RSFSR government responded in 1991 with legislation creating a system of universal obligatory medical insurance; this legislation reached its final form in April 1993. Its primary goal was to channel more money into the health care system, in particular through new regional, quasi-governmental, off-budget insurance Funds that would not have to compete politically with other budget priorities. It was also hoped that the insurance mechanism would encourage market-based efficiency and quality through competition between insurers and between health care providers.

Here is how the system was designed to work.[2] A basic, though not clearly specified, level of health care benefits is mandated to be covered for all insured citizens. Money for these services is funneled in from two sources: employers pay a 3.6 percent payroll tax on behalf of their workers, and local governments pay a per capita contribution set at the regional level for nonemployed persons (students, pensioners, the unemployed, housewives, etc.). These revenues flow into the appropriate one of 89 new quasi-governmental, territorial health insurance Funds, with a small percentage of the employers' payroll tax going into an analogous federal-level Fund whose job is primarily to equalize financial circumstances across the regions. The regional Funds then make payments to one of a number of competing private insurance companies licensed to work in the obligatory medical insurance system, based on claims submitted on behalf of patients treated in similarly licensed clinics or hospitals. The intention is for insurance companies to compete with one another for business from individual patients or employers enrolling large numbers of workers, with competition centered around the companies' success in affiliating with the highest-quality clinics and hospitals and maintaining high standards of quality control and defense of patients' rights. Health care providers compete for recognition of these quality standards by the insurance companies and by individual patients. Clearly, then, patient (or employer) choice of insurance company and provider is a central feature of this new system.

Insurance: Success or Failure?

Has obligatory medical insurance achieved its stated goals? The reviews are mixed. In terms of revenue generation, there is little question that the financial situation in the health care sector is significantly better with obligatory medical insurance than it would have been in its absence. A comparison with other social programs is instructive. Budget funding for education and cultural purposes, for example, fell by 27 percent and 31 percent respectively from 1992 to 1995; health care suffered from similar budget cuts, but the impact of those reductions was muted by the presence of the off-budget insurance contributions, such that health care spending as a whole declined by only 10 percent during that same time period.[3] The years 1993–1995 were particularly "fat" ones for health care, as insurance contributions began to supplement budget expenditures. By all accounts, however, around 1995 local and regional legislatures began to "notice" the presence of the insurance revenues, and responded by cutting government health budgets by a commensurate amount. In essence, therefore, the insurance money has replaced rather than augmented budget financing for health care, but at least it has done so via an earmarked pool of funds ostensibly untouchable for non-health-related purposes.

According to data provided by the Federal Obligatory Medical Insurance Fund, almost 80 percent of the medical care facilities in the country are currently working within the insurance system,

supported by a network of 376 licensed health insurance companies. Over 130 million Russian citizens, or more than 82 percent
of the population, have been issued obligatory medical insurance
policies. In 1998 alone, insurance revenues accounted for almost
25 percent of the total financing of the health care system.[4]

The trouble begins when adherence to the revenue generation
provisions of the insurance law is examined closely. Neither employers nor local governments are making their full required contributions into the system, although the former are much less guilty of
this form of tax evasion than the latter. In an era of scarce resources,
and in a situation where the law is quite vague in its specification of
the per-citizen contribution required of the municipalities for those
who are not employed, it is not surprising that these localities suc-
cumb to the temptation to skimp on their payments. As of early
1999, the total debts of local governments to the insurance system
amounted to 11.5 billion rubles (expressed in 1999 ruble values),
with no payments at all being transferred by 15 regions by the middle of the year.[5] The resulting problem, of course, is that employers
cannot pay enough into the system to compensate, particularly
when nonworking people constitute around 60 percent of the population and are the demographic group (children, the elderly) most
likely to consume health services. (See table 3.1 for the overall structure of revenues flowing into the regional Funds.) This financial situation is exacerbated by Russia's overall health crisis; as the
morbidity of working-age people increases, their relatively reliable,
employer-based medical insurance contributions go down. The federal Fund has sent to the Duma a draft piece of legislation that
would cover municipal payments on behalf of their nonworking citizens as a protected article of local budgets, but the proposal has
gathered little support or momentum.

These revenue generation problems have been tackled aggres-
sively by the regional Funds whose job it is to collect the money.
More than half the employees of some of the Funds are assigned to
tax collection, and in many cases these efforts have paid off. In the
city of Moscow, for example, 90–95 percent of legally mandated
medical insurance payments are actually made on time; this is a significantly better success rate than that achieved by the state tax service.[6] Other regional Funds are compensating for enterprises' and
local governments' financial difficulties by accepting in-kind payments or promissory notes in lieu of ruble payments. A coal mine, for

Table 3.1   Structure of Income of the Territorial Medical Insurance Funds, 1997

Source	Income, Millions of Rubles	Percentage of Total Income
Insurance taxes on employers	17,280.6	60.7
Payments from municipal governments for nonworking citizens	6,540.2	23.0
Investment income	112.9	0.4
Fines and penalties assessed on noncompliant insurance companies and employers	1,804.8	6.3
Other sources	2,721.6	9.6

Source: Annual Report of the Federal Obligatory Medical Insurance Fund, published in Meditsinskiy vestnik, no. 24 (115), 1998, 7–10.

example, might pay the miners' insurance contributions in coal, which the Fund then allocates to the heating needs of various hospitals and clinics. A substantial amount of enterprise debt to the insurance Funds has been covered this way since the beginning of 1998.

But, despite scattered success stories and budgeting innovations, the overall picture is one in which the resources paid into the health care system, from government budgets at all levels and from insurance, do not even approach the level necessary to cover the Russian constitution's promise of free health care to all citizens (Article 41). According to one estimate, the insurance Funds collected in 1997 only 37.5 percent of the total amount necessary to finance all the "free" care promised under the insurance program.[7] It is the health care workers and the patients who feel the squeeze. Patients are increasingly required to purchase their own medications (which are supposed to be provided free for inpatient treatment), hospital food, and even linens, gauze, and bandages. Doctors, nurses, and other medical workers are heroically continuing to treat patients, sometimes for months, without being paid.[8] Anecdotal accounts of wages paid in barter have become increasingly common, with the barter payments occasionally taking on such inappropriate forms as coffins and vodka. Physicians' strikes have begun to emerge in particularly desperate regions such as Vladivostok. And head physicians in major-city clinics and hospitals are beginning to complain of understaffing problems, as talented professionals continue to abandon a disintegrating profession and medical schools have trouble attracting qualified applicants.

The federal-level obligatory medical insurance Fund has attempted to douse the fire of crisis in the most desperate regions, with subsidies going out to 79 regions in 1998. But its share of the employers' payroll tax simply does not provide enough money to go around. Early drafts of the 1998 federal government budget tried to address this problem with 8 billion rubles (drawn from the total amount allocated for assistance to the regions) earmarked specifically for health care, to be distributed throughout the country according to regional needs by the federal insurance Fund, but the governors scuttled the proposal; they did not want restrictions placed on their federal subsidies. The federal and regional Funds have further suffered from occasional illegal raids of their coffers. In 1994–1995, for example, an unknown number of rubles were taken from the federal Fund to pay for Russia's military action against Chechnya; in 1998, money was diverted to pay back wages to striking coal miners.[9]

Uneven Impact of the Insurance Mechanism

Even if all the legally mandated resources were successfully channeled into the obligatory medical insurance system, however, persistent questions remain about whether that system is appropriately organized to achieve its structural goal of enhancing the quality and efficiency of the health care system. The most important dynamic here has been the dramatic variation in the evolution of the insurance mechanism among Russia's 89 regions. It would not be inaccurate to describe Russia as currently operating under 89 distinctly different systems of health care. But it is possible to group the modes of implementation of the insurance legislation into four categories:[10]

1. The insurance company model, in which the law is followed essentially as written. As of early 1998, this model encompassed 14 regions, serving about 26 percent of the total Russian population.

2. The Fund-as-insurer model, in which insurance companies do not exist, and instead the regional quasi-gov-

ernmental Fund and its affiliates fulfill their role. Thirty-two regions finance health care through this scheme, serving about 30 percent of the population.

3. A mixed model, in which some people hold policies issued by insurance companies, and others find their health care paid for directly by the regional Fund. The mixed model is in place in 37 regions, covering nearly 41 percent of the population.

4. The noncompliant model, in which a regional Fund may or may not have been established, insurance companies are nonexistent, and the vast majority of health care monies flows directly from government budgets to clinics and hospitals. Where the Funds do exist, they are routinely bypassed or ignored. Noncompliance with the insurance law is in effect in six regions, affecting only a little more than 3 percent of Russia's population.

The implications of such diverse application of the obligatory medical insurance law are clear. First of all, it results in a dramatic divergence in per capita health expenditures among the regions, with Moscow and some of the eastern areas of the country enjoying levels four to six times higher than in most of the North Caucasus and Central Chernozem regions.[11] More importantly, it means that the structural changes intended by the insurance system cannot possibly take hold evenly and systematically. Even if the incentive structure dictated by the insurance scheme were perfect, it would have the opportunity to offer those incentives to only a minority of hospitals and clinics in a minority of regions. But the problem lies even deeper than that, since even in those 14 regions where all insurance contributions flow through insurance companies, a significant portion—in most cases, the majority—of resources devoted to health care still comes from government budgets. In other words, even under the best-case existing scenario, medical care providers receive money from two sources—insurance companies, and the budget—and so their incentives for improving efficiency and quality of care are mixed (see table 3.2).

This mixed budget/insurance model of financing has simply not been adequate to produce the structural changes necessary to encourage market-based incentives. Competition between insurance

Table 3.2   Structure of Russian Health Care Expenditures, 1996

Funding Source	Amount, Millions of Rubles	Percentage of Total
Federal budget	6,083	7.5
Local budgets (not including obligatory medical insurance payments)	44,568	54.9
Obligatory medical insurance	20,040	24.7
Out-of-pocket payments	5,510	6.8
Payments by enterprises	4,963	6.1
Total	81,164	100

Source: V.P. Korchagin, *Finansovoye obespecheniya zdravookhraneniya* (Moscow: *Epidavr,* 1997), 46, taken from official Russian government data.

companies is impossible, of course, in those regions that do not have them, and its impact is negligible in the many areas that are served by only a few. It is difficult to convince private insurance companies to operate in some of the more sparsely populated parts of Russia, where high logistical costs would eat into already slim profit margins. The system operates as intended in a few regions such as Samara and Kemerovo, where a handful of companies compete to attract new business, but this is not the case even in some areas operating under the "insurance company" model and generally labeled as progressive in their health care reforms. The city of Moscow, for example, enjoys the services of six companies licensed to provide obligatory medical insurance, but those six firms carved up the city geographically when the system was first born, and they continue to claim distinct territories within the city, never competing directly against one another.[12]

Competition between physicians, between clinics, and between hospitals is virtually unheard of as well, largely because of the resilience of the Soviet practice of assigning patients to primary care-givers strictly according to residence or workplace. Doctors' salaries are largely set according to government-specified scales, with wage differentiation only for level of specialization and length of service. Even when head doctors at various treatment institutions are given leeway to reward health care workers under their supervision for exceptional performance, these rewards usually take the form of one-time bonuses. Head doctors are reluctant to commit surplus resources to wage payments when unexpected increases in the prices of medicines and utilities are so common, and may need to be addressed at any time. Clinics are reluctant to try to attract new patients, since by definition those new enrollees would live outside their neighborhood area, and physicians do not want to travel far for house calls (still a significant feature of Russian medical practice). Physicians within clinics actually experience an incentive not to attract new patients, since their only reward is an increased personal work load. And patients, even within those few areas in which they are granted the freedom to choose their own polyclinic physician (and are well informed about this opportunity), respond indifferently; the common sentiment is that all physicians have similar levels of education, and therefore they are essentially "all the same."[13]

The only hope for competitive incentives therefore lies in the alteration or abolition of those rigid salary scales, and in the longer term, in the birth of a private health care sector granted the right to participate on equal terms in the system of obligatory medical insurance. Recent health ministers have made preliminary overtures toward dealing with the politically thorny salary issue. Most health care workers are reluctant to exchange a guaranteed wage for the uncertainty of a merit-based system in which some might lose their jobs.

Several other recent proposals have been aimed at correcting the perceived defects in the obligatory medical insurance system and the general structural problems in Russia's health care system. One, which first emerged in late 1996, would abolish private health insurance companies, subsume the quasi-governmental insurance Funds back into the health ministries at the federal and regional level, and essentially return the country to an entirely budget-financed model. This proposal, backed initially by the Communist Party but also supported by important elements in the government, gained considerable political currency after the August 1998 financial collapse that caused the health care system to lose substantial revenues due to failed banks and investments in state securities. It stems from a widespread perception that the insurance companies are nothing but greedy middlemen, siphoning money away from health care needs and making huge profits from "administrative expenses" and the investment of insurance revenues, but providing little in the way of benefit to the system. The proposal in the form of a draft law passed a first reading in the State Duma on June 11, 1999 by a vote of 318–2, but considerable controversy will continue to surround this radical change to the insurance mechanism before any final passage takes place.[14]

Another prominent suggestion would retain the insurance concept, but merge the medical insurance and social insurance off-budget Funds. Since social insurance covers sick leave, health professionals generally favor this idea in principle as likely to promote administrative efficiencies. But they reject it in practice for two reasons: first, because of the likelihood that the combined Funds would be assigned a lower payroll tax than the sum of their separate current levels (3.6 percent for medical, 5.4 percent for social insurance); and second, because the merger would place tax collection into the hands of the state tax collection service, which as a rule has not performed its primary function nearly as effectively as the medical insurance Funds.[15] This latter fear also moved a step closer to realization with a 31 December 1998 government proposal to turn tax collection for all of the off-budget Funds, including medical insurance, over to the state tax service on an experimental basis in three regions: the Republic of Bashkortostan, Khabarovsk Kray, and Orlov Oblast.[16] Critics warn that this change is designed simply to give the government access to the supposedly off-limits, earmarked pools of money currently flowing into these Funds, channeling that revenue inevitably back into the general budget pool, and that the resultant raiding of social programs could result in genuine widespread social unrest.

Even these proposals, however—abolishing insurance companies, and merging medical and social insurance—focus exclusively on mechanisms of revenue generation and revenue flow. They do not tackle the structural issues essential to encourage intensive growth, efficiency in resource consumption, and improved quality of health care. In this way, they would at core abandon any intention of instituting real insurance as the mechanism for financing Russian health care, instead replacing the insurance concept with an all-encompassing form of social security. The proposals also seem insufficient to address the most urgent issue facing Russian health care, the dramatic mismatch between available resources and the amount of health care promised by the Russian constitution and the perceived spirit of the insurance legislation.

It has been estimated that, in order to fully finance the amount of medical care currently provided to Russian citizens, the obligatory medical insurance payroll tax would have to be raised to 9 percent—a level that health care advocates lobbied for when the insurance legislation was written, but that proved utterly infeasible politically. Under a September 1998 government proposal, this problem will be solved through the annual generation of a new list of specific types of medical services to be provided free of charge. This list will correspond directly to obtainable health care funding and resources, taking into account existing health care facilities and the state of the population's health, and will be financed primarily through the insurance system at the regional level. Individual regions will be permitted to offer benefits beyond, but not less than, this federally mandated list, ensuring that local officials cannot siphon off health insurance money to non–health-related purposes. Only emergency medical care and ailments deemed to be "socially significant"—sexually transmitted and other infectious diseases, mental illness, and others—will be financed directly from the federal budget. A specific list of pharmaceutical products, consisting of 415 mostly domestically produced medicines, is also included in the scope of mandated coverage.[17]

Given current resource levels, if carried out as written, this scheme will dramatically shrink the number and types of services covered by the insurance system and therefore granted to the population "for free." A substantial percentage of medical care will have to be transferred to legal, paid services, with payments made either out of pocket at the point of service or through the purchase of additional, voluntary medical insurance beyond the mandated government insurance system. Health officials have discussed the situation as though the only forms of care to be removed from the realm of free benefits will be "optional" services such as massage, cosmetic surgery, private hospital rooms, and the like. Even under the most optimistic levels of funding, however, significant paring of coverage will be necessary in order truly to match the medical treatment carried out with the money available to pay for it. Dental services, for example, are certain to be removed entirely from the list of benefits. The realization of this "guarantee" also presupposes significant transfer payments to the regions in order to equalize spending across the country. It is unclear how the legislature's rejection of the 8 billion rubles in subsidies for 1998 have affected the plan's conceptualization and implementation, although in principle it seems certain that these proposals will remain in the realm of good intentions without some additional money. Under the best-case scenario, this plan will result in a replacement of the current form of de facto rationing—better health care goes to those with the better ability to pay—with a system that directs expensive care to those in the greatest medical need, regardless of their personal resources.

Structural Reform of the Health Care System

Even sensible rationing and reduction of free benefits, however, do not address the litany of structural deficiencies that continue to limit intensive growth, discourage efficiency in resource consumption, and restrict improvements in quality of care. To that end, the most important elements of current reform proposals focus on the rigidities and perverse incentives still in effect from the Soviet period. One of those is the marked tendency to direct patients toward treatment by highly specialized physicians under inpatient hospital conditions, when much more cost-effective clinic visits to a general practitioner would do. Between 65 and 70 percent of treatment resources are currently spent on hospitals, with another 10–12 percent going toward expensive emergency ambulance calls.[18] The outpatient physician of first contact, the workplace or neighborhood physician to whom each Russian citizen is assigned, currently works more as a dispatcher than as a caregiver. In recent years, she (the vast majority of these clinic physicians are women) has rendered care to only 40–42 percent of the patients she has seen, referring the rest to almost entirely hospital-based specialists for further tests and consultations.[19] As a result, patients suffer from long queues for tests and surgical procedures, with the waits often taking place after admission to a hospital even though tests have not yet been performed. They are therefore unnecessarily exposed to hospital-based infections and other complications. The average length of hospital stay is currently 16–17 days, one of the longest in the world.[20]

Breaking these habits will require a number of structural reforms: replacing expensive hospital care with outpatient clinic visits, tests, procedures, and even surgeries, where appropriate; shifting the thrust of medical education and practice to include widespread introduction of general practice or family doctors; and allowing, even encouraging, patients to choose which clinic or hospital to go to for treatment, instead of adhering to rigidly assigned catchment areas, in order to realize the benefits of competition. Russian commentators boast that progress has been made nationwide in this regard, with a reduction in the number of total inpatient hospital beds, from 13.8 per 1,000 population in 1990 to 11.9 in 1998.[21] But this kind of action alone will not result in significant cost savings, since most hospital resources go toward payments for staff wages and communal services (heat, electricity, etc.) that will not change simply by reducing the number of beds on a ward. Not just beds, but entire areas of hospital space must be reprofiled, so that personnel and material resources are redirected toward less expensive and resource-intensive, but still medically appropriate, types of outpatient care.

Although these kinds of ideas have been paid lip service for years, the current financial woes of the health care system seem to be encouraging more serious consideration in some quarters of a shift from extensive to intensive growth. The World Bank has spent 270 million dollars in 39 oblasts on a recent project to develop Russia's polyclinic network, facilitating the shift away from inpatient-based health care. The Russian health ministry cautions that this transition should take place not mechanically or haphazardly, but with specific goals in mind: 15 percent of the total number of hospital beds must be eliminated, and of those remaining, 15 percent should be allocated for medical-social purposes (care for the homeless, indigent, etc.), 20 percent for long-term treatment of patients with chronic illnesses, 20 percent for intensive care, and 45 percent for recovery from surgery and other short-term rehabilitation. Specific goals have also been set for hospitalization rates. In 1996, Russian citizens averaged 3,560 bed-days (days occupying a hospital bed) per 1,000 population. For 1998, the target was a reduction of this figure to 2,900 per 1,000 population, with the remaining 660 transferred to treatment in an outpatient setting.[22]

In some regions, where World Bank pilot projects are in effect, implementation of this idea is working. In Tula, for example, polyclinic and other hospital-replacement care is slowly but surely emerging to follow the spirit of the recommendations. Small but growing percentages of resources formerly devoted to inpatient treatment are now directed toward more cost-effective alternatives: 6 percent of hospital funding now goes toward day hospitals, where patients needing long-term treatment come during daylight hours but return home at night; 3 percent funds newly formed hospital departments essentially equivalent to Western nursing homes, where treatment for the elderly can be provided much more cheaply than in a regular hospital; and 0.6 percent goes toward hospitalization at home, where long-term care is delivered by nurses' visits to patients' apartments.[23] Centers for ambulatory surgery are also being established.

Hospitals are also, under some domestically funded initiatives, beginning to retool. Moscow's City Clinical Hospital No. 31, under a project dubbed "The Creation of the Clinic of the 21st Century," is now offering its own array of outpatient services, in essence blurring the previously strict boundaries between outpatient clinic care and inpatient services in hospitals. Since virtually all of even the most rudimentary diagnostic and treatment equipment is located in hospitals anyway, this would seem to be a more efficient route than building, equipping, and staffing brand new clinic facilities. This hospital now offers ambulatory endoscopic diagnostics and treatment, radiation diagnostics, physical therapy and other rehabilitative services, a clinical laboratory, and a pharmacy, all previously available only on an inpatient basis. Still designated as an "experiment," the hospital's new directions of activity have been funded both by budget and insurance revenues and by private investors. With appropriate political support, and if it proves financially profitable for its private backers, this demonstration project could be replicated in cities across Russia; similar success stories are already beginning to sprout up in the Ulyanovsk Oblast and other regions.[24]

Another Moscow facility, the Spasokukotskiy Clinic, has established itself as a model for conducting outpatient surgeries. In its new Center for Ambulatory Polyclinic Surgery, not only resident surgeons but also physicians employed by other hospitals have performed 3,500 operations since the facility opened, in fields ranging from gynecology and urology to ophthalmology and otolaryngology. In the vast majority of cases, these patients have suffered few or no complications, enabling them to return home the day of surgery, and to return to work an average of 3.5 times faster than if they had been treated under inpatient conditions.[25]

The expansion of hospital-replacement techniques will not work without appropriate incentives for all of the players involved. These kinds of specifics regarding implementation are, unfortunately, absent from current official reform proposals. World Bank and private investor funding is not going to touch most Russian health care institutions; some kind of systemic change in the structure of financing and payments to clinics and hospitals is needed, whether those resources come from the budget or from medical insurance companies. The current incentive system, which in the vast majority of cases continues to pay hospitals according to numbers of occupied beds and clinics according to numbers of patient visits, is certain to scuttle attempts to alter the superstructure of health care delivery. In the late 1980s, a few of Russia's regions experimented with a system of capitation financing for polyclinics, in which clinics were paid according to the number of patients enrolled as part of their service network, regardless of whether or how often those patients actually sought care. The clinics then acted as exclusive fundholders, referring patients to hospitals only when medically necessary and paying for that hospital care out of their own coffers. During its short life span, this arrangement resulted in dramatic reductions in average length of hospital stay and total numbers of hospital beds in Samara and Kemerovo oblasts. The economic reforms of the early 1990s, however, caused the system to crash, as inflationary real hospital costs bankrupted the still budget-financed clinics. Under more stable inflationary conditions and a guaranteed level of funding from the insurance mechanism, many Russian analysts will call for a return to this or a similar scheme of payments to health care providers. If successfully implemented and coupled with active patient choice of physician and clinic, with higher wages going to individual caregivers and treatment facilities offering higher quality services and therefore attracting more consumer demand, the inefficiencies resulting from perverse incentives held over from the Soviet era might finally become a thing of the past.

Family Practice and Privatization

The shift to more cost-effective outpatient medical care will also not work without a parallel expansion of the activity of general practice or family physicians. Conceptually, the family doctor did not exist in the Soviet Union. Virtually all physicians chose a narrow specialty from the beginning of their medical school training programs. Currently there are over 100 designated specialties, far more than virtually anywhere else in the world, with lines distinguishing medical expertise drawn along a wide variety of boundaries: specialists in the treatment of specific illnesses; physicians trained in one particular diagnostic method or apparatus (without the license to treat the diagnosed malady); specialists in various age groups of the population (neonatal, pediatrics, adolescents, geriatrics); surgeons trained to care for one particular organ or system (for example, heart specialists cannot perform heart surgery—only cardiosurgeons can); and physicians licensed to practice only in one specific type of environment (neighborhood clinic, workplace, emergency room or vehicle, health resort or sanitarium, sports medicine, etc.). One Russian physician, fearing a continuing trend in this direction, predicts sardonically that soon the health ministry will follow the lead of the resort city of Mineralny Vody in designating a new "physician-enema therapist" specialty, trained specifically to treat intestinal problems with the mineral waters of the Caucasus.[26]

In theory, the spread of general medical practice will enable more broadly trained physicians to treat patients more cost-effectively at the clinic level; rationalize the number of and procedures for referrals to specialists; facilitate the building of more personalized, long-term relationships between doctors, patients, and their families; and encourage a cost-effective shift toward preventive health maintenance and away from emergency care. The emergence of well-trained general practitioners will be particularly welcome in rural areas, where low population densities make it difficult to maintain a wide array of specialists in residence.

Current clinic-level physicians are likely to resist these changes unless retraining is made widely and easily available. So far, reforms in medical education have instead focused on the production of new generalists. In the last two years, again funded largely under World Bank auspices, Russian medical schools have established new departments and programs to train general practitioners. In Moscow, St. Petersburg, and the Tula, Samara, Leningrad, and Kemerovo oblasts, a total of around 400 family doctors are already serving almost a million patients.[27]

Private health care is even more politically controversial. This issue was rancorously debated in the Duma in 1998, as legislators considered the draft law "On Private Health Care."[28] Introduced by deputy Gamid Askerkhanov, the proposed draft was straightforward. It would have given private practice doctors the right to participate in the obligatory medical insurance system and to lease space not currently actively used in existing state clinics and hospitals (including the sizable number of facilities badly needing repair, or on which original construction was never completed). Private practitioners would be prohibited only from treating "socially significant" illnesses (again, such as STDs, infectious diseases, mental illnesses, etc.) and carrying out other "sensitive" procedures such as harvesting tissues and organs for transplantation. The law would also have placed under regulation the substantial and growing amount of questionably legal payments for medical care rendered in state health care institutions. Its proponents intended it to boost quality in the state sector through the promulgation of genuine competition, encourage state institutions to pay their best doctors and nurses higher wages to prevent them from defecting to the private sector, and place under regulation and taxation the almost 100,000 traditional and "alternative" providers already working outside the umbrella of the government's health care network. In Askerkhanov's words, "The patient suffers from the monopoly of state medicine."[29]

After heated discussion on the floor of the legislature in March 1998, however, it became clear that the draft in its current form was doomed. Askerkhanov withdrew it from consideration, in the hopes that an amended version to be presented later might enjoy more support.[30] The arguments against legal legitimization of a private health care sector were predictable, as was their source in the Communist and Liberal Democratic parties. Several deputies argued that the draft law provided for unacceptably weak regulation and even preferential tax provisions for private practitioners, and at its core was intended to "shove aside" patients toward private physicians and therefore permit even further reductions in budget allocations toward health care. In other words, the predominant fear was that competition would destroy state health care, leaving the poor and middle-class without access to any health care at all. One deputy repeatedly called the draft law "a cancerous tumor on the decrepit body of state and municipal health care."[31]

The deputies opposing the law on private health care, however, are ignoring one important fact: current estimates hold that "private," out-of-pocket payments for medical care, either to unlicensed practitioners or as side payments to established physicians, amount to 1.25 percent of GNP, or about one-third of all health care expenditures.[32] One anecdotal account claims that rooms at Moscow's public hospitals are available only for a $200–300 side payment, with patients otherwise lying on beds placed in corridors; that nurses require "installments" of $2–4 per day in order ensure that they do not "forget" patients; and that physicians frequently ignore or intentionally misdiagnose serious conditions until a "fistful of dollars" prods them to become "more attentive" to the need for appropriate treatment or surgery.[33] The chair of the Duma's Committee on Health Protection, Dr. Nikolay Gerasimenko, has cited research showing that people earning below minimum wage spend 35–50 percent of their own personal resources on medical services paid for out-of-pocket.[34] Meanwhile, on the other side of the socioeconomic spectrum, hundreds of thousands of more well-off citizens currently routinely purchase private voluntary medical insurance, amounting to an estimated total of five to seven percent of total Russian health care expenditures.[35] In other words, the reality of the situation is that people are already systematically denied the comprehensive "free" health care guaranteed to them by the Russian constitution, and some regulation of this spontaneously emergent set of side payments is needed.

Proposals have emerged to acknowledge that people are paying for their own health care, but to systematize these payments and simultaneously cover the "budget gap" by introducing official co-payments for treatment provided under obligatory medical insurance. Proponents argue that mandatory co-payments would also encourage people to pay more attention to their own health status, perhaps to take preventive measures such as improving their diets, curbing the use of alcohol and tobacco, and increasing their level of exercise, if they knew that they would have to make legal and predictable out-of-pocket payments every time they accessed the health care system. So far, these arguments have achieved little significant political currency.

Conclusion: Impact of the August 1998 Financial Crisis

The August 1998 economic crisis in Russia had a dramatic impact on the health sphere. Government-channeled financing of health care, including both budget allocations and employer payments into obligatory medical insurance, was slashed by 18 percent in 1998 compared with 1997.[36] These decreases were felt most harshly by health care workers, whose wage arrears were almost five times larger at the end of 1998 than at the beginning. The supply of medications and medical equipment to clinics and hospitals also suffered, as inflation drove prices up and general financial instability caused a production drop-off in 32 of the 80 major pharmaceutical enterprises in the country.[37] Price increases in food and medicines for patients, and also for water, fuel, and electrical services, further squeezed hospital and clinic budgets (not incidentally exacerbating an already existing imbalance in the structure of those facilities' budgets, where too much money is spent on communal services and not enough directly for medical treatment).

The insurance system itself also suffered direct financial hits, with insurance companies losing a significant amount in insurance taxes that were "frozen" in state securities, and the level of collection of insurance taxes decreasing by about 10 percent.[38] This exacerbation of the existing financial crisis in health care has carried direct, and possibly long-term, political consequences, as actors across the political spectrum have begun to question the utility of obligatory medical insurance as a whole. In essence, the insurance scheme has become conceptually discredited. Former proponents of maintaining the role of private insurance companies in the system, for example, have jumped ship and now support the draft law to return all health care financing to government hands; the crisis has prompted many observers not only to label the insurance companies wasteful "middlemen," but also to examine more critically their limited success in reducing health care costs and promoting resource efficiencies. The August 1998 crisis dramatically increased the probability that the insurance system will undergo dramatic, systemic legislated change in the near future.

The financial crisis has also contributed to other nodes of political instability directly affecting health care. Along with the game of musical chairs played by the dizzying turnover of Russian prime ministers, for example, has come a succession of new ministers of health—now amounting to six new ministers in the last four years. Without stable leadership, and most importantly without a consistent and effective voice on behalf of health and medical care in the government, not only medical insurance but all of health care financing and structural reform has suffered.[39] The government, for example, put forward in 1998 a proposal to reduce the health insurance tax on employers from 3.6 percent to 3.4 percent, despite repeated insistence from representatives of the health sector that movement in the opposite direction is desperately needed.[40] Without a strong central presence in the ministry of health, it is also clear that the regions will continue to go their own way, with haphazard, uncoordinated formation of health policy and reform that is unlikely to produce consistent, effective intensive growth.

In sum, the financial situation in Russian health care is bleak. There is simply not enough money to pay for all of the free medical care promised to Russian citizens as part of their constitutional birthright. While credible proposals exist on paper to make more effective use of the resources on hand, an absolutely necessary strategy given the virtual impossibility of new monetary infusions in the foreseeable future, the health care system has exhibited neither the political inclination nor the financial will to move toward systematic, country-wide implementation of these ideas. International assistance and private investments do not have the reach required for widespread long-term change. Until the political momentum is gathered to move forward with serious structural reforms, patients and health care workers alike will continue to suffer from the collapse of the Soviet health care safety net.

NOTES

This research was assisted by a grant from the Eurasia Program of the Social Science Research Council with funds provided by the State Department under the Russian, Eurasian, and East European Training Program (Title VIII), and a Fellowship Grant from the National Council for Eurasian and East European Research, also under the authority of a Title VIII Grant. The author would like to thank the SSRC and the NCEEER for their generous support.

1. Christopher Williams, "Russian Health Care in Transition," in *Russian Society in Transition,* eds. Christopher Williams, Vladimir Chuprov, and Vladimir Staroverov (Aldershot, England: Dartmouth Publishing Company, 1996), 185.

2. Judyth L. Twigg, "Balancing the State and the Market: Russia's Adoption of Obligatory Medical Insurance," *Europe-Asia Studies* 50, no. 4 (1998): 583–602.

3. Igor Sheiman, "From Beveridge to Bismarck Model of Health Finance: A Case Study of the Russian Federation" (paper presented at the conference "Innovations in Health Care Financing," Washington, D.C., 10–11 March 1997), 4–5.

4. A. M. Taranov, V. Yu. Semenov, and K. Yu. Lakunin, "Razvitiye sistemy obyazatel'nogo meditsinskogo strakhovaniya v Rossiyskoy Federatsii," *Zdravookhraneniye,* no. 3 (1999): 7–13; "Sistema OMS protivostoit krizisy," *Meditsinskaya gazeta,* no. 49, 30 June1999, 4.

5. Taranov, Semenov, and Lakunin, "Razvitiye sistemy."

6. Il'ya Lomakin-Rumyantsev, then Executive Director of the Moscow City Obligatory Medical Insurance Fund, interview by author, Moscow, May 1997.

7. S. V. Shishkin, "Problemy i vozmozhnyye stsenarii razvitiya sistemy meditsinskogo strakhovaniya," *Zdravookhraneniye,* no. 5 (1999): 53–61.

8. Vladimir Starodubov, "Podvedem itogi, posmotrim v budushchyeye," *Meditsinskiy vestnik,* no. 1(116), 1999, 3.

9. Yevgeniy Goryunov, Chair of Medical Insurance Subcommittee, State Duma Committee on Health Protection, interview by author, Moscow, June 1998.

10. N. A. Kravchenko, "Regional'nyye finansovyye modeli razvitiya sistemy OMS v Rossii," *Zdravookhraneniye,* no. 2 (1998): 41–57.

11. Yuri Komarov, "Kak posravnit' da posmotret'," *Meditsinskiy vestnik,* no. 8(123), 1999, 6–7.

12. Maria Ivanova, Director for Work with Federal Medical Establishments, MedStrakh Medical Insurance Company, interview by author, Moscow, June 1998.

13. Galina Skvirskaya, Head of Department of Organization and Control of Medical Care for the Population, Ministry of Health of the Russian Federation, interview by author, Moscow, June 1998.

14. Mariya Shchetinina, "Vse bedy ot posrednika?" *Meditsinskiy vestnik,* no. 12(127), 1999, 3; Leonid Perelietchikov, "Zakony po vesne i oseni schitayut," *Meditsinskaya gazeta,* no. 52, 9 July 1999, 1, 3.

15. Vladimir Semenov, then First Deputy Executive Director, Federal Obligatory Medical Insurance Fund, interview by author, Moscow, June 1998.

16. Nikolay Dolenko, "Otchayannyy eksperiment, ili kak v odnochas'ye mozhno razrushit' sistemu obyazatel'nogo meditsinskogo strakhovaniya," *Meditsinskiy vestnik,* no. 3(118), 1999, 4.

17. Tatyana Dmitrieva, "Natseleny ne na slova, a na delo," *Meditsinskiy vestnik,* no. 21(88), 1–15 November 1997, 3.

18. Deputy Minister of Health Anatoly Vyalkov, "Programma gosgarantiy stavit zhestkiye usloviya," *Meditsinskaya gazeta,* no. 100, 16 December 1998, 4.

19. The analogous figure in Great Britain, for example, is 80–82 percent of patients treated entirely at the level of the primary care physician. See the interview with Oleg Shchepin, "Semeynyy vrach. Zachem gorodit' zabor?" *Meditsinskaya gazeta,* 25 February 1998, 4.

20. Shchepin, "Semeynyy vrach," 4.

21. Shishkin, "Problemy i vozmozhnyye," 53–61.

22. Tatyana Dmitrieva, "Ryadom, vmeste, na yedinuyu tsel'," *Meditsinskiy vestnik,* no. 19(86), 1–15 October 1997, 2.

23. Elena Chernienko, "Chtoby kontseptsiya ne stala dogmoy," *Meditsinskiy vestnik,* no. 20(87), 16–31 October 1997, 12.

24. "Otkrytyy razgovor o zdorov'ye Rossiyan," *Meditsinskaya gazeta,* 27 February 1998, 4–5.

25. Galina Konstantinova and Tat'yana Alikperova, "Khirurgiya odnogo dnya," *Meditsinskaya gazeta,* 3 April 1998, 6.

26. Igor Derevyanko, "Dozhdemsya li 'klizmoterapevtov'," *Meditsinskaya gazeta,* 20 February 1998, 5.

27. Dmitrieva, "Natseleny ne na slova," 3.

28. Published in its entirety in *Meditsinskaya gazeta,* 1 April 1998.

29. "Za i protif," *Moskovskiye novosti,* 15–22 February 1998, 23.

30. Gamid Askerkhanov, member of State Duma Committee on Health Protection, interview by author, Moscow, June 1998.

31. "Rakovaya opukhol' na odryakhlevshem tele zdravookhraneniya . . .," *Meditsinskiy vestnik,* no. 8(99), 16–31 March 1998, 12.

32. Shishkin, "Problemy i vozmozhnyye," 53–61.

33. "Patients Cough Up For 'Free' Treatment," Agence France Presse, Moscow, 27 April 1999.

34. Cited in "Kodeks zdravookhraneniya," *Meditsinskiy vestnik,* no. 3(118), 1999, 3.

35. Nadezhda Mart'yanova, "Sredniy klass privykayet k kachsetvu," *Meditsinskiy vestnik,* no. 12(127), 1999, 9.

36. Shishkin, "Problemy i vozmozhnyye," 53.

37. Starodubov, "Podvedem itogi," 3.

38. Leonid Perepletchikov, "Yesli deneg nyet, no ochen' khochetsya," *Meditsinskaya gazeta,* no. 87, 30 October 1998, 1.

39. See Nikolay Naglyy, "Reformy otrasli: pochemu oni buksuyut?" *Meditsinskaya gazeta,* no. 85, 23 October 1998, 4.

40. Fedor Smirnov, "OMS skoree zhivo, chem mertvo. No yego nuzhno lechit'," *Meditsinskaya gazeta,* no. 4, 20 January 1999, 6.

CHAPTER 4

Negotiating the Post-Soviet Medical Marketplace: Growing Gaps in the Safety Net

Julie V. Brown and Nina L. Rusinova

SOVIET ERA CONSTITUTIONS PROCLAIMED THE FUNDAMENTAL right of their citizenry to essential medical care that would be free at the point of delivery. That commitment was renewed in the early 1990s by the new constitution of the post-Soviet Russian Federation. Among the many problems facing the Russian government since the breakup of the USSR has been figuring out how to finance and rehabilitate the troubled medical care system it inherited from the former regime. Sharply negative trends in national health statistics have served as a constant reminder of both the extent and the urgency of the problem. As other chapters in this volume amply demonstrate, those macro-level indicators present a disturbing picture of a system in deep crisis. Many commentators have questioned whether the medical care system is currently capable of providing adequate care to the Russian people. As for the extent to which medical care (irrespective of quality) can be had free of charge, that also remains open to question.

All of these matters have been broadly discussed in the Russian mass media, and the general population is well aware of them. "There are no healthy people here," is a recurring refrain in the conversations of ordinary Russians about health and illness in their homeland, and their assessments of the overall condition of the medical system are similarly pessimistic.[1] Nonetheless, these same people are also users of the system, and, as is true in other societies, the conclusions they draw from their own direct experiences tend to be more complex and variegated than their global assessments of its effectiveness. In this chapter we focus on the experiences of Russian citizens who find themselves in need of medical attention. Where do people with poor health go for help? What do they encounter when they enter the system? How well does the medical care system meet their needs? And, most importantly, to what extent are people who need medical attention deprived of it because the constitutional guarantee of access to care remains unfulfilled? How significant, in other words, are the gaps in the medical care safety net and who is slipping through them?

These are broad and complex questions, and experiences certainly differ somewhat from region to region. The data on which the present analysis is based come from mass surveys and intensive interviews with ordinary Russians (the consumers of medical care) and with medical practitioners. All of this research has been carried out by the authors in the city of St. Petersburg, Russia's second largest city, throughout the 1990s. Our earliest survey (N=1,500) took place in the spring of 1992, just a few months after the dissolution of the Soviet Union. Between 1993 and 1995 we conducted intensive interviews with carefully selected samples of both physicians (N=80) and middle-aged *Peterburgtsy* from different levels of the urban social structure (N=44). In the spring of 1998 we completed another mass survey (N=1,198) of the entire adult population.[2]

St. Petersburg, the former imperial capital, has traditionally been reasonably well supplied with medical institutions and highly trained medical experts. For that reason, the experiences of *Peterburgtsy* are doubtless somewhat different from those of Russians in rural and other medically underserved regions. However, examining the "best" the system has to offer serves as a significant indicator of both the nature and the scope of the problem at the national level.

Paying for Medical Care

Our research indicates quite clearly that, in the late 1990s, medical treatment in urban Russia is rarely completely free of charge. On the contrary, very few people avoid spending at least a few rubles when they enter the medical care system, and quite a few end up paying significantly more than that. Of the *Peterburgtsy* who had sought medical attention during the thirty days preceding our most recent interviews with them, fewer than one in ten said that all aspects of their treatment had been free. Not surprisingly, the highest expenditures were reported by those who sought care in "pay" clinics. However, almost half of the people who were treated at their neighborhood polyclinics also paid for physician visits (48.9 percent), for medical tests (44.4 percent), and/or for medical procedures (43 percent). Patients who went to polyclinics affiliated with their place of work paid even more. While free care at such institutions was a highly valued perquisite in the Soviet period, in early 1998, more than two-thirds (69.5 percent) of the people who went to their workplace polyclinic had to pay to see a physician, and at least half also paid for diagnostic tests (50 percent) and/or medical procedures (58.3 percent). As can be inferred from their name, "pay" (*platnaia*) polyclinics do not provide free care. Everyone in our study who elected to visit such an institution was charged a fee to be seen by a physician. More noteworthy is the fact that all of the *Peterburgtsy* who took their medical problems to a physician friend (*znakomyi vrach*) during this same period also paid for the privilege. It appears that the informal "barter" medical economy that played such an important role in the Soviet era is being transformed by larger market forces. Virtually all physicians in St. Petersburg provide some medical care to their friends and families.[3] In the past many of these interactions involved informal exchanges of goods and services. Transactions apparently now commonly involve more formal cash reimbursements. Having "connections" may still be an important determinant of access to good quality medical care, but being well connected does not appear to protect people from the necessity of paying for the services they receive.[4]

Almost a quarter (24.2 percent) of our respondents paid more than 100 rubles for their most recent medical encounter. Given that the median per capita monthly income in this sample of *Peterburgtsy* was only 430 rubles, that figure is hardly trivial. Medications remain one of the most costly items in the medical care budgets of this population. More than one in five (21.8 percent) of the people who had needed medications within the last month told us that they had paid in excess of 100 rubles for their drugs alone. The proportion of *Peterburgtsy* paying at least that amount for dental care is even higher (53.7 percent). Only one person in five (22.5

percent) paid nothing for their most recent visit to a dentist, and far fewer (7.8 percent) were able to find free medications.

Thus, being sick in St. Petersburg can be a costly enterprise. Expenditures of the magnitude just described would make a serious dent in the budget of the majority of Russians. Unfortunately, the problem of paying for medical care is all too often complicated further by economic deprivation. As is true in societies around the world, poor health in Russia is strongly associated with poverty. More than seventy years of Soviet rule and the oldest "universal access" national health care system in the world failed to eliminate socioeconomic status differences in health. These differences were quite evident in 1992, and, if anything, they became more pronounced by 1998.[5] By far the strongest predictor of level of health among *Peterburgtsy* is material well-being. People with poor health do tend to be older than the population as a whole and poverty is more common among the elderly; however, the correlation between poverty and ill health is evident in *all* age groups.

Peterburgtsy *in Poorest Health*

The scope of the problem (and the extent to which urban Russians are falling through the social and medical service safety net) becomes evident when we focus on the experiences of those who have the poorest health. In our 1998 survey we assessed health using the *SF-36,* an instrument that has been widely used internationally and measures several distinct dimensions of health.[6] For the purposes of the discussion here, we have identified *Peterburgtsy* whose scores on the General Health scale are in the lowest 25 percent.[7] This group has a much greater than average need for medical and other support services, and, as we shall see, these needs are all too often inadequately met.

Peterburgtsy with the lowest levels of health are disproportionately older and female. Almost half (47.8 percent) are over the age of sixty and more than two-thirds (68.4 percent) are women. They also have less education than other members of the population, and they are less likely (regardless of age) to be gainfully employed. More than a quarter (28.3 percent) have completed less than a secondary education. This is twice as many as in the general population. While older *Peterburgtsy* tend to be less educated than their younger counterparts, this pattern cannot be attributed to age alone. The correlation between poor health and lack of education is evident among people as young as 30 years of age.

The most striking characteristic of the members of this group, however, is the extent to which they are suffering various kinds of deprivation. Almost half (46.8 percent) told us that they just barely get by from one payday to the next and are often forced to borrow money in order to buy basic necessities. The situation of most of the others is scarcely better. Another third (38 percent) described their incomes as just barely sufficient to provide for necessities. Even purchasing clothing is difficult, i.e., they either have to borrow money or scrimp and save to be able to buy things to wear. In other words, more than four in five of St. Petersburg's unhealthiest residents are forced to devote much of their energies to the struggle for mere economic survival. The majority (61 percent) of them have made no major purchases in the 1990s (almost twice as many as in the population as a whole). While younger *Peterburgtsy* tend to be much more active consumers overall, even among those in their twenties, people with poor health are far less likely than their age peers to be buying newly available durable goods, such as televisions, refrigerators, furniture, and washing machines.

These much lower levels of consumption are only one indicator of the deprivation experienced by this group of *Peterburgtsy*. Their incomes are significantly lower than the population median, and most say that lack of money restricts them in many ways, including their ability to go to the movies or the theater (89.7 percent), to take a vacation (87.3 percent), to invite friends and family to their homes (79.9 percent) or to make such visits themselves (82.9 percent). Given the vast international literature on the importance of social and emotional ties to health, it seems reasonable to suggest that these kinds of deprivations may contribute to the ill health these people are experiencing.[8] Perhaps even more significant is the fact that they also often find themselves unable to buy basic foodstuffs. As many as one in four indicated that lack of money for food is a constant problem.

Adequate diets are essential to the maintenance of health. For people whose health has already been compromised, nutritional deprivation is even more problematic. Significant proportions of *Peterburgtsy* with poor health are regularly unable to purchase meat and fish (75.1 percent), eggs (36.4 percent), dairy products (54.5

percent), and fruit (53.5 percent). There are even a few (8.8 percent) who told us that there are times when they cannot afford to buy bread. For one in twenty (4.7 percent) that is a continual problem.

The fact that so many *Peterburgtsy* report depriving themselves of food they consider to be essential serves as clear evidence that the system is not adequately protecting vulnerable groups. Although much attention has focused on the dislocations and suffering associated with the post-Soviet economic transitions, our interviews with a cross-section of this urban population indicate that for many people these deprivations are not a totally new experience. In 1992, more than a quarter of our respondents attributed their personal health problems to deprivation they had experienced earlier in their lives. Among the factors they mentioned were inadequate diets (32 percent), low incomes (42 percent), and poor living conditions (33 percent). Furthermore, significant numbers of *Peterburgtsy* told us in 1998 that the levels of economic well-being in their families of origin were not qualitatively different from the ones with which they are coping at the present time. This is particularly common among people with poor health, one in five (22.4 percent) of whom described childhoods characterized by economic deprivation so severe that at times they did not even have enough to eat. The parents of more than half (58.8 percent) of them had chronically faced the same dilemma that our respondents are currently experiencing: how to find enough money to buy basic clothing for themselves and the other members of their family.

Limited Options for Medical Care

Given their recurring experiences with economic deprivation, limited access to medical care is probably not the most important explanation for the health problems these *Peterburgtsy* are currently experiencing. Nonetheless, most of them do now need and seek out expert medical help on a regular basis. All too often they find that the promise of free care remains a hollow one. Instead, they encounter obstacles that seriously limit their ability to get the kinds of help they believe they need.

Almost three-quarters (74.9 percent) of these unhealthy *Peterburgtsy* told us that they had at least considered consulting a physician within the previous 30 days, and almost half of them actually did so. Of those who did not, very few indicated that concerns about cost had kept them home. More often, the problem either seemed to resolve itself or else the individual had other more pressing priorities and ultimately decided that he or she could manage the situation without medical assistance. That response seems to be particularly characteristic of people suffering from chronic conditions, who everywhere learn to recognize and handle many of their recurring symptoms.

Thus, the most serious problem is not that economic deprivation prevents many *Peterburgtsy* from crossing the thresholds of medical institutions. Most people do take their problems to the medical system. Fewer than one in twelve of these people with particularly weak health gets no medical care, and that minority avoids the medical system for a variety of reasons, only one of which is cost. Rather, the problem is that financial constraints significantly limit the options open to them, both in terms of where they are able to go for help and the content of the medical care that is offered to them and/or available at a price they can afford to pay.

People with poor health are far more likely than healthy *Peterburgtsy* to seek care only within the state medical system, where the costs are usually the lowest. While the oldest members of the population are more prone to utilize the state system no matter how healthy they are, even young people with serious medical problems mostly end up taking them to their neighborhood polyclinics. This is not because they are particularly satisfied with the care they receive there. Indeed, the people who use neighborhood polyclinics are almost twice as likely to cite cost (66.2 percent) as a primary factor in their decision as they are to say that they go there because they have had good experiences in the past (34.8 percent).

The options are particularly limited for women. Men are far more likely than women to choose to get their medical care at either workplace medical institutions (30 percent vs. 10.1 percent) or from physician friends (17.4 percent vs. 12 percent), and those who do are much happier with their overall experiences than the people who go to neighborhood polyclinics. The people who use workplace polyclinics, for example, are almost twice as likely to describe the care they have received as unqualifiedly "good" than are people who frequent neighborhood polyclinics (31.9 percent compared with 16.9 percent). Furthermore, more than half (51.1 percent) of the latter describe their polyclinic experiences as mostly or all "bad," while fewer than one in five (19.4 percent) workplace poly-clinic users are that negative.

In other words, the heavy use of the state system by women with poor health is not due to their greater confidence in it but rather to the fact that they have less access to alternatives.[9] Women are less likely to have worked in those economic sectors that provide workplace medical care. They also have less substantial "connec-tions" to the medical care system (including physician friends). While women are somewhat more likely than men to report that they know someone who works in the medical care system and at least in principle is in a position to assist them, close examination reveals that their contacts are often less helpful than those described by men. Fewer women, for example, say that their "connections" can help them to consult with a highly qualified physician, to find medications, or even to secure useful advice in general.[10] Last, but hardly least, women of all ages have incomes that are significantly lower than those of their male counterparts, so they have less dis-cretionary income they can choose to allocate to medical treatments.

Even restricting oneself to the care available from the state sys-tem, however, is not sufficient to keep medical costs manageable for many *Peterburgtsy*. Almost half of the people with poor health (45.9 percent) told us that paying for medical care has become a major item in their family budget. Far more (68.9 percent) indicated that they sometimes deny themselves necessary health care because they cannot pay for it. Fully half (50.5 percent) told us that they perpet-ually find themselves in that situation! In short, medical deprivation is a widespread phenomenon.

Access to Medications

One of the greatest problems reported by *Peterburgtsy* is access to medications. Even under the Soviet system people commonly paid for prescription medications. Thus, the idea that one should do so is not new to most people. However, in the Soviet era certain cate-gories of drugs were free, and there were large groups in the popu-lation for whom the prices were either eliminated or greatly reduced. As late as 1992 the primary worry of the people in this par-ticular urban population was how to *find* essential medications, *not* how to pay for them. The unavailability of medicines was a serious problem in the early 1990s. More than half of the people we surveyed reported problems getting medications they needed. However, only a very small minority (3 percent) attributed this to their excessive cost. Far more people said that the medications they needed were simply not available or they had been unable to locate them. Pensioners were actually more confident in 1992 than the rest of the population that medications (and medical care in general) would be affordable for them, because at that time they retained a measure of confidence in the promise that their costs would be subsidized by the state.

By early 1998 the situation had changed radically. The proportion of the overall population reporting at least occasional difficulties procuring needed medications had dropped slightly (from 57 percent in 1992 to 48.8 percent in 1998). However, those people who *are* having problems attribute them to escalating costs. The medications they need have simply become too expensive. The prices that *Peterburgtsy* report paying for prescription drugs are quite high, especially considering per capita income levels. Almost two-fifths (39.8 percent) of the people who had been treated for a medical problem within the last month had paid in excess of 50 rubles for medications alone, and as indicated previously, more than one in five (21.8 percent) had paid twice that much for this single illness episode.

The group most gravely affected by the high cost of medications is people who have serious and/or recurring health problems and low incomes. A disproportionate share of *Peterburgtsy* with these characteristics are pensioners, who have learned that their status no longer affords them much protection from high drug prices. Almost half (46.5 percent) of our unhealthy group had paid in excess of 100 rubles for the medications prescribed at their most recent medical visit. Only one in ten (10.5 percent) had been able to find all of the drugs prescribed at that visit cost-free. In consequence, the health problems experienced by these people often remained untreated. Indicative of this is the fact that only one in four (25.9 percent) told us that they are almost always able to get all the medicines they need. Nearly half (47.4 percent) said that they hardly ever can.

Physician-Patient Interaction

Medical practitioners are well aware of the financial constraints under which many of their patients operate. Most of the physicians we interviewed in the mid-1990s indicated that they believe it is important for them to familiarize themselves with the personal and economic circumstances of their patients. They also conceded that they take these circumstances into account in making treatment decisions. "If I see that [a patient] is not in a position to acquire a particular medication," commented a surgeon who works in a polyclinic, "then I try to select something else." While many of these doctors were hesitant to acknowledge openly that economic realities are compelling them to make compromises in the quality of the care they provide low-income patients, their remarks on the subject suggest that this concern is ever present in their minds. As another polyclinic physician noted, "There are some families where I know that if I prescribe an expensive medication it just won't get purchased.... So always, before I write a prescription, I think about how realistic it would be for them to buy the medication." One doctor, who is employed by a workplace polyclinic, spoke very directly about the extent to which the Russian medical system had already taken on the dual-class character so common in other parts of the world: "It is imperative now to determine [patients'] material situation. Some medications are very expensive. You have to choose: there's medicine for the wealthy and there's medicine for the poor."[11]

In short, the evidence strongly suggests that the quality as well as the quantity of medical care provided to *Peterburgtsy* varies according to their financial circumstances. Doctors make treatment decisions based on their perceptions about the ability and willingness of their patients to expend precious resources on their health. The comments cited above suggest that these particular doctors are reasonably familiar with the life-styles and attitudes of at least some of their individual patients. Unfortunately, that is all too often not the case. Although the doctors of St. Petersburg mostly concur with the view of the international medical community that health care tends to be more effective when it is provided within the context of an ongoing relationship between physician and patient, that type of relationship is the exception rather than the rule in urban Russian medical practice. Fewer than one in three *Peterburgtsy* with poor health told us that he or she has a "regular" physician (32.3 percent). In other words, these decisions about "rationing" of care are commonly reached as a result of short-term encounters between strangers. Given the predominance of paternalistic attitudes among

Russian physicians (not to mention their heavy patient loads), it is reasonable to assume that many of those decisions are made without a great deal of input from the patient.

The character of those physician-patient interactions may be one reason why so many ailing *Peterburgtsy* are convinced that the medical treatment they have received has not only failed to improve their health but has actually made it worse. This was reported by approximately half (53.5 percent of women; 48.9 percent of men) of the people we surveyed. Even more striking is the fact that almost one-third (33.5 percent of women; 28.2 percent of men) described their experiences with harmful medical care as a recurring problem rather than a single isolated incident of medical error. It is worthy of note that this perception has been a persistent one, i.e., *Peterburgtsy* were just as likely to blame bad medical care for their current health status in 1992 as they are in the late 1990s.

One must keep in mind that these accusations of medical mistakes do not come from the official reports of formal morbidity and mortality reviews conducted by medical professionals. Rather, they are lay people's subjective assessments of the impact of medical care on their own health. This is not to suggest that those assessments are necessarily invalid; however, research in other societies has demonstrated that perceptions about physician competence and quality of care can be influenced by the structure of the interaction. For example, people who have little control over the selection of their medical care providers, and whose contacts with those providers are time-limited and sporadic, tend to be more critical of the quality of their care.[12] A great many doctor-patient interactions in the medical systems of urban Russia have these characteristics.

Nonetheless, many of the people who were critical of medical decisions that had been made on their behalf could cite the opinion of another physician in support of their accusations. More than a third (35.9 percent) of the people we surveyed in 1998 indicated that on at least one occasion the treatment they had been prescribed by one physician had been directly criticized by another physician. Multiple experiences of this type are especially common among people with poor health, who spend more time interacting with a variety of doctors as they negotiate their way through the highly specialized medical care system. Thus, at least some of those people who are convinced that they have fallen (or been pushed) through the safety net that is supposed to ensure the quality of medical care base their conclusion not solely on their own assessments of how they are feeling but on the professional judgments of medical experts as well.

Given their overall discontent with the quality of the medical care they have received over the years, it seems remarkable that so many *Peterburgtsy* have relatively favorable recollections of their most recent medical encounters. Fewer than a third (28.8 percent) of those who had visited a neighborhood polyclinic in the month prior to our survey in early 1998 indicated that they had been dissatisfied with that particular experience, and even fewer (16.6 percent) expressed displeasure with the way they had been treated by the doctor who took care of them. The people who had seen medical providers in other settings were even less likely to have negative feelings about their encounters.

These findings are actually not quite as incongruous as they may seem on the surface. Research in other societies has consistently shown that people tend to be far more critical of the medical care system in the abstract than they are of their own personal care. This has certainly been characteristic of *Peterburgtsy* throughout the 1990s.[13] Those people who have been thoroughly alienated from the medical care system simply do their best to avoid it. (That perspective was summed up by a skilled worker we interviewed in the mid 1990s who remarked: "You know, it's torture for me to go to the doctor. I see those lines and I feel awful. Next time I'm not going to go, even if I really get sick.") As for those who do seek medical help, merely being seen by a physician and receiving some kind of diagnosis and treatment recommendation may have positive effects on well-being—at least in the short run. Nor can we discount the possibility that criticism of the system has been so intense and people's past experiences so negative that *Peterburgtsy* now simply have very low expectations for their outpatient encounters with it. Since they do not expect much they are less likely to be disappointed.

There can be little doubt that inadequate incomes dramatically increase the probability that *Peterburgtsy* will not receive all the medical care that they need. This problem is almost certainly aggravated to some degree by the structure of medical practice. The fact that medical practitioners and their patients frequently do not know each other very well almost certainly limits the respect and trust they feel for each other. It would be nothing short of extraordinary if this interaction pattern did not adversely affect the content of their communication about potentially sensitive topics, such as the social and economic circumstances of the latter.

Formal Safety Nets for the Most Vulnerable

In theory, physicians are not supposed to have to worry about such matters. Their task is to diagnose and treat rather than to worry about whether the care they recommend is affordable for their patients. There are, in fact, formal safety nets, one purpose of which is to protect those who are likely to have greater than normal needs for medical care and lower than average incomes. Since early in the Soviet period, for example, certain categories of people with limited ability to support themselves because of a physical and/or emotional condition have been legally classified as having a disability (*invalidnost'*). That status entitles them to a variety of benefits, including (but not limited to) access to inexpensive or even free medications, medical equipment, and medical services.[14]

Determining eligibility for disability status has historically been assigned to so-called medical-labor expert commissions (*Vrachebno-Trudovye Ekspertnye Komissii*), and the procedures have been highly bureaucratized with regularly scheduled reviews of eligibility. Anecdotal reports from physicians in the post-Soviet era have suggested that in practice there has been some liberalization of the eligibility criteria. The primary goal has been to expand the safety net to cover more of those having trouble making ends meet and taking care of their health. Our research provides some support for their contentions. In 1992 fewer than one in ten (9 percent) of the people we surveyed were legally classified as disabled. In 1998 the number was twice as high: 18.5 percent. All of the increase has been in Category II, defined as those people "who have lost the capacity to work efficiently in their former or any other occupation but may be able to work in specially created conditions."[15] Sixteen percent of our 1998 sample bears this legal classification, more than three times as many as in 1992. The majority of Category II *invalidi* are elderly women. That economic as well as medical need has been taken into account in determining their eligibility is strongly suggested by the fact that their health problems seem to be less debilitating than was true of Category II *invalidi* in 1992. Far fewer of them, for example, report that their health is so bad that they require continual assistance in managing the demands of daily life.

Thus, there have apparently been some efforts to extend existing safety nets to protect more of the vulnerable. Unfortunately, these efforts have not been particularly helpful. Almost half (47.8 percent) of *Peterburgtsy* with the poorest levels of general health are classified as disabled. However, having the status clearly has not begun to solve their problems. Indeed, the people who are disabled are just as likely as those without the status to report that they are often unable to pay for medical care they need, and only one in five (21.3 percent) say that they can usually get the medications they need. Although they are entitled to subsidized medications, they often cannot find them at the reduced prices, and they cannot afford to pay the regular prices. While the nonmedical benefits of disability status, such as subsidized housing and transportation costs, doubtless help to ensure these people a minimal level of subsistence, the vagaries of the medical marketplace limit its effectiveness as a guarantor of access to medical care.

As suggested above, the help needed by the most seriously ill and disabled members of the population extends far beyond financial assistance for rent, food, and medical treatment. The physical condition of some *Peterburgtsy* is so impaired that they need constant help even with such routine daily chores as shopping, cooking, cleaning, bathing, and getting dressed. Approximately one in ten of our respondents describes his or her own health in these terms; however, this almost certainly underestimates the scope of the problem in the population as a whole. As a matter of fact, more than a quarter (27.1 percent) of the households we surveyed include at least one individual who requires *continual* assistance because of health-related limitations. Historically, much of the responsibility for the care of the chronically ill and disabled has fallen on the shoulders of family members. In the past, however, it was easier for physicians to "prescribe" extended hospital stays for such patients. While the official reason for the hospitalization might be a formal course of treatment, a latent consequence was to lessen the physical and emotional burden on members of the patient's household.

Hospitals are now both less willing and less able to take on this responsibility. The net effect is a marked increase in the burden borne by family and friends, the so-called "hidden health care system."[16] The positive news is that only half as many of the people needing constant help in 1998 said that they do not get it as was true in 1992. More than one in five (21.3 percent) said they had no assistance at the time of our initial survey; only 10 percent now make that claim. The great bulk of this day-to-day care is provided by close relatives and friends; however, neighbors also participate occasionally, particularly in communal apartments. Very few families can afford to pay for private home health care workers, although there has been a growing market for this kind of service. There has also been some expansion in the system's efforts to reach such people outside of institutions, as is indicated by the fact that far more people now report that they receive assistance from social workers and other medical assistants than was true early in the decade. Almost half of the people needing ongoing care in 1998 told us that they sometimes (47.4 percent) or even regularly (34.1 percent) get this kind of help.

Nonetheless, the greatest burden is clearly shouldered by members of the patient's immediate household. Research elsewhere has well documented the health risks to which informal caretakers are subjected when they must continually care for a seriously ill or disabled family member.[17] Crowded living conditions and economic uncertainty (not to mention the absence of labor-saving home health products, such as disposable products for incontinent adults) certainly elevate stress levels in many such households in urban Russia.[18] Thus, in this instance, the gaping holes in the medical and social services network affect not only the patients but members of their extended families as well.

Conclusion: "I Wouldn't Want to Get Sick"

In conclusion, getting adequate medical care remains seriously problematic for many *Peterburgtsy*. Relatively little care is available for free, and people lack confidence in the quality of much of the care they do receive. Not surprisingly, this is a source of concern. Healthy people tend to fret about other problems, but for *Peterburgtsy* with poor health worry about whether they will have access to medical care is an ongoing preoccupation. They think about it a great deal, and in the long run this anxiety may be almost as great a threat to their well-being as the flaws in the system itself.

The citizens of Russia's second largest city no longer understand how their medical system operates. More than half of the people we surveyed know little or nothing about what medical services they are legally entitled to receive. Heavy users of the medical system, including *invalidi,* are no more knowledgeable than anybody else. Very few *Peterburgtsy* are confident that they will be able to get almost any kind of medical help that they might need. Overall, only one in ten (10.6 percent) is that optimistic, and among people who have health problems the percentage is even lower (5.7 percent). Three-quarters of the latter fear that they are not going to be able to get competent medical care, to have access to a hospital bed or to afford necessary medications. Two-thirds doubt that adequate emergency care will be available in the event of a crisis. For the most part, the only people who are relatively unconcerned about these problems are those who are young, healthy, and reasonably well off financially. For the rest of the population the situation is perceived to be much more tenuous. The safest solution, as one of the people we interviewed several years ago remarked, is simply to do your best to stay healthy: "I wouldn't want to get sick. That would be terrifying . . . really terrifying. Unless something changes I think I would just go ahead and buy myself white slippers (*belye tapochki,* i.e., burial garb). Yes, I am afraid."

NOTES

Financial support for this research has been provided by the Ford Foundation, the American Philosophical Society, the American Sociological Association, the Center for East-West Trade, Investment and Commerce at Duke University, the Soros Foundation, and the UNCG Excellence Foundation.

1. This comment was made repeatedly by people we interviewed in St. Petersburg, although many of them insisted that they were exceptions to that rule. In addition to the findings of our research, which are discussed later in this chapter, reports of popular opinion surveys assessing attitudes toward the medical care system are summarized in K. Muzdabaev, *Dinamika urovnia zhizni v Peterburge 1992–1994* (St. Petersburg: SMART Publishers, 1995).

2. These data were collected as part of an ongoing research project examining the relationship between health and social inequality in post-Soviet Russia. Both surveys involved multistage sampling procedures that controlled for gender, age, and type of residence.

3. N. L. Rusinova and J. V. Brown, "Women's Work and Women's Careers: Effects of Gender Expectations on Female Physicians in St. Petersburg, Russia" (paper presented at the International Congress on Women, Work, Health, Barcelona, Spain, 1996).

4. J. V. Brown and N. L. Rusinova, "Russian Medical Care in the 1990s: A User's Perspective," *Social Science and Medicine* 45, no. 8 (1997): 1265–1276.

5. Martin Bobak, et al., "Socioeconomic Factors, Perceived Control and Self-Reported Health in Russia: A Cross-Sectional Survey," *Social Science and Medicine* 47, no. 2 (1998): 269–279; J. V. Brown and N. L. Rusinova, "Health Inequalities in Post Soviet Russia: A Case Study of St. Petersburg" (paper presented at the Annual Meeting of the Southern Sociological Society, New Orleans, 1997).

6. A thorough description of this instrument can be found in J. E. Ware, Jr., *SF-36 Health Survey: Manual and Interpretation Guide* (Boston: The Health Institute, 1993).

7. A minimal score on the General Health scale indicates that the individual "evaluates personal health as poor and believes it is likely to get worse." See Ware, *SF-36 Health Survey*. In other words, this scale is based on respondents' subjective assessment of their overall health. The scale is constructed from answers to four questions. Research has consistently indicated that such assessments are very good predictors of future mortality and medical care utilization. See, for example, I. McDowell and C. Newell, *Measuring Health* (New York: Oxford University Press, 1987).

8. See, for example, M. Pilisuk and S. Parks, *The Healing Web: Social Networks and Human Survival* (Hanover, NH: University Press of New England, 1986).

9. Another factor encouraging use of the state system is simply that people are more familiar with it.

10. The only exception to this pattern is that more women than men say that their "connections" can help them get admitted to a good inpatient facility.

11. Herbal remedies tend to be cheaper than chemical ones, and more than half of *Peterburgtsy* utilize them to some extent. Cost is not the only reason why many people prefer these "natural" medications, however, and people with poor health are not more likely to do so than healthy people.

12. See, for example, J. A. Clark, et al., "Bringing Social Structure Back into Clinical Decision Making," *Social Science and Medicine* 32, no. 8 (1991): 853–866; and J. A. Hall and M. C. Dornan, "What Patients Like about Their Medical Care and How Often They Are Asked: A Meta Analysis of the Satisfaction Literature," *Social Science and Medicine* 27, no. 9 (1988): 935–939.

13. Even in 1992, when criticism of the medical care system was so high that 88 percent of the population believed it to be in need of fundamental reform, only 40 percent were critical of the polyclinic care they themselves had received, and even fewer (9.2 percent) were critical of their personal experiences with the hospital system.

14. The USSR's disability programs are described in some detail in Bernice Madison, "Programs for the Disabled," *The Disabled in the Soviet Union*, eds. William O. McCagg and Lewis Siegelbaum (University of Pittsburgh Press, 1989), 167–198.

15. Cited in Madison, "Programs for the Disabled," 171.

16. L. S. Levin and E. I. Idler, *The Hidden Health Care System: Mediating Structures and Medicine* (Cambridge, MA: Ballinger, 1981).

17. See, for example, E. Brody, *Women in the Middle: Their Parent-Care Years* (NY: Springer, 1990).

18. E. K. Abel, *Who Cares for the Elderly?* (Philadelphia: Temple University Press, 1991) discusses the positive aspects of care giving. We are also grateful to E. S. Pushkova, head geriatric physician of St. Petersburg, for her contributions to our understanding of the difficulties for families posed by the absence of social supports and home health products.

CHAPTER 5

The Politics of Health Care in Russia: The Feminization of Medicine and Other Obstacles to Professionalism

Kate Schecter

Introduction

IN THE CURRENT ECONOMIC TURMOIL EMBROILING RUSSIA, the health care system is in a particularly precarious position. Physicians have not been able to improve their financial or professional standing. This chapter will examine the underlying causes of the professional predicament that Russian physicians face. Numerous forces are holding physicians back from developing an autonomous political voice to advocate for their profession.[1] The legacy of Soviet socialized medicine and the feminization of the medical field are important contributing factors. More recent impediments to professionalism such as lack of institutional capacity and economic resources to support reforms are also contributing to the problem.

A revitalization of the professional stratum is necessary for Russia, not only for medicine to survive, but also to contribute a significant element of a stable democracy.[2] The medical profession is an essential group that, on an immediate level, if it were functioning better, could be helping to stave off the worsening health crisis. Seen on an even broader level, physicians represent the broken and stunted middle class that has barely emerged since the fall of the Soviet Union in 1991. If physicians are unable to reinvigorate their profession, and organize as an interest group to make demands for

increased expenditures for health care, the health care system and
health indicators will continue to decline.

Professionalism in Historical Perspective

Terms used to denote the concept of a middle class in socialist societies are "the professional class," "the intelligentsia," and "the technical intelligentsia." All of these categorizations refer to a skilled,
educated stratum of society that lives above poverty level.[3] Russian
society is currently experiencing the consequences of an impoverished and atomized middle class. In making the transition to democracy and a market economy, policy makers and political analysts
both in Russia and in the West have focused primarily on political
and economic models for democratization. Much of the democratization literature on Russia is about the development of legislative institutions, the presidency, the parliament, constitutional
development, market reforms, and privatization.[4] The early economic reforms of "shock therapy," the privatization of state enterprises, and much of the machinations of the Russian government
since 1991 show that the transition process has evolved unevenly.
The most neglected areas of reform have been in the nurturing of a
middle class, which is the wellspring of a new and viable economy,
and the restructuring of the welfare system. The result of this uneven or lopsided reform is an extremely stratified society with a
small wealthy elite and a majority of the population living in or
close to poverty.

Health statistics indicate a population in deep crisis. Outbreaks
of epidemics, murder, suicide, drug abuse, and alcoholism are all on
the rise. Life expectancy, particularly for male adults, is declining
rapidly (from 64 years in 1989 to 57.3 in 1994).[5] Russian mothers
and children are vulnerable to these health threats, and this is evident in the increasing maternal and infant mortality rates.

Why were these areas of morbidity and mortality neglected?
Health care in Russia has never been a high priority. Throughout the
Soviet period, health care (which includes stomatology, or dentistry,
sports and recreation, and sanitation, not just medical care) never
warranted more than 6 percent of the GNP, and for most of the 75
years it received 3 percent of the GNP. In post-Soviet Russia the
budgetary allocation dropped to 1 to 2 percent of GNP in the early

1990s and rose slightly to 4.9 percent by the middle of the decade.[6] While the United States spends more than any other industrialized nation (14 percent) on health care and is striving to lower this amount, the former Soviet Union still suffers from neglect of this crucial aspect of life.

During the Soviet period, autonomous professional groups were considered a threat to the central leadership, and they were systematically eliminated.[7] Russia entered the post-Soviet era with a huge proportion of its population deprofessionalized and disenfranchised. The professions had operated with no autonomy and in complete isolation from the West, and thus they had become extremely dependent on the state. During the Gorbachev era, an awareness that a strong professional class was lacking spurred Gorbachev to encourage more creativity in the sciences and other professions:

> Scholasticism, doctrinaire thinking and dogmatism have been shackles for any genuine advance to knowledge. They lead to stagnation of thought, put a solid wall around science, keeping it away from real life and inhibiting its development. The atmosphere of creativity is particularly productive for the social sciences. We hope that it will be used actively by our economists and philosophers, lawyers and sociologists, historians and literary critics for a bold and innovative formulation of new problems and for their creative theoretical elaboration.[8]

This idea of supporting and nurturing a professional class fell victim to the tumult of the transition and has yet to recapture the attention of the central leadership. President Yeltsin and his cabinet were aware of the extreme stratification and alienation of Russian society, but with fiscal and political crises constantly taking center stage, the Yeltsin administration was unsuccessful at stabilizing social policy.

The concept of the professions has engendered a large literature in the West, with definitions that are not easily transferred to the Russian context.[9] The problems of ethnocentrism and cultural bias are inescapable. In the Russian context, the highly educated specialists who make up the professional class have by and large not been able to fully exercise their group autonomy to improve their status and political power. Not all professions have had the same experience. The legal profession has had a very different trajectory than the medical profession. Lawyers have benefited greatly from the influx of foreign business and capital. Many professions have been unable to function in the new political and economic climate, however, and the result has been stagnation and in some cases desperation. In the natural sciences, several well-known scientists have committed suicide, drawing attention to the plight of these specialists, who were privileged in the former system and now find themselves completely disenfranchised.[10] Formerly fully state-supported, this sector of society now faces no pay, no jobs, no support from the state, and a competitive, corruption-filled market.

The Soviet government touted its health care system, with more physicians per capita and more women physicians than anywhere else in the world, as proof of the success of socialism. Reading between the lines revealed a very different world. Physicians received inadequate medical educations that often left them unprepared to practice. Mandatory rural duty left hundreds of physicians stranded in rural outposts with little or no equipment. Isolation from other medical communities left Soviet physicians unaware of new discoveries and technologies. Despite the impressive numbers of physicians and hospital beds, the quality of Soviet health care actually suffered greatly from isolation and neglect.[11]

The collapse of the Soviet Union brought on a wave of Western literature about the Soviet legacy and how difficult the transition would be.[12] There is no question that the legacy of the Soviet period crippled the medical field from the beginning of the new state. It was only in the fall of 1996 that the American Medical Association (AMA) expressed an interest in helping its Russian counterparts. The purpose of the AMA program is to help develop leadership in Russian medicine, and to establish a method for granting credentials and licenses to physicians. The president of the Russian Medical Association, Dr. Ashot Sarkisyan, is hoping that this alliance will help support a "fragmented, disorganized, and severely underfunded medical system."[13]

Other Western medical groups and individual physicians have been involved in helping Russians with their health care system, but few of these efforts have had a systemic impact.[14] Of course, Western aid is not the cure for what ails the Russian health care system, but Russian physicians can learn the processes of professionalization and relationship to government from their Western counterparts. A stable, viable medical profession can only emerge through self-generated initiatives; Western aid cannot fill this vacuum. In addition, it is essential for Russian physicians to form their own corporate entity that will work in the Russian context. Russian physicians may want to emulate or borrow from other models, but they will need to tailor their goals to operate within the confines of the Russian political and economic system.

The social contract between the state and the workers during the Soviet era entailed cradle-to-grave security for Soviet citizens in exchange for their individual freedom. This "bargain" created a society where workers became extremely state-dependent. The intelligentsia and technical specialists also suffered from their dependence on the state, and this led to a "culture of employees" that thwarted risk-taking and independence. Instead of envisioning a future where they might break away from their bosses and become self-employed or develop associations to protect their rights, even the most innovative scholars and scientists saw the future as predetermined by the nature of the communist system.

Physicians in Russia are still caught in this state-dependent, employee model. When they want to redress a problem, often the first response is to strike for higher pay. The concepts of corporate unity or professional mobilization have not taken hold. Striking against the state may bring a temporary solution of a small pay increase or payment of back wages, but it does not address the more serious and broader issues plaguing the health care system.

In this author's interviews with 12 physicians in a variety of hospitals and polyclinics throughout Moscow and in the suburban town of Zelenograd (often referred to as the Silicon Valley of Russia), a number responded similarly to the issue of independent doctor's associations. An older woman, chief pathologist at a large suburban hospital, responded to the idea of an independent doctors' association by saying, "We don't have the money to pay our physicians. Who has money to create an association? You know it takes money. We need to rent a hall, someone has to organize the association. We simply don't have the funds for this kind of extra activity. We are barely able to subsist, let alone think about creating a professional association. There is an association, but they don't do anything." Another doctor, Dr. Vasily Balazov, who runs the largest pediatric hospital in Moscow, the Republican Children's Clinical Hospital, responded similarly, "No, we don't need associations . . . our only problem is money."

Despite the hardships that physicians endure (many months of wage arrears, lack of equipment and funding, long hours, and lack of respect from patients),[15] a large exodus into private medicine has not occurred. Why are physicians staying in the state-run system? Why are they not flocking to the few small private clinics that pay very well? One possible explanation is the employee mentality of dependency described above. Physicians have no entrepreneurial training or experience, and they are not venturing into risky private enterprises. State dependency developed certain attitudes toward work, whether one was an industrial worker or a scientist. One of the primary characteristics of all Soviet workers was a disinclination to risk personal initiative. The same problem is evident in the study of environmental pollution in the former Soviet Union. Throughout the Soviet period, workers and Soviet citizens in general seemed to be oblivious to the terrible pollution surrounding them. Political initiatives to curb deadly pollutants only began in the late 1980s after the Chernobyl accident, and to this day, public awareness and activism regarding these health threats remains minimal.

Physicians also do not have any capital to invest, nor do they have any training in running a business or dealing with the market. Another disincentive to starting a private practice is that most private businesses need to pay "protection" money to criminal groups. The majority of Russia's physicians are low-paid women who are unlikely to become private entrepreneurs. They are immersed in their state-sponsored positions and despite months of unpaid wages, they cannot envision leaving the system. Instead, many physicians work part time in the shadow economy or moonlight in order to survive. All those interviewed for this study worked in the shadow market, although most people were reluctant to discuss what they did on the side to make ends meet. Men are driving their cars as taxis or helping repair cars and homes; women are knitting and sewing or tutoring privately.

More controversial is the matter of physicians' qualifications. Even if physicians want to open a private clinic, they do not have the expertise of a general practitioner to offer their patients. Soviet state-controlled medical education and central planning left a legacy of specialists in Russian medicine who often have such a narrow education that they can only perform one task. Many of these physicians realized the limits of their education only when they had exposure to medicine outside of the former Soviet

Union. In Israel, Russian immigrant physicians often find they are severely handicapped by their insufficient training and their narrow specialization.[16]

Women in Russian Health Care

One of the most unusual aspects of Russian medicine is the preponderance of women physicians. Women accounted for 10 percent of the physicians in Russia in 1913; by 1950 they made up 76 percent of all physicians (in the Soviet Union), and today women make up about 80 percent of all physicians in Russia.[17] Women in Russia (and women physicians are no exception) remain second-class citizens, shunted to the side, forced into unemployment, low-wage semi-employment, or prostitution. Women's groups and nongovernmental organizations (NGOs) run by women are slowly emerging in Russia, and there are few success stories. Despite economic and political reforms, little has been done to assist this large section of the population. Seventy percent of Russia's unemployed population are women, and most of them are over 30 years old.[18] In addition, women make up the majority of the hidden unemployed—workers who officially have jobs, but are not being paid. Given the huge redundancies in the Russian workforce, women are the first to be laid off. Adrift in a society that is becoming increasingly competitive, violent, and male-dominated, women find themselves trapped. The confluence of increasing poverty and the development of Russia's underclass are becoming more solidified in the current climate. Health care in Russia is an occupational sector that has also been largely feminized and marginalized. Rarely have the two problems of women's poverty and the crisis within the health care system been linked together in recent analyses. Much evidence exists to suggest that they are interrelated.

The neglect of women and children and the dismissive attitude toward health care in Russia are dangerous trends. Women are a frightened and silenced half of the population. In this author's interviews with women physicians in the spring of 1997, respondents repeatedly declined to discuss the issues of women or women's health separately from the general issues facing Russia and the health care system. One woman gynecologist refused to discuss the problem of women's health in Russia, insisting that there were no problems with sexually transmitted diseases (STDs), teenage pregnancy, or lack of birth control. For many, including physicians, these are still shameful taboo subjects even though they are clearly widespread social crises.

Russia is a society divided, not just by income brackets, but along gender lines as well. A regression is taking place, wherein women are reverting back to traditional gender roles, and many are willingly participating in their promotion as sex objects. The prevalence of prostitution and pornography is growing, exacerbating the sexist and abusive gender relations among many men and women.[19] In health care, this trend is evident in the lack of focus on birth control and the elimination of STDs and AIDS. Both STDs and AIDS have reached epidemic proportions, and the Russian people remain largely uninformed about how these diseases are transmitted or how to practice safe sex. Men are the group most at risk, but the trend of high adult male mortality and a disregard for women's reproductive health bode ill for Russian society as a whole.

The rise in crime has had a devastating effect on the Russian population and, from a public health standpoint, it is an important contributing factor to the health crisis. Crime is taking a significant toll on Russian women. Eighty percent of violent crimes in Russia occur in the home; 15,000 women are killed by husbands every year. Divorce rates are on the rise, and there is little or no legal protection for women. Organized crime's trafficking in prostitutes is a huge, profitable business that only encourages the idea of women as commodities. Men who operate prostitution rings are rarely punished and carry on international crime rings with near impunity.[20]

The problems facing Russian women today are not new phenomena of the transition period. The degradation of the female portion of the population has a gradual and protracted history. A brief historical examination of women in Russian and Soviet medicine reveals that women have been utilized or discarded as a convenient labor source repeatedly over the years, and the present period is a low point, but not an anomaly. In addition, it is important to note that women have not just been willing victims, pushed wherever the government or the male leadership has directed them. They have played an instrumental role in determining their participation in certain occupational sectors, most prominently in the field of medicine.

The process of women entering Soviet medicine had its roots in pre-Revolutionary Russia. Traditionally, women were regarded as healers in Russian culture. From the sixteenth century to the nine-teenth, peasant women were consulted for witchcraft healing and midwifery. Numerous forces prevented women from studying med-icine in imperial Russia. Nevertheless, women fought traditional so-cietal values, tsarist legislation, and prejudice within the medical community, and this persistence prevailed; by 1882 there were 227 women physicians in Russia, compared to France's seven and En-gland's ten.[21] By 1910 there were 1,500 women physicians in Rus-sia, outnumbering any other European country.[22]

The political agenda of the Bolsheviks called for the complete socialization and centralization of Soviet medicine; with those changes came the proletarianization of the profession. Women were the available labor source to carry out the Bolshevik agenda, and they became the "surrogate proletariat" for the transformation of health care.[23] Industrialization, modernization, and military strength were the priorities of the new state. Jobs in medicine opened for masses of uneducated or slightly educated women. Labor was divided into productive and nonproductive categories, and industrial and military workers ranked high as productive labor. Social services such as health care and child care were considered nonproductive labor; these had lower status and were allotted lower priority accordingly.

The Feminization of Poverty

More women worked outside the home in the Soviet Union than in any other industrialized country in modern history. In 1925, women made up 25 percent of the work force; by 1987, this had more than doubled to 51 percent of the labor force. This means that 92 percent of Soviet women worked outside the home.[24] The unfortunate repercussion of such an enormous influx of women into the Soviet workforce was that women worked in most of the unskilled and manual jobs in industry, construction, and agriculture, and they were less likely to be promoted or allocated as much responsibility as their male coworkers.[25] The Soviet economy became dependent on this female labor source to perform the undesirable jobs that the better-educated labor force avoided. In many cases, rural women, desperate for any kind of work they could find in the city, took dan-gerous and unhealthy jobs so they could remain in an urban setting.

With the fall of the Soviet Union, these women manual workers lost their jobs first.

The jump in the number of women participating in the work force, and in medicine in particular, can obfuscate the impact of such a large social upheaval. Never before in modern history had so many women started working so rapidly. In retrospect it is clear that medicine was not a high priority field for the Bolsheviks or their successors, and that women physicians were not accorded the privileges that male professionals enjoyed. The best contrasting example is engineering. Men were encouraged to enter a profession that would entitle them to the traditional benefits associated with professionalism. They would receive high salaries, prestige, specialized training, and a corporate collegiality developed among the engineers who had reached the higher echelons of society. Of course, the state still retained control over the engineers' professional group autonomy, but in return they received high status and high-paying jobs.

Social upheaval and transformation of the type occurring in Russia in the 1990s has historically been to the detriment of women.[26] Conditions during the 1920s, despite the revolutionary atmosphere and the experimentation of this decade, were actually harder on the female population than might be expected. Legally, the Revolution helped women immensely, compared to their former status under the tsar. The Revolution enabled women to expand their formal legal rights concerning insurance, labor, maternity leave, divorce, holidays, education, and suffrage. In addition, after the Revolution a minimum wage for all working people was set. Although not all of these new laws were heeded, they nevertheless established a precedent of developing women's rights.[27] However, on a less visible level, women's burdens only intensified after the Revolution. Now they were expected not only to perform all their traditional roles, but also to work long, hard hours outside the home. The discussion and propaganda spouted about women's emancipation and equality only helped to hide the reality of life for women. Women doctors faced the same conundrum throughout the Soviet era. The increased number of women in the work force did not bring them a higher level of professionalism in the 1920s nor in the 1990s.

The great social and political upheaval of the 1990s in Russia has had many of the same effects as the social transformations following the Revolution of 1917. Most of the women did not have the access or the desire to participate in the contestation for power and money. Despite the historical precedence of the early women's liberation movement in Russia and the Soviet Union, there are few signs of such a movement today. Feminism, as it developed in the United States, has not taken root in Russia. A number of explanations for this significant social difference include: (1) women were forced to work and now want to have a choice to work or stay at home; (2) poverty and scarcity of material goods have made women subordinate their desire for equality and respect to access to consumer goods; (3) women want to raise their children and not have to put them in state-run day care centers at an early age; and (4) free, legal abortion is not a hotly contested issue and therefore not a right that women need to rally around to protect. The daily grind of trying to survive has left little energy to organize. During the present stormy period in Russian politics and society, the press and popular attitudes are emphasizing the traditional beacons of stability while women stress their femininity.

Conclusion

The 1993 Russian constitution states that medical care will remain free and accessible, and the majority of the population still expects free state-sponsored medical care as a basic human right. Although all children, elderly, and unemployed citizens are covered by state-sponsored health insurance, at this juncture, the insurance system has not been able to alleviate the problem of wage arrears for medical workers. In Russia, the established socialized clinics and hospitals struggle to operate alongside emerging private practices that cater to the wealthy elite. The nationalized compulsory health insurance plan is in effect, but it has not solved the primary problem of lack of financing.

Another obstacle preventing physicians from breaking out of the state system is that they know the majority of their patients cannot pay for services. Physicians would have to leave their patient pool behind and serve only a small wealthy clientele. Russia remains a far less mobile society than the United States, and in most cases, a neighborhood doctor has been working with the same patients all of his or her life. There are strong ties between physicians and patients, and many favors are bartered. Many physicians spend the majority of their working hours making house calls. Opening a private clinic with high fees for services means catering to a very small percentage of the population, and this would necessitate abandoning the majority of patients.

The Soviet legacy of isolationism and neglect of the health care sector has led to continued problems in the level of education and access to current medical technology. For the 70 years of Soviet rule, medicine remained cut off from interaction with the West, and medical textbooks remain extremely outdated throughout the education system. To this day, physicians do not have access to medical journals from the West, and when they do receive a few, many face language barriers because the majority do not read a foreign language.

In the West, medical technology accelerated in complexity in the post–World War II years. The Soviet Union was left out of this leap forward in the medical world. Much of the technology used in Russian hospitals is either extremely antiquated or it has been exported piecemeal to individual hospitals where Russian physicians do not have experience working with high-tech machinery and are dependent on foreign physicians to show them how to operate the new technology.

The health crisis in the former Soviet Union is extreme; it is part of a systemic crisis affecting the entire political and social system. The lack of medical professionalism and inadequately trained physicians are clearly not the primary reasons for the crisis. Epidemics of infectious and other diseases are spreading rapidly. Vaccination rates are decreasing because parents are afraid to expose their children to unsanitary needles. Newspapers carry stories daily of spoiled or contaminated foods, poisoned water, and children afflicted with conditions typical in wartime situations such as rickets, stunted growth, malnutrition, tuberculosis, polio, dysentery, and salmonella poisoning.

Numerous explanations can be found for this critical situation. Poverty, stress, poor diet, environmental pollution, alcoholism, smoking, and a general psychological malaise regarding the future are all contributing to the escalating death rate. During the Cold War, despite harsh living conditions, people had a sense of security provided by the socialist welfare state. With the fall of the Soviet Union, millions of citizens are in shock. An extreme stratification of society has developed, with a large proportion of the Russian population living in poverty. The decaying health care system is not the only, nor even the primary, cause of the health crisis, but a revitalization of this sector could help alleviate the problem.

Until the economy stabilizes, most medical support must come from state-sponsored national insurance. Privatization is not the answer at present, because physicians do not have the tools nor the capital to start their own practices, and the majority of the population cannot afford to pay for health care. The medical corps is demoralized, and one clear part of the solution is an elevation of physicians to a professional level.

Unemployment, hidden unemployment, prostitution, high numbers of abortions, epidemics of STDs, and deeply entrenched poverty all paint a dismal picture of the status of Russian women. Depicting Russian women as purely victims of the economic and social transformation creates an extreme impression. Of course many have found ways to survive in the new economy, learning to patch together unofficial work. Efforts to train women in entrepreneurial skills are making small inroads.[28] Resourceful, educated younger women learn to use the Internet and other new technologies, educate themselves in the methods of the political and economic environment, and tap into new opportunities, but the majority of Russia's women are struggling to survive.

The main problem facing Russia's women is hidden unemployment. Women were required to work outside the home, and now they are dependent on this income and the network of barter arrangements that has developed around places of work. This factor alone explains why so many women physicians continue to work in state-run hospitals and clinics even though they suffer months of wages in arrears.

In addition to labor and health problems, Russia has one of the highest divorce rates in the world, and the majority of families are run by single mothers, many of whom cannot escape bringing their children up in poverty. Both of these issues—the breakdown of the health care system and the impoverishment of women in Russia— are not drawing attention partly because they are not new problems. These social ills have been simmering for many years, but it is precisely because they have reached crisis proportions that they must be addressed. Continued marginalization of these two socio-economic areas will only mean further deterioration of the social fabric of Russia as a whole.

NOTES

The research for this paper was made possible by a generous grant from The National Council for Soviet and East European Research. The author would like to thank NCSEER for its support and Ari Roth, Jerrold Schecter, and Leona Schecter for their helpful editorial comments.

1. For the purposes of this paper, a professional occupation is defined as a self-regulating occupation that requires training, specialization, and an orientation toward a code of ethics that entails corporate responsibility. This definition combines a few basic criteria that appear in many Western definitions of professionalism and that have come to be generally accepted. Two books that clearly define the term are Paul Starr, *The Transformation of American Medicine* (New York: Basic Books, Inc., 1982), 15, and Samuel Huntington, *The Soldier and the State: The Theory and Politics of Civil-Military Relations* (Cambridge, MA: Harvard University Press, 1959), 8–10.

2. Barrington Moore Jr., *The Social Origins of Dictatorship and Democracy: Lord and Peasant in the Making of the Modern World* (Boston: Beacon Press, 1966), and Harold Perkins, *The Rise of Professional Society: England Since 1880* (London: Routledge Press, 1989).

3. There is a small literature on the middle class and its importance in socialist societies. For a discussion of the terms and applicability, see Michael Kennedy, "The Constitution of Critical Intellectuals: Polish Physicians, Peace Activists and Democratic Society," CSST Working Paper #46 (Ann Arbor, MI: The University of Michigan, April 1990), and Michael Kennedy, *Professionals, Power and Solidarity in Poland* (Cambridge, UK: Cambridge University Press, 1991). For an in-depth discussion of the history of the middle class in the Soviet Union, see Harley Balzer, ed., *Russia's Missing Middle Class: Professions in Russian History* (London: M. E. Sharpe, 1996). Also, the last Open Media Research Institute publication of the journal *Transition* (21 March 1997) is devoted to the issue of the middle class in Russia.

4. A few examples include Jeffrey W. Hahn, ed., *Democratization in Russia; The Development of Legislative Institutions* (New York: M. E. Sharpe, 1996); Nicolai N. Petro, *The Rebirth of Russian Democracy; An Interpretation of Political Culture* (Cambridge, MA: Harvard University Press, 1995); and David Remnick, "Can Russia Change?" *Foreign Affairs* (January/February 1997).

5. L. K. Levashov, et al., *Kak zhivesh Rossiya?* (Moscow: Russian Academy of Sciences, 1995).

6. S. Ia. Chikin, "O finansirovanii zdravookhraneniia za gody Sovetskoi vlasti," *Sovetskaia meditsina*, no.11 (1990): 41–42. This article
provides the following figures for percentage of GNP allotted in the
1930s: between 2.1 and 6.6 percent, in 1940: 5.2 percent, and in the
1960s: between 3.8 and 4.2 percent. This trend of between two and
four percent has continued up to the present.
7. Kendall Bailes, *Technology and Society Under Lenin and Stalin: Origins of the Soviet Technical Intelligentsia, 1917–1941* (Princeton,
NJ: Princeton University Press, 1978).
8. From Gorbachev's speech to the party congress in February, 1986,
quoted in Martin Walker, *The Waking Giant* (New York: Pantheon
Books, 1986), xxiv-xxv.
9. The problem of comparing professions in socialist and capitalist
countries is analyzed in Anthony Jones, ed., *Professions and the
State; Expertise and Autonomy in the Soviet Union and Eastern Europe* (Philadelphia, PA: Temple University Press, 1991). The professional power of doctors in the United States and Western Europe is
examined in the following works: Elton Rayack, *Professional Power
and American Medicine* (Cleveland, OH: World, 1967); Eliot Freid-
son, *A Study of The Sociology of The Profession of Medicine* (New
York: Dodd, Mead, 1970); Jeanne Brand, *Doctors and the State: The
British Medical Profession and Government Action in Public Health,
1870–1912* (Baltimore, MD: Johns Hopkins University Press, 1965);
Harry Eckstein, *Pressure Group Politics: The Case of the British
Medical Association* (Stanford, CA: Stanford University Press,
1960); Talcott Parsons, *The Social System* (New York: Free Press,
1951); Jeffrey Berlant, *Profession and Monopoly: A Study of Medicine in the United States and Great Britain* (Berkeley, CA: University
of California Press, 1975); Deborah A. Stone, *The Limits of Professional Power: National Health Care in the Federal Republic of Germany* (Chicago: The University of Chicago Press, 1980).
10. Ludmila Ruvinsky, "As Prestige and Funding Wane, Siberian Scientists Struggle to Survive," *Transition*, 21 March 1997, 11–14; and
Loren Graham and Andrew Kuchins, "Scholars in Peril," *The Washington Post*, 19 November 1998, A29.
11. For more on problems in Soviet health care see Mark Field, *Doctor and Patient in Soviet Russia* (Cambridge, MA: Harvard University Press, 1957); Kate Schecter, "Professionals in
Post-Revolutionary Regimes: A Case Study of Soviet Doctors,"
Ph.D. dissertation, Columbia University, 1992; Michael Ryan,
Doctors and the State in the Soviet Union (New York: St. Martin's
Press, 1990); and William A. Knaus, M.D., *Inside Russian Medicine* (Boston: Beacon Press, 1981).

12. See Timothy J. Colton and Robert Legvold, eds., *After the Soviet Union: From Empire to Nations* (New York: W. W. Norton and Company, 1992); David Lane, ed., *Russia in Transition: Politics, Privatisation and Inequality* (London: Longman, 1995); and Gail Lapidus, ed., *The New Russia: Troubled Transformation* (Boulder, CO: Westview Press, 1995).

13. K. P. Foley, "Russia: American Medical Association Offers Aid To Physicians," RFE/RL, Washington, D.C., 5 March 1997.

14. There are a few significant exceptions to this phenomenon of sporadic Western aid: the American International Health Alliance (AIHA), two World Bank loans to bring technical assistance and systemic reform, and the Soros matching grants that have begun to bring the WHO DOTS tuberculosis therapy to a few seriously infected regions.

15. Dr. Galina Salova, a physician in a large suburban hospital, explained the lack of respect toward doctors by saying, "During the Soviet period we were required to run to a patient's home for even a slight mishap. Patients had free, accessible health care, and they used it frequently, even when they didn't really need it. This led to a disrespectful attitude towards doctors: we are free and plentiful. This disrespect prevails and we still are required to go on a house call whenever we are called."

16. In interviews conducted for a comparative study of Russian immigrant physicians in three countries, we found that this issue of narrow specialization hindered doctors from practicing or retraining in their new country. See Judith Shuval and Judith Bernstein, et al., *Immigrant Physicians: Former Soviet Doctors in Israel, Canada, and the United States* (Westport, CT: Praeger Press, 1997).

17. *Zhenshchiny i Deti v SSSR*, 1985.

18. Sue Bridger, Rebecca Kay, and Kathryn Pinnick, *No More Heroines? Russia, Women and the Market* (London: Routledge, 1996), 51. See also Valerie Sperling's chapter in this volume.

19. For more on the rise in prostitution and pornography, see Igor Kon, *The Sexual Revolution in Russia* (New York: The Free Press, 1995); Igor Kon and James Riordan, eds., *Sex and Russian Society* (Bloomington, IN: Indiana University Press, 1993); and Mary Buckley, ed., *Perestroika and Soviet Women* (Cambridge, UK: Cambridge University Press, 1992).

20. Swanee Hunt, "Women's Vital Voices; The Costs of Exclusion in Eastern Europe," *Foreign Affairs* (July/August 1997): 4, 5.

21. Christine Johansen, "Medical Courses for Women," in *The Modern Encyclopedia of Russian and Soviet History*, ed. Joseph L. Wieczynski, vol. 21, 1981, 174.

22. Knaus, *Inside Russian Medicine,* 69.

23. I have borrowed this term from Gregory Massell, *The Surrogate Proletariat: Moslem Women and Revolutionary Strategies in Soviet Central Asia, 1919–1929* (Princeton, NJ: Princeton University Press, 1974).

24. Annette Bohr, "Resolving the Question of Equality for Soviet Women—Again," *Radio Liberty: Report on the USSR* 1, no.14 (7 April 1989): 11.

25. Zoya Pukhova, *For a Better Life and More Good Will* (Moscow: Novosti Press Agency Publishing House, 1988), 7, cited in Kathleen Mihalisko, "Women Workers and Perestroika in the Ukraine and Belorussia—A Problematic Relationship Unfolds," *Radio Liberty: Report on the USSR* 1, no.15 (14 April 1989): 31.

26. For more on women during revolutionary crises or massive social change, see Darline Gay Levy and Harriet Branson Applewhite, "Women and Political Revolution in Paris," pp.279–308; Laura Levine Frader, "Women in the Industrial Capitalist Economy," pp.309–334; and Richard Stites, "Women and the Revolutionary Process in Russia," pp.451–472, all in Renate Bridenthal, Claudia Koonz, and Susan Stuard, eds., *Becoming Visible: Women in European History* (Boston: Houghton Mifflin Company, 1987). See also Joan Kelly, *Women, History and Theory* (Chicago: University of Chicago Press, 1984), 1–18.

27. Buckley, *Perestroika and Soviet Women,* 35.

28. Hunt, "Women's Vital Voices," 6.

CHAPTER 6

Drug Abuse in Post-Communist Russia

John M. Kramer

> Drug addiction is a door that only opens one way. It is very rare
> for people to return. In short, this problem can eliminate us as a
> nation in the very near future. We are talking about self-preserva-
> tion. This metaphor suggests itself here: AIDS and Chernobyl
> taken together.
>
> —*Oblastnaia gazeta* (Ekaterinburg), March 19, 1996, p. 2.

SUGGESTING THAT NONALCOHOLIC DRUG ABUSE can eliminate the Russian nation "in the very near future" is undoubtedly hyperbolic, but
the available data on the evolving status of this pathology in the
Russian Federation are indeed worrisome. Thus, the findings from
one of the most comprehensive surveys to date, conducted in 1992,
on drug abuse among residents of urban centers in Russia, reportedly "exceeded all expectations," with 11.5 percent of the respondents (and 23 percent of them in Moscow) admitting that they had
consumed unspecified illicit "narcotics" at least once, whereas researchers had hypothesized that the respective figure would be between 2 and 3 percent.[1] Overall, this survey concludes that a
"fundamentally new narco-situation" has emerged in Russia.[2]

More impressionistically, public opinion polling data indicate
that ordinary Russians themselves—whether rightly or wrongly—
believe that drug abuse represents a growing threat to their welfare.
In one poll among residents of Russia, more than two-thirds of the
sample felt that physical extinction threatens the Russian people,

with 57 percent of the sample blaming alcoholism and drug addiction for their relatively low life expectancy.[3] Another poll reportedly found that the percentage of Russians who now believe that their progeny will grow up to become "drug addicts" (28 percent of the sample) was almost as high as the respective percentage (29 percent of the sample) who felt that alcoholism, historically the preeminent social pathology among Russians, would afflict their offspring.[4]

Officials are especially concerned about the reported link between drug abuse and several infectious diseases. Thus, official data indicate that 23 percent of the reported cases of hepatitis B and 34 percent of the respective cases of hepatitis C involve intravenous drug abusers who contracted their disease through the use of shared syringes.[5] Particularly striking is the officially reported link between such drug-related behavior and Human Immunodeficiency Virus (HIV), the precursor to Acquired Immune Deficiency Syndrome (AIDS): this behavior reportedly accounts in Russia for over 90 percent of all the newly registered cases of individuals testing positive for HIV in 1997 and 1998.[6]

While some link undoubtedly does exist between intravenous drug use and HIV and AIDS, the official data may actually reveal more about which groups in society the authorities are testing for these maladies rather than the precise factors that are causing them. Such a hypothesis appears warranted when one examines official data reporting that between 1987 and 1995 not one registered drug addict appeared among the 1060 individuals officially testing positive for HIV, while in 1996 this figure suddenly increased to 920 of the 1495 individuals registered in that year as HIV positive.[7]

To be sure, drug abuse in Russia existed under both tsarist and Soviet rule,[8] but a cluster of variables associated with the postcommunist period has increased substantially the incentives and opportunities to engage in this behavior: psychological, material, and social dislocations attendant upon the transition to capitalism; enhanced personal freedoms and a concomitant diminution in communist-style regimentation and surveillance; greater economic wherewithal among some segments of the population to purchase drugs; the widespread exposure of the citizenry, especially youths, through the mass media, tourism, and economic intercourse to Western life-styles that include the glamorization of the illicit drug culture; and easily penetrated borders that international drug cartels exploit to make Russia both a target country to market their wares and launder their illicit monies, and a transit country to smuggle narcotics to Western Europe and the United States.

Yet the following analysis also demonstrates that the legacy of communist misrule in the Russian Federation manifestly continues its pernicious impact on the overall scope of, and capacity to combat, drug abuse.

The Indigenous Situation

No country in the world possesses definitive data on the extent of drug abuse within its borders. In the United States, for example, the Department of Health and Human Services conducts an annual survey of drug use that government officials themselves admit could understate the actual number of cocaine addicts by as much as 400 percent and that has failed in recent years to reflect the increasing use of heroin that many experts report.[9] Most obviously, this circumstance derives from the seemingly universal professional and personal incentives many drug users have to conceal their affliction from public view. In Russia, these incentives are especially compelling both because drug addicts are subject to compulsory treatment for their condition in prison-like facilities run by the police, and because an unknown, but undoubtedly large, number of drug abusers reside illegally without requisite official documentation in Russia's urban centers, particularly Moscow, from which they can be summarily expelled if their existence becomes known to the authorities. Then, too, terms such as "addiction," "abuse," and "dependency" are inherently ambiguous and consequently insusceptible to precise quantification. Russian sources themselves—unfortunately emulating their Soviet predecessors—often exhibit this imprecision by referring to all drugs—regardless of their pharmacological properties—as "narcotics" and all users as "addicts." Thus, in a recent interview former Russian President Boris Yeltsin rejected any distinction between different types of drugs—whether "hard" or "soft" drugs—because "they are still drugs, they still cause dependence, suppress personality, destroy the mind."[10] The legacy of communism in the Russian Federation only compounds the difficulty of assessing the evolving status of drug abuse. The ideological taboo against admitting even to the existence of drug abuse under communism meant that the Soviet regime gathered no comprehensive national data on this pathology that could provide a statistically valid baseline against which to compare current, and thereby reveal emerging trends in, drug-related behavior. Given these uncertainties, the following materials can serve, at best, only to illuminate the approximate state of drug abuse in Russia.

Official statistics depict a steady increase, albeit with considerable regional variations, in drug addiction and drug abuse. The number of individuals newly diagnosed as "drug addicts" annually between 1991 and 1997 illustrates this trend (see table 6.1). According to the Russian Ministry of Health, the number of individuals registered with medical institutions as drug addicts between 1991 and 1997 increased nearly fourfold and totaled 120,606 at the beginning of 1998, or 82.4 registered drug addicts per 100,000 population. This latter index was exceeded in 25 of Russia's 89 regions, with the four regions registering the highest number of drug addicts per 100,000 population all located in Western Siberia: Tomsk Oblast (283.8), Republic of Tuva (276.7), Altai Krai (211.3), and Tiumen Oblast (199.3). In 1997, medical institutions registered 72,478 individuals, or 49.5 persons per 100,000 population, as abusing, but not addicted to, "narcotics," 3.7 times higher than the respective figure for 1991. Here again, 25 of Russia's regions—led by the Republic of Tuva, which registered 177.6 drug abusers per 100,000 population—exceeded the respective national average for this index.[11] Yet responsible officials openly admit that these data substantially understate the actual dimensions of drug abuse—a common "rule of thumb" is by upwards of 90 percent—given that most drug abusers are not officially registered with the authorities and many of the psychotropic substances they abuse remain legal. As a deputy minister in the Ministry of Health bluntly contends about official data on drug abuse, "Take any statistic and multiply it by five or ten times, then you may be a little closer to the truth."[12] The ministry itself estimates that at the end of 1997 there were between 500,000 and 700,000 "actual addicts" in the Russian Federation.[13]

The numerous estimates on the scope of drug abuse in Russia vary widely and are terminologically imprecise. Commentaries for several years have been reporting the same estimate of 4 million people who have "experimented" with illicit drugs. Reports also show approximately 1.5 million to 2 million individuals in the Russian Federation who some sources say "regularly use" drugs, while other sources use the qualitatively different term "addict" to characterize

Table 6.1 Newly Diagnosed Drug Addicts in the Russian Federation, 1991–1997 (per 100,000 population)

Year	Number of Individuals	Percent Increase over Preceding Year
1991	3.9	—
1992	3.5	−9.9
1993	6.4	82.9
1994	9.5	48.4
1995	15.5	63.2
1996	20.7	33.5
1997	28.4	37.2

Source: Voprosy narkologii, no. 3 (1998): 7 (data from official Russian government sources).

their condition.[14] An official publication of the Ministry of Health uses the 1.5 million figure to denote the number of Russians who "systematically consume for nonmedical reasons narcotics and powerful acting substances"[15]—a characterization that presumably lumps together such otherwise diverse psychotropic substances as hashish (which produces no physical and, usually, no psychological dependence) with sundry opiates (which produce both physical and psychological dependence).

It strains credulity to claim that the overall scope of illicit drug use has remained essentially unchanged in the Russian Federation for several years. Not surprisingly, some estimates on this subject are far higher than the prevailing ones. Thus, a research project conducted on the subject between 1993 and 1998 among selected demographic groups in several of Russia's regions estimated that at the beginning of 1998 there were upwards of 11 million drug addicts— approximately 7 percent of the population. Another source places the number of illicit drug users in the country at between 10 and 15 million individuals.[16] If the survey's sample is statistically representative of the urban population of the Russian Federation in that year, then upwards of 10.7 million residents of urban areas aged 10 and above had already consumed illicit narcotics by 1992. Naturally, this estimate could prove hyperbolic, but even if one assumes that it overstates the actual situation by 50 percent, the 1992 estimate would still exceed the respective 1998 estimate on the same subject made by the Ministry of Internal Affairs (MVD) by upwards of 33 percent.[17] In contrast, the survey might well *understate* the actual extent of illicit drug use especially because it completely excluded from its sample any representatives of the 39 million people resident in rural areas in 1992.

The 1992 survey similarly reported rates of illicit drug use in cities such as Moscow and St. Petersburg far higher than official data indicated. Its findings suggest that there could have been upwards of 2.6 million residents aged 10 and above in these two cities who had consumed illicit narcotics at least once as early as 1992. The survey also found fairly widespread use in Moscow of the black market either regularly or occasionally to procure unspecified "narcotics": 8.2 percent of its respondents in Moscow admitted they engaged in this activity and another 4.5 percent of the respondents refused to answer the question, thereby prompting the survey's analysts to label them "potential" users of the black market.[18] Other sources report similarly extensive drug abuse in these two cities. For example, a respected Western publication categorically contends that there are upwards of 500,000 "drug addicts" in Moscow alone.[19] In St. Petersburg, the chief narcotics officer estimates that there are upwards of 100,000 drug addicts in the population and another 200,000 individuals who abuse illegal drugs regularly.[20]

Drug abuse among the young is eliciting particular concern. In a 1997 address to the nation devoted to the troubled state of Russia's youth, President Boris Yeltsin singled out drug abuse among teenagers, which is escalating so rapidly that "we have not had time to even prepare for this," as one of the most pernicious pathologies besetting the young.[21]

The limited data available on this subject suggest that illicit drug use among youths in Russia may be substantially higher than the respective usage found in the United States, where in 1997 11.4 percent of youths aged 12–17 surveyed said that they had consumed illicit drugs at least once in the last year.[22] Thus, senior officials in the Ministry of Health, citing unpublished epidemiological surveys conducted under their auspices, reported that 15–30 percent of the respondents admitted that by the age of 16 they had "sampled" (*proba*) "narcotics and other psychoactive substances."[23] Similar surveys on this subject conducted in Moscow among students in secondary schools and vocational-technical schools found that 44 percent of the male students and 25 percent of the female students had "used drugs or other psychoactive substances" at least once and that, among students who had used such drugs, 36 percent of them had done so more than 10 times. Another report, based in part on survey research among school-aged children, estimates that there are approximately 300,000 "drug addicts" in Moscow aged 16 and younger, and that nationally there are close to 2 million such youths aged 10–18, i.e., approximately nine percent of the individuals in that age group.[24]

While these data may appear exaggerated, consider that as early as 1992, according to the "calculations of specialists" as reported in an official publication of the Ministry of Health, upwards of 5 million students had already tried unspecified "narcotics" at least once and 500,000 of them consumed these substances "regularly."[25] That the number of youths involved in drug-related crimes in Russia is escalating sharply lends credence to the sense of widespread youthful drug abuse. According to August 1997 data from law enforcement agencies, the number of youths apprehended for drug-related crimes had increased by 12 times since 1996, and during this same period 25 percent of the teenagers apprehended for all crimes were in a state of narcotic or alcoholic intoxication when they committed them.[26] The data in table 6.2 convey a similar impression. The chairwoman of the Movement for the Health of the Nation sought to explain why so many youths engage in drug-related behavior and other crimes by noting that upwards of 1.5 million Russian children and teenagers neither work nor go to school, and that in 1996 alone 2,000 children committed suicide, 200 children were murdered by their own mothers, and over 17,000 children experienced threats on their lives: "Treated inhumanely, children do what is being done to them," she contends.[27]

The Drug Market

Available materials suggest that a "two-tier" drug market exists in Russia's cities, especially Moscow and St. Petersburg, consisting of a "high-end" group of increasingly affluent drug abusers—the so-called New Russians—with the economic wherewithal to purchase expensive, often imported, drugs such as cocaine, high quality heroin, and synthetic "designer" drugs, and a far larger and economically less well-off group of "low-end" drug abusers whose

Table 6.2   Individuals Registered in Psychoneurological and Narcological Clinics in Russia (by type of diagnosis)

Year	Narcotic Addiction		Narcotic Abuse		Nonnarcotic Substance Abuse	
	Number	Per 100,000 Population*	Number	Per 100,000 Population*	Number	Per 100,000 Population*
1993	719	11.2	4,627	71.6	7,147	112.6
1994	1,319	20.4	6,593	102.0	6,872	106.3
1995	3,027	46.5	8,813	135.5	8,596	132.2
1996	4,840	73.3	10,934	165.6	10,637	161.1
1997	5,902	89.7	14,104	213.5	13,474	203.9

Source: Data for 1993–1996 from *Voprosy narkologii*, no. 4 (1997): 32. Data for 1997 from *Voprosy narkologii*, no. 3 (1998): 6–8. All data are from official Russian government sources.
* Aged 5–34.

psychotropic substances of choice include such traditional staples of the Russian drug scene as hashish, sundry opium-based derivatives, various synthetic drugs, and legally available volatile substances, including glue and paint remover. Especially alarming, an official U.S. government report issued in 1997 finds that the "high-end" drug trade in cocaine, heroin, and synthetic drugs is expanding beyond its traditional consumers and becoming "increasingly popular with all economic groups, particularly among urban youths." That hitherto prohibitively expensive drugs are now becoming more affordable to those of limited means—the MVD reports that in Moscow the price for one gram of heroin declined from $200 in 1995 to between $50 and $80 in 1998—is a key factor promoting this development.[28]

The "division of labor" among organized drug traffickers operating in the RF similarly reflects this two-tier drug market. According to the MVD, nationals from Afghanistan, Pakistan, and former Soviet republics of Central Asia control the "high-end" market in heroin and ethnic Russians and Nigerians the respective market in cocaine, while at the "low end," Ukrainians control the market in cannabis and nationals from Central Asian states the market in raw opium.[29] The MVD estimated, without amplifying publicly on its methodology for doing so, that the value of this illicit drug trade exceeded $1.2 billion in the first half of 1998 alone.[30] The Collegium of the Federal Security Service (FSB) has labeled drug trafficking a "threat to the national security" of Russia, and in July 1999 the Russian Security Council, on instructions from President Yeltsin, devoted a session exclusively to examining ways to combat this illegality.[31]

Both external and internal sources supply the drug market. Officials estimate that imported drugs now account for upwards of two-thirds of the illegal drugs on the Russian domestic market.[32] While this estimate must be treated cautiously given the manifest difficulties involved in its computation, it does seem clear that international drug traffickers increasingly view the Russian Federation as a target country for their wares besides fulfilling its more traditional role as a conduit to bring narcotics to markets in Western Europe. Several factors promote the international drug trade in Russia: a geographic position astride producers of illegal drugs in Central Asia and Southwest Asia and their export markets in Western Europe, increasingly open and porous borders attendant upon the dissolution of the USSR, the partial dismantling of police state controls on freedom of movement and entry from abroad, poorly trained, understaffed, ill-equipped and notoriously corrupt law enforcement agencies, and a potentially huge, and still mostly untapped, domestic market for illegal drugs.

Abusers also utilize domestic sources to satisfy their illicit drug habits. The vast areas—upwards of 2.5 million acres—where hemp and poppies grow wild are a major source of raw materials for hashish, marijuana, and opium-based derivatives. Elderly people, known colloquially as "narcogrannies" and "narcograndads," often traffic in such drugs, as well as in analgesics legally obtained through prescription, to supplement their meager incomes.[33] Underground commercial laboratories, at times the offshoots of formerly state-owned chemical facilities that have now been privatized, have become a major source of sundry synthetic drugs. In 1997, law enforcement officials closed 848 such laboratories—an 18 percent increase over the respective figure for 1996.[34] Russia's underground drug producers have now developed their production capacities sufficiently to enter international markets: U.S. officials have reported several seizures in the United States "of large quantities of Russian produced amphetamines."[35] An undetermined, but undoubtedly large, number of drug abusers with limited economic wherewithal satisfy their habit through various homemade psychotropic substances based on cheap and often legally obtainable analgesics and even poppy seeds sold at local markets. One source refers to this home-based drug culture as "Russia's forgotten drug problem—too underground to appear in official statistics, too fragmented to be of interest to the police, too hopeless for the government to tackle."[36]

The Response

Under communism, the Soviet regime promoted the specious ideological claim that drug abuse was a pathology alien to socialism that could flourish only amidst the spiritual vacuity and material deprivation of capitalism. To the extent that the regime did anything to combat drug abuse, it did so primarily through coercive means by treating drug abusers as social miscreants engaged in criminal behavior.[37]

Consequently, Russia faces an uphill battle against drugs, having inherited almost no efficacious drug-control measures from its communist predecessor. This circumstance dictates pursuing the following desiderata if the Russian Federation is to begin mitigating its drug problem:

- fostering frank public discussion regarding the causes of, and appropriate responses to, drug abuse and drug-related crime;
- mounting a credible campaign to alert the citizenry, especially youths, to the dangers of drugs;
- promoting civil society as a key partner in the fight against drugs;
- developing an effective corpus of drug-related legislation and its enforcement;
- allocating the necessary human, physical and material resources to the treatment of drug abuse and addiction; and
- forging strong links with concerned foreign governments and international organizations to combat international drug trafficking and drug-related crimes such as money laundering operations.

To date, the Russian Federation has made some progress in realizing these desiderata. Perhaps most significantly, a lively public debate is ensuing about how best to combat drug abuse and drug-related crime. The contending approaches in this debate will evoke déjà vu among American observers, for they bear a striking resemblance to respective approaches found in the United States. One approach seeks primarily to limit the supply of drugs through stringent legal penalties for both the consumers and suppliers of illegal drugs. The 1997 law "On Narcotics and Psychotropic Substances" that criminalizes the possession and use of illicit drugs and mandates the compulsory treatment of drug addicts is emblematic of this approach.[38] The law stipulates prison terms of up to three years for the possession for personal use of such "hard" drugs as heroin or cocaine, while the intent to distribute these same drugs in "large" or "specially large" quantities entails imprisonment for 3 to 7 years and 7 to 15 years, respectively. Advocates of the supply-side approach are found primarily among law enforcement officials, politicians seeing it as a politically appealing position, and ranking officials in the State Narcological Service, of whom many are holdovers from the same agency under the Soviet regime. Representatives of this latter group, employing rhetoric reminiscent of Soviet times, publicly have endorsed as "necessary" the compulsory treatment of "drug addicts" who exhibit "asocial aims or anti-societal conduct" in "special establishments of the MVD."[39]

The contending "demand-side" approach seeks primarily to reduce both the demand for drugs and the adverse social and physical consequences attendant upon those already abusing drugs. It advocates therapeutic programs to treat drug abusers, so called "harm reduction" initiatives such as providing intravenous drug users with clean needles to reduce the dangerous consequences of their actions, educational efforts to prevent more people, especially youths, from becoming drug abusers by alerting them to the costs of doing so, and perhaps the legalization of some drugs (e.g., marijuana) that are not considered particularly harmful or even all drugs as a way to fight drug-related crime, including that of police corruption. Its advocates often cite the USSR as an example of how, in the words of one prominent drug-treatment specialist, it is "absolutely useless" to try to combat drug abuse primarily through punitive means.[40]

Polling data suggest that public opinion in Russia is split between demand-side and supply- side approaches to drug abuse. Thus, responding to the question in one poll, "What action should be taken?" against "drug addicts," 49 percent of the sample responded either "eliminate them" or "isolate them," but 38 percent of the sample responded "help them," 5 percent wanted to "leave them alone," and seven percent of the respondents were undecided on a course of action.[41] In another poll conducted among residents of Moscow, almost half of the respondents advocated tougher laws to fight the "drug mafia," but approximately one-third of the overall sample, and 41 percent of the teenagers within it, supported distributing disposable syringes free of charge to drug users.[42] The aforementioned 1992 poll on drug abuse among urban residents in Russia found a much greater consensus on the issue of whether "narcotics" should be legalized, with 71 percent of the sample unalterably opposed to legalization and overwhelming majorities in the sample who felt that legalization would increase the number of drug addicts (84 percent), threaten the overall health of the nation (76 percent), promote AIDS (73 percent), and engender a complex of other pernicious phenomena. President Yeltsin stated in a July 1998 interview that he himself is unequivocally "opposed to the legalization of drugs."[43]

Support for or opposition to the 1997 drug law clearly reflects the divide between these respective approaches to drug abuse. Supply-side proponents have hailed the measure as "an extremely important step in the direction of freeing Russia from the wave of narcotics sweeping the country."[44] Explicitly endorsing the provision in the law mandating compulsory treatment for drug addicts, the chief of the MVD Administration on Illegal Drug Trafficking argued that if a drug addict refuses treatment, he needs to know "we will put him in prison."[45] Demand-side proponents equally adamantly oppose this legislation, variously assailing it as "amoral," "ludicrous," "openly punitive," "inconsistent with the constitution," and creating a "feeding trough" to extract monies and staff for the agencies charged with its implementation.[46] The ranking official in the Ministry of Health dealing with narcotics-related issues admitted that the ministry is "not delighted" with all aspects of the new law.[47] That the police might consider it illegal under the law to combat AIDS by distributing sterile syringes to drug abusers elicits particular concern. "We're trying, with the Interior Ministry, to find a way to minimize the negative effects when the law is implemented," a first deputy in the ministry stated, "but the fact that we need to do this shows there could be problems."[48]

Besides the 1997 drug law, the Russian Federation has taken other legal and organizational measures to combat drug abuse. The government has published with great fanfare several federal programs to this end (in 1992, 1993, and 1995, respectively), all of which contain essentially the same measures and have suffered the same fate of receiving almost none of the requisite monies for their implementation. The government announced that it would promulgate by the end of 1998 yet another federal program to combat drug abuse, but it had failed to do so as of July 1999.[49] That the government recently established both a Main Administration on Illegal Drug Trafficking within the MVD and an "experimental police force . . . outside the MVD" with the identical bureaucratic mandate to combat the drug trade further reinforces the impression of an antidrug program lacking conceptual clarity, exhibiting no clear sense of direction or priorities, and relying more on form than substance to achieve its goals.[50]

In 1998, the MVD registered 190,000 drug-related crimes in the Russian Federation—only a marginal increase over the respective figure for 1997 of 185,000. In contrast, the latter figure represented increases over the figures for 1996 and 1995 of 90 percent and 130 percent, respectively.[51] Of course, these data are susceptible to very different interpretations: that by 1998 (1) the police were finally beginning to win the war against drugs; (2) drug-related criminality was overwhelming the police, who were no longer able to cope with the upsurge; and/or (3) official statistics on this subject were as flawed as ever and reflected, at best, as a senior MVD official expressed it, only "the tip of the iceberg" in the actual state of affairs.[52]

Certainly, critics remain unimpressed with these results, contending that law enforcement agencies rarely apprehend major drug traffickers and often seemingly permit the local drug trade to proceed with impunity. "Government agencies either cannot or do not want to catch the real drug traders," argues a Moscow trial court judge. "Everybody knows that drugs are on sale . . . in my neighborhood, but you can count the people arrested for that on the fingers of one hand."[53] The well-documented corruption that pervades law enforcement agencies and often makes them accomplices to, not guardians against, illegality likely explains much of this ineffectual response to the drug trade. As one critic bluntly expressed it, law enforcement personnel often behave "as if their salaries are paid by the international drug mafia rather than the treasury."[54] Many ordinary Russians seemingly share this perception: in one government-sponsored poll in Moscow, 33 percent of the sample overall, and 50 percent of the teenagers in the sample, "are convinced that the police have links with the drug mafia."[55]

There have been only limited demand-side initiatives to combat drug abuse enacted to date. To mitigate what appears to be pervasive ignorance among youths to the dangers of drugs—in one survey of 17 and 18 year olds, less than 2 percent of the sample possessed "satisfactory knowledge" about the nature of drug abuse and AIDS[56]—several television stations and newspapers participated in a campaign entitled "Mass Media Against Drugs" that publicized these issues.[57] To the same end, the Moscow city government supports several school-based programs, including one modeled on a similar U.S. program for use in primary schools that emphasizes parental involvement and small group discussion of physical health and drug-related issues.[58] Another potentially promising initiative in Moscow entails efforts by two nongovernmental organizations (NGOs) to establish so-called Rehabilitation Zones within the city where they will rely upon extensive interaction with the public to combat drug abuse among the young by disseminating information about the dangers of drugs and offering therapeutic services to those already abusing them.[59] In Sverdlovsk Oblast, the NGO "Youth Against Drugs" sought to foster public awareness about the dangers of drugs "so that people talk about it and cry out at every step" by initiating a campaign to collect 200,000 signatures on an appeal to the authorities to fight drug addiction.[60] In Krasnodar, the youth group "Eastern Wave" organized rock concerts where youthful attendees received copies of the group's pamphlet "Say No to Drugs" and other materials detailing the risks of contracting infectious diseases through sexual and drug-related behavior. Eastern Wave also disseminates these materials to area schools, youth groups, and governmental agencies.[61] At the governmental level, the Ministry of Health in 1996 convened "The All-Russian Conference on Problems of Preventing the Spread of HIV Among Drug Addicts," whose participants, inter alia, learned about "positive international experience" in pursuing "harm reduction" measures to limit the spread of HIV among drug abusers, including providing them with disposable syringes for intravenous injection.[62]

To be sure, these demand-side initiatives remain limited in both scale and impact, but they do represent at least a beginning in changing the almost exclusively punitive approach to drug abuse that existed under the Soviet regime and in enlisting civil society in antidrug initiatives.

The next great challenge—one that will not be overcome easily or quickly—involves trying to expand dramatically both the quantity and quality of drug-treatment clinics to meet requisite demand for their services. To date, the existing state-run clinics mostly offer "treatment" that differs minimally from that offered by their predecessors in Soviet times, wherein drug abusers were placed in prison-like conditions to undergo a "cold turkey" separation from their dependency. Not surprisingly, drug abusers avoid such "treatment" however possible, while those with the inclination and economic wherewithal are turning to the few existing private clinics to treat their affliction.[63] However, the future status of these private clinics is uncertain. On the one hand, a senior official in the Ministry of Health recently contended that "these private centers can take on much of the work with addicts."[64] In contrast, the 1997 law on drugs (Article 55) explicitly states that "only state and municipal" clinics can treat drug addicts and abusers—a provision that, if implemented strictly, would doom the private clinics and severely compromise demand-side efforts to combat drug abuse.

Finally, the Russian Federation has pursued bilateral and multilateral initiatives with other governments and international organizations to combat international drug trafficking and, of manifest importance, to project an image among Western states as a responsible member of the international community worthy of full-fledged participation in its activities and institutions. Multilateral measures include adherence to the three principal United Nations Conventions on narcotics: the *1961 UN Single Convention on Narcotic Drugs,* the *1971 UN Convention on Psychotropic Substances* and the *1988 UN Convention on Illicit Traffic in Narcotic Drugs and Psychotropic Substances.* Russia's efforts to participate in the UN Drug Control Program suffered a major setback in April 1997 when UN officials determined that it possessed insufficient material and technical means to execute the responsibilities that accompany participation. However, the UN did pledge to provide financial assistance to mitigate the deficiencies that it identified in Russia's counter-narcotics programs.[65] The Russian Federation also participates in sundry multilateral initiatives to combat drug trafficking under the auspices of the Commonwealth of Independent States (CIS) with other former Soviet republics who are also members of this organization. To date, these initiatives have proven little more than rhetorical declarations of intent—victims of the diverse and often conflicting national interests of the CIS states and the widespread fear among the non-Russian members that Russia views the CIS primarily as a means to reestablish its hegemony over them.

Russia has also concluded numerous bilateral agreements to combat drug-related criminality both with former Soviet republics, including Kazakstan, Kyrgyzstan, Ukraine, and Uzbekistan, and such diverse Western states as Austria, Chile, Colombia, Germany, and Switzerland.[66] Bilateral cooperation to this same end with the United States has been expanding. Both the U.S. Federal Bureau of Investigation and the U.S. Drug Enforcement Agency maintain offices in Russia whose staff cooperate with their Russian counterparts to combat organized crime, including drug-related crime. The Russian Federal Border Service and the U.S. Coast Guard have concluded a *Memorandum of Understanding* that includes agreement to interdict drugs on the high seas. In February 1996, a *Mutual*

Legal Assistance Agreement entered into force between the United States and the Russian Federation that specifically designates illicit traffic in narcotic drugs and psychotropic substances and money laundering as offenses covered by the agreement. The United States has also provided material assistance for drug-related initiatives (e.g., to establish drug rehabilitation centers under the auspices of the Ministry of Health) and training programs for law-enforcement personnel. By the beginning of 1999, the United States had provided training programs in combating organized crime, narcotics trafficking, and financial crimes to over 5,000 Russian officials and students at sites in the United States and Russia and at the U.S.-sponsored International Law Enforcement Academy in Budapest, Hungary.[67]

These initiatives represent a welcome volte-face from the minimal cooperation that the USSR, especially before Mikhail Gorbachev came to power in 1985, extended to other governments in the fight against international drug trafficking and drug-related crime. Yet it is equally true that the potential for cooperation between the Russian Federation and other governments to combat these illegalities remains far from exhausted. That a draft agreement to provide expanded U.S. drug-related assistance to Russia remains, in the words of an official State Department report, "stalled" because Russia refuses to exempt the assistance from import duties and taxes is emblematic of this latter circumstance.[68]

Conclusion

Surveying the spread of drug abuse and drug-related crime in the RF, authorities there may well reflect, as Thomas Jefferson once did of political corruption, that "the time to guard against it is before it shall have gotten hold of us, it is better to keep the wolf out of the fold than to trust to drawing its teeth and talons after he shall have entered."[69] Indeed, data presented in this study, e.g., on illicit drug use among youths, suggest that the "teeth and talons" of drugs may actually in certain key respects be more embedded in Russian society than in its respective counterparts in the West—although definitive generalizations cannot be made given the paucity of epidemiological data in the Russian Federation and elsewhere on this subject.

What the materials in this study do make clear is that it is precisely several of the successes that Russia has accomplished in its transformation from communism—dismantling many police state controls, opening borders, increasing the economic wherewithal of at least some of its citizenry—that have created propitious conditions for the promotion of drug abuse. Yet this study similarly demonstrates that the legacy of communism endures in Russia, both exacerbating the propensity to abuse drugs and inhibiting efforts to mitigate this pathology. Both encouraging and troubling trends exist in the response to drug abuse. Especially encouraging is that a lively public debate is transpiring about how best to combat drug abuse, and civil society is emerging from its dormancy under communism to play an increasing role in this effort. In contrast, provisions in the 1997 drug law mandating the compulsory treatment of drug addicts and prohibiting private clinics from dispensing drug therapies are throwbacks to Soviet times, likely to be as ineffectual today as they were then. Then, too, efforts to combat drug abuse suffer from a perennial shortage of funds as the bankrupt Russian government devotes little attention and even less resources to what it considers a relatively low priority problem even under optimal economic circumstances, let alone those it experienced in 1998, which led it essentially to default on its domestic and foreign debt.

The drug problem in Russia likely will worsen considerably if the current economic crisis persists, both because monies to fund drug-related initiatives will become even scarcer and because more individuals will likely seek solace from their economic and social deprivation in drugs. Under these inauspicious circumstances, can the Russian Federation overcome the legacy of indifference to this pathology inherited from its communist predecessor, learn from both the successes and failures of Western polities in combating it, and develop its own effective response to mitigate the threat of drug abuse and drug-related crime to its public welfare? Answers to these questions will substantively affect the quality of life in Russia and in other states affected by its drug problems as they enter the next millennium.

NOTES

1. *Sotsiologicheskie issledovaniia*, no. 6 (1994): 138–145. All subsequent references in the text to this poll are from this source. The poll

itself appears to be one of the most methodologically sophisticated surveys conducted to date on this subject in the Russian Federation. The sample for the survey comprised 2,245 individuals resident in 12 cities of varying sizes throughout Russia who either were interviewed directly or completed a questionnaire on their drug-related activities and socioeconomic background. See page 139 for an explanation of the sampling techniques and mode of analysis employed in the survey.

2. *Sotsiologicheskie issledovaniia,* no. 6 (1994): 139.

3. The All-Russian Center for the Study of Opinion conducted the poll as reported in *The Moscow Times,* 5 November 1995, 23. The article provided insufficient information to assess the methodological sophistication and validity of the poll.

4. Data reported in *The San Diego Daily Transcript,* 22 November 1995.

5. *Voprosy narkologii,* no. 4 (1997): 66.

6. Data from the Russian Federation Ministry of Health, cited in *Zdravookhranenie Rossiiskoi Federatsii,* March/April 1999.

7. *Voprosy narkologii,* no. 4 (1997): 6.

8. For information on this subject, see Mary Schaeffer Conroy, "Abuse of Drugs Other than Alcohol and Tobacco in the Soviet Union," *Soviet Studies* (July 1990): 447–480.

9. As reported in a summary of the 1994 study in *The New York Times,* 29 July 1994.

10. *Komsomolskaia pravda,* 3 July 1998.

11. All data on registered drug addicts and drug abusers from *Voprosy narkologii,* no. 3 (1998): 6–7.

12. Quoted in *Russia Review,* 10 February 1997, 17.

13. According to the "chief narcotics expert" of the ministry, reported in an interview with *Novoe vremia,* 12 October 1997.

14. For representative examples of such terminological imprecision, see, for example, *Voenno-meditsinskii zhurnal,* no. 9 (1988). See the interview with the minister of the interior, carried by *INTERFAX,* 4 June 1999, for a recent example of where the standard figure of 2 million is used to denote the number of individuals who "regularly use drugs" in the RF.

15. *Voprosy narkologii,* no. 1 (1994): 21.

16. The estimate of approximately 11 million drug addicts in the RF is made in Aleksandr Kolesnikov, "Narkomaniia v Rossii: Sostoianie, tendentsii, puti preodoleniia," *Informatsionnyi sbornik "Bezopasnost,"* no.11–12 (December 1998): 8. The estimate of between 10 and 15 million illicit users is in *Literaturnaia gazeta,* 5 November 1997.

17. The MVD estimates that in 1998 there were approximately four million individuals in the RF who have "experimented" with unspecified "narcotic" substances. The data are contained in a report submitted

to the Russian State Duma, as reported in Radio Free Europe/Radio Liberty, *Newsline*, no. 42, part 1 (3 March 1998).

18. Sotsiologicheskie issledovaniia, no. 6 (1994): 142.

19. *Russia Briefing*, 22 December 1994, 7.

20. Data cited by Radio Free Europe/Radio Liberty, *News Service*, 2 May 1997.

21. *Ekho Moskvy*, 24 October 1997.

22. Derived from data in the National Household Survey on Drug Abuse, as reported in *The Washington Post*, 21 August 1996.

23. *Voprosy narkologii*, no. 4 (1997): 33. To place these data in context, the same surveys reported that 70–85 percent of the respondents by the age of 16 had already consumed alcohol.

24. *Voenno-meditsinskii zhurnal*, no. 9 (1998); Kolesnikov, "Narko-maniia v Rossii," 45.

25. *Voprosy narkologii*, no. 2 (1992): 57.

26. *INTERFAX*, 31 August 1997.

27. *INTERFAX*, 31 August 1997.

28. U.S. Department of State, Bureau for International Narcotics and Law Enforcement Affairs, *International Narcotics Control Strategy Report, 1997* (Washington, D.C.: 1998). Estimates on drug prices in Moscow from the Ministry of the Interior reported in *Moscow News*, 4–10 February 1999.

29. International Narcotics Control Strategy Report, 1997.

30. Cited in Moscow News, 21–27 January 1999.

31. Reported by *ITAR-TASS*, 29 June 1999.

32. Data from an interview with a ranking official in the State Customs Service, carried by *ITAR-TASS*, 14 January 1999.

33. See, for example, *Rabochaia tribuna*, 16 March 1996; *The Moscow Times*, 12 November 1995, 39.

34. Data from an official report by the minister of the MVD, reported in *Moskovskaia pravda*, 18 March 1998.

35. *International Narcotics Control Strategy Report, 1997*.

36. *The Moscow Times*, 12 November 1995, 39.

37. For a detailed analysis of the status of drug abuse in the USSR and the responses of the Soviet regime to it, see John M. Kramer, "Drug Abuse in the USSR," in *Soviet Social Problems*, eds. Anthony Jones, Walter D. Connor, David E. Powell (Boulder, CO: Westview Press, 1991), 94–118.

38. *Voprosy narkologii*, no. 4 (1997): 11–15, publishes those articles in the law that are relevant to drug abuse and addiction.

39. *Voprosy narkologii*, no. 1 (1994): 13.

40. Quoted in *Ogonëk*, no. 15 (April 1997). The speaker is chief physician at a Moscow drug clinic and chairman of the NGO "No to Alcoholism and Drug Addiction."

41. *Segodnia,* 24 January 1995. The All-Russian Center for Studying Public Opinion, under the direction of Yurii Levada, one of Russia's most prominent pollsters, conducted the poll. The sample for the poll comprised 2,957 individuals from sundry "regions of Russia."

42. Data reported in *Moscow News,* 28 November–4 December 1996, from a poll conducted among 880 residents of Moscow, 169 of whom were relatives of individuals with known drug problems, by the Institute of Social Research at the Russian Government Academy, which allegedly "reports directly to the president."

43. Quoted in an interview with *Komsomolskaia pravda,* 3 July 1998.

44. *Ogonëk,* no. 15 (April 1997).

45. *Ogonëk,* no. 15 (April 1997). The quotations are taken from, respectively, *Obshchaia gazeta,* 17–23 April 1997, and *Ogonëk,* no. 15 (April 1997). The critics contend that "top police officials" played key roles in drafting the Duma legislation, which in their opinion accounts for its punitive character. For an elaboration on this argument, see *Ogonëk,* no. 15 (April 1997).

46. *Novoe vremia,* 12 October 1997.

47. *Novoe vremia,* 12 October 1997.

48. *Novoe vremia,* 12 October 1997.

49. See *ITAR-TASS,* 29 December 1998, for a report on President Yeltsin's directive to elaborate a new antidrug program. For a discussion of earlier antidrug programs adopted, but never implemented, in Russia, see Penny Morvant, "Drug Market Expands in Russia," *Transition,* 20 September 1996, 22–23.

50. U.S. Department of State, Bureau for International Narcotics and Law Enforcement Affairs, *International Narcotics Control Strategy Report,1996* (Washington, D.C.: 1997) notes the establishment of the MVD Main Administration on Illegal Drug Trafficking. See *INTERFAX,* 17 September 1998, for the announcement of the newly established "experimental police force."

51. Data on drug related crime for 1998 are from the interview on this subject with the deputy secretary of the Russian Security Council, *ITAR-TASS,* 29 June 1999. Respective data for 1997 from the minister of the MVD are reported in *Moskovskaia pravda,* 18 March 1998. *ITAR-TASS,* 1 October 1996, provides data on such criminality in 1995 and 1996.

52. Quoted by *ITAR-TASS,* 1 October 1996.

53. Quoted in *The Christian Science Monitor,* 5 October 1995.

54. *Moskovskii komsomolets,* 3 November 1998.

55. As reported in *Moscow News,* 28 November–4 December 1996. Lending credence to the public's beliefs, a "Clean Hands" campaign to root out pervasive corruption within the MVD led to the dismissal in 1996 of 10,000 officials, including three deputies to the minister

of the MVD and the deputy head of the ministry's main directorate in the Moscow region, on charges of passing classified information to a criminal organization. Open Media Research Institute, *Daily Digest,* 20 January 1997.

56. Reported in *Voprosy narkologii,* no. 1 (1994): 86. This source provided no information on the methodology employed in conducting the poll, including the composition of its sample.

57. For a discussion of this initiative, see *Interfaks-AiF,* 16–22 February 1998.

58. *Voprosy narkologii,* no. 1 (1994): 78–82.

59. For an extended discussion of this initiative, see *Voprosy narkologii,* no. 4 (1998): 67–69.

60. *Oblastnaia gazeta,* 19 March 1996.

61. *Agentsvo sotsialnoi informatsii biulleten,* no. 13 (3–9 April 1998).

62. Details on the proceedings of the conference are provided in *Voprosy narkologii,* no. 3 (1996): 4–7.

63. As a doctor at one of Moscow's government-run clinics admitted, "People only bring their children here as a last resort, or the militia does it for them. . . . In any case, we succeed in curing very few." A colleague at a respective clinic for underage addicts explained, "We try to get them out of here as fast as possible, before they learn too much from the others or become a bad influence." At her clinic, the typical "treatment" lasts one to two weeks, during which time the youngsters are locked up and heavily sedated as they go "cold turkey." *The Moscow Times,* 12 November 1995, 41. For a stinging indictment of the present state of treatment at government-run drug clinics, see the interview with the ranking official in the Ministry of Health responsible for narcotics-related issues, published in *Novoe vremia,* 12 October 1997.

64. *Novoe vremia,* 12 October 1997

65. *ITAR-TASS,* 17 April 1997.

66. See the report by the minister of the MVD that includes a discussion of these initiatives, as published in *Moskovskiaia pravda,* 18 March 1998.

67. U.S. Department of State, Bureau for International Narcotics and Law Enforcement Affairs, *International Narcotics Control Strategy Report, 1998* (Washington, D.C.: 1999).

68. *International Narcotics Control Strategy Report, 1998.*

69. Thomas Jefferson, "Notes on Virginia (1782)," cited in H. L. Mencken, *A New Dictionary of Quotations on Historical Principles* (New York: Knopf: 1946), 223.

CHAPTER 7

The Problem of AIDS

David E. Powell

Time does not wait, and history will not forgive.

—*Meditsinskaia gazeta,* 11 November 1994

It is obvious that, at the present time, both the government and parliament find it more interesting to discuss how to help the victims of financial pyramid schemes than the victims of HIV-infection.

—*Meditsinskaia gazeta,* 5 November 1997

A SPECTER IS HAUNTING RUSSIA—the specter of AIDS (Acquired Immune Deficiency Syndrome) and HIV (the Human Immunodeficiency Virus, which generally leads to AIDS). HIV/AIDS has put the people of the Russian Federation at grave risk, and both the government and ordinary citizens are doing far too little to combat this problem. The only question today is whether the country is on the brink of an epidemic or, instead, is in the midst of one.

The AIDS phenomenon, while relatively new, has already proved to be one of the twentieth century's greatest cataclysms. Because carriers of HIV almost always develop the disease itself, and because there is currently no cure for the latter and little prospect that an affordable one will be found in the near future, this scourge will continue to affect more and more people. As of December 1998,[1] a total of 33.4 million people around the world were HIV-positive, a figure almost 10 percent higher than the 30.6

million reported for December 1997. Altogether, since HIV first appeared two decades ago, the virus has infected more than 47 million people, approximately 13.9 million of whom have died.

More than 95 percent of all HIV-infected people live in developing countries, and these same nations have experienced 95 percent of all deaths to date from AIDS. Sub-Saharan Africa is especially afflicted: 70 percent of persons who became infected in 1998, and 80 percent of those who died during that year, live or lived in the southern half of the continent. And what of the situation in Russia? Largely isolated from the rest of the world until the collapse of communism in 1991, that nation is unprepared for the "plague of the twentieth [and soon the twenty-first] century." But the plague has already arrived, and all evidence suggests that what is currently a problem of manageable proportions will soon be a situation that is out of control.

The Magnitude of the Problem

The Problem of "Official" Statistics

Although there are official statistics on the incidence (the number of new cases) and the prevalence (the total number of cases) of both HIV and AIDS, no one—either in Russia or in the West—knows with certainty what the current situation is. Official agencies and experts on infectious diseases, as well as the press, frequently confuse the notion of incidence with that of prevalence, and they often fail to distinguish between those who are HIV-positive and those who have developed full-blown AIDS.[2] Communications issued by the State Committee on Statistics (Goskomstat) note that the actual number of infected individuals is at least ten times higher than the number registered. Ignorance about this disease is widespread within the medical community, many members of high-risk groups avoid being tested, diagnostic equipment and techniques are notoriously poor, and the authorities are only beginning to face up to the need to gather and publish accurate information about the disease.

Although the first cases of HIV/AIDS appeared in the USSR in the mid-1980s (or possibly earlier), government spokesmen were certain that they were anomalies. The Soviet leadership dismissed AIDS as a problem of the decadent West or the third world: the only persons at risk of becoming infected, they said, were homosexuals, bisexuals, prostitutes, drug addicts, those who led a "disorderly" sexual life (i.e., were promiscuous), and, most important, black Africans.

As of 30 June 1999, some 15,819 HIV-positive cases, of whom 526 were children, had been detected in Russia. The overwhelming majority of adult virus carriers (74.9 percent) are men.[3] Vadim Pokrovskii, director of the Russian Scientific and Methodology Center for the Struggle With AIDS (the AIDS Center), a corresponding member of the Russian Academy of Medical Sciences and the country's leading expert on AIDS-related matters, attributes the spread of the disease to the rapidly developing market for narcotics, the flourishing of prostitution, mass migration, the commercialization of the blood donor system, and ignorance among medical specialists and the population as a whole, as well as their propensity to engage in behavior that puts them at risk of becoming infected.[4]

A year earlier, First Deputy Health Minister Gennadii Onishchenko told a parliamentary hearing that Russia might be forced to spend its entire health budget on people with the HIV virus, "unless steps are taken now to stop the disease from spreading."[5] Something like $1.5 million is needed to take care of only the officially registered 16,000 infected persons, but with expenditures for drugs to cover only those with HIV estimated at only $1,000 a month, in Russia neither the government nor HIV patients themselves can afford to buy the most effective medicinal preparations, such as protease inhibitors. (In the United States, in contrast, $10–20,000 is spent annually on each HIV patient.)[6]

The Rapid Spread of HIV and AIDS in the 1990s

In June 1997, Mikhail Narkevich, head of the health ministry's Public Health and Epidemic Monitoring Department, declared ominously, "In the first five months of this year, the number [of HIV cases] doubled. We expect it to double again over the summer. . . . If the present rate of increase continues, we can expect 800,000 to a million HIV-infected Russians by the end of this decade."[7]

Where did this figure of 800,000 come from? Presumably, it involved multiplying official numbers of "recorded" cases by a factor of about ten. Thus, in November 1997, Pokrovskii said that "at the moment, there are some 60,000 HIV-positive people in Russia, or roughly tenfold as compared with the total of reported cases." Like

Narkevich, he declared that "there could be up to one million infected Russians by the year 2000, most of them drug users."[8]

The areas with the largest numbers of infected people are
Moscow and Moscow Province, followed by Kaliningrad Province,
Krasnodar, Tver, Rostov-on-Don and Nizhnii Novgorod, but even
the remote West Siberian Khanty-Mansy Autonomous District reported 125 HIV-positive cases in November 1998. In the first six
months of 1999, some 2,627 new HIV cases were recorded in
Moscow and Moscow Province—12 times more than were recorded
in the same period in 1998.[9]

A Brief History

The first public mentions of the disease in the period 1985–86, in
Trud, Literaturnaia gazeta, Meditsinskaia gazeta, Sovetskaia kultura
and other mass-circulation newspapers, consisted of little more than
an outpouring of slander, fabrications, and distortions. Commentators emphasized two themes. The deadly virus was described as a creation of the U. S. military and the Central Intelligence Agency as part
of an ongoing bacteriological warfare program aimed at the "socialist camp."[10] But before the Americans would feel confident about
using it, the official view went on, the virus first had to be tested—
and it was tested, on particularly vulnerable groups such as drug addicts and homosexuals. Thus, Soviet propagandists were able to
"explain" the prevalence of the virus among these groups.

But even while they were denouncing the U. S. government, officials in Moscow began to realize that Soviet society, too, was
about to confront grave risks. Thus, while asserting that the USSR
was not affected by the "social conditions" that would lead to the
spread of AIDS, Viktor M. Zhdanov, Director of the Academy of
Medical Sciences' Ivanov Institute of Virology and an authority on
AIDS, suggested that the "vast flow of tourists into the Soviet Union
and close contacts with foreign countries make it possible that AIDS
will penetrate here."[11] People were warned, in particular, to avoid
sexual relations with foreigners.

The Tragedy in Elista

That Russia was not immune to developments occurring elsewhere
in the world became painfully apparent in 1989. At the beginning of

that year, it was revealed that 27 babies (the figure was subsequently raised to 49 children and nine mothers) in the town of Elista, 150 miles south of Volgograd near the Caspian Sea, had been infected with the AIDS virus while in the local children's hospital.[12] A nurse, it seems, had come to provide the children with vaccinations; she had taken seven needles with her, but only one syringe, and while giving the children their injections, she changed the needles but used the same syringe. (In communist times, nurses routinely used the same syringe and/or needles when taking blood samples from, or giving injections to, patients under their care.)[13]

A similar, though less lethal, outbreak occurred in Volgograd in May, when the AIDS virus was discovered in 49 children in a local hospital. Once again, the problem was attributed to a shortage of disposable syringes and inadequate sterilization of instruments.[14] In July 1989, yet another outbreak of AIDS among hospitalized children was reported in Rostov-on-Don, where four children became infected and died.[15] In all likelihood, other episodes were hushed up and not reported, or were revealed in sources to which few Westerners have access (e. g., provincial newspapers). At the beginning of 1998, some 102 of the 268 cases of AIDS in Russia involved youngsters 0–14 years of age.[16]

Causes and Consequences

The Role of Intravenous (IV) and Other Drug Users

When HIV first appeared in Russia, it was spread by Russians—primarily by nurses who used the same syringe or needle more than once. There followed a period during which foreigners (students, sailors, etc.) were viewed as the principal means for transmitting the virus. Today, the country has come full circle, with Russians once again bearing primary responsibility for infecting one another. This time, however, the virus is being spread by homosexuals, bisexuals, prostitutes, and, most important, IV drug users and their sexual partners.

Why are people turning to drugs? The reasons are numerous, but youthful curiosity, increased availability of banned substances, and the nation's continuing economic difficulties have been the major factors behind the upsurge in drug abuse.[17] A nationwide conference of health care specialists, held in Moscow in May 1999, put the number of drug users in the Russian Federation at "close to 2 million," two-thirds of whom were under the age of 30.[18] For the year 1996 as a whole, the sharing of syringes among IV drug users was said to be the main cause of HIV infection, occurring in 80 percent of cases. This dramatic shift was explained by a sudden increase in the number of persons using psychoactive drugs, chiefly those that were injected intravenously, as well as an equally dramatic upsurge in STDs, a circumstance that facilitates the transmission of the AIDS virus.[19]

Thus, the epidemiological situation allegedly underwent a remarkable change during 1996. Almost all new infections, it was said, were brought on by IV drug users employing nonsterile syringes. But even though there clearly has been an explosion of drug use in Russia in recent years, attributing the spread of HIV/AIDS almost exclusively to this phenomenon violates even an elementary understanding of epidemiology and thus lacks credibility. In all likelihood, the authorities have known, and still know, very little about the true situation.[20]

The most common way for people to contract HIV involves drug users ingesting "Russian heroin," a cheap home-made mixture of liquid opium and vinegar or acetic anhydride. The drug often has a cloudy, muddy color; to make it more attractive physically, users typically mix several drops of their own blood in it.[21] Other addicts add their blood to "flush out" particles of narcotics left either in used syringes or in the original pot. Then they inject it back into their own bodies, along with HIV or traces of any other communicable disease present in the group.[22]

The Role of Prostitution

In recent years, the number of prostitutes working in such major tourist centers as Moscow and St. Petersburg, various port cities, and elsewhere in Russia has grown markedly. In 1997, a Western reporter described "the garish throngs of prostitutes, pimps, madams and crooked police who have made central Moscow their business center since the collapse of Communism."[23] Very few practice "safe sex." Asked by a journalist in 1997 if they used condoms, three prostitutes in the capital laughed. "This is my job," one of them said. "And those guys in the cars are my bosses. . . . Now do you think I can tell my bosses to wear a condom?"[24] Not surprisingly, the city's AIDS

Center estimates that at least 10 percent of the 50,000 prostitutes operating in downtown Moscow are HIV-positive.[25]

A survey carried out in late 1996 found that only 23.5 percent of all Russian women said they or their partners used contraceptives. One clinic polled 300 women, most of them prostitutes, each of whom had been with more than 20 sexual partners in a year. Ten percent said they never used condoms; the rest said they used them only occasionally. Not a single woman said she always used a condom. Part of the explanation for this situation is traditional male chauvinism; partly it involves poor-quality Russian goods.[26]

Homosexuality and the Spread of HIV

As the USSR began to unravel, Soviet citizens were allowed to travel abroad, businessmen from the capitalist world sought out investment opportunities in Russia, and thousands of foreigners—students, professors, bankers, dancers, rock musicians, etc.—flocked to Moscow and other Russian cities. Soon the country's borders became porous, illicit drugs were easier to obtain, prostitutes felt freer to ply their trade, and more and more homosexuals "came out of the closet."

For most of the Soviet period, the Criminal Code had made male homosexuality a crime punishable by up to five years in prison or a term in a labor camp. (Female homosexuality was never addressed by Soviet legislation.) Although the law was seldom applied—in 1992, for example, approximately 400 homosexuals were jailed, only 25 of whom had engaged in consensual acts[27]—it kept gay men from publicly acknowledging their sexual preference. More important, it deterred these men from seeking any form of medical assistance. In April 1993, parliament voted to repeal the law, and President Yeltsin signed the bill shortly afterward.

Nevertheless, one continues to encounter fatalism among large numbers of homosexuals. Surveys show that gay men in Russia are as aware of the risks of contracting AIDS as their counterparts in the West. One poll conducted in 1997 found that 80 percent considered unprotected anal sex "potentially dangerous," but only 32 percent of those individuals regularly used condoms. As an American source pointed out, "It is that sense of helplessness, as much as anything, that will make the age of AIDS in [Russia] every bit as deadly as it has been anywhere else."[28]

The Prison System as a "Culture Medium" for the Spread of HIV/AIDS

According to the Ministry of the Interior, in March 1998 Russia's penal colonies and pretrial detention centers housed almost a million people, 1,179 of whom were HIV-positive.[29] The figures are small, but they are growing rapidly; because the number of people incarcerated in Russia is unusually large, because they are confined to special units, and because homosexual acts are commonplace, prisons are likely to serve as "incubators" in which the virus will spread rapidly. In 1997, the head of the penal system said that only 36 percent of the system's estimated financial needs were being met, and very little money was available to protect the inmates' health. The incidence of HIV infection, he went on, had doubled or tripled since 1993.[30]

In 1997, the Russian Ministry of Internal Affairs announced plans to set up the first of several camps for convicts who were infected with the virus. The idea was to send these individuals as far from civilization as possible. According to one journalist, "the corrective-labor camp in Pechora [in the northwestern part of Siberia] is supposed to become a concentration camp [kontsentratsionnyi lager] for all Russian prisoners with AIDS." At the time this information was released, the camp, a conventional corrective-labor institution designed for 2,500 persons, already was being used to house prisoners suffering from tuberculosis.[31] At the same time, the government announced plans to establish a special prison colony in the town of Ardatov, in Nizhnii Novgorod Province, for convicts who had contracted the virus. (As we have seen, Nizhnii Novgorod has a high incidence of HIV infection; roughly 100 of the prisoners located there were HIV-positive.)[32]

Sexually Transmitted Diseases (STDs)

Although the recent rise in reported cases of HIV infection in the former Soviet republics has been most prominent among IV drug users, the disease has already begun to spread to people who are drug-free. The alarming rise in rates of STDs indicates a rise in unsafe sex: the presence of STDs, then, is both a barometer and a herald of AIDS, since they indicate the level of sexual activity in a population and also help to spread HIV. Further complicating matters is the fact that the people most apt to contract STDs are men and women between the ages of 15 and 24, the very individuals who are most sexually active. Worldwide, 50 percent of all HIV infections are found in people of this age bracket.[33]

The prevalence of syphilis, gonorrhea, and herpes has risen dramatically in Russia, and it is now far greater than the rate in Western Europe or North America. A new era of sexual freedom has caused these diseases to spread especially rapidly in Russia. Between 1989 and 1997, the rate of syphilis rose by 40 times, and among children by 45 times. In the latter year, Russia had 217 cases of syphilis per 100,000 people, more than 50 times the rate in the United States or Europe. The prevalence of gonorrhea was 173.5 per 100,000 people.[34] But the published figures do not adequately reflect the real situation: a substantial (but unknown) number of sick people are not listed on official registers. Some attempt to treat themselves by means of "alternative" medicine, others are unaware that they are infected, and still others are too ashamed or afraid to seek medical help.

Ignorance, Fear, and Loathing on the "HIV/AIDS Front"

Just as in some parts of the West, one can find medical personnel in Russia who refuse to handle AIDS patients out of fear of contracting the disease or out of contempt for patients they consider moral reprobates. Precisely how widespread these phenomena are is unclear, but press references, along with anecdotal evidence provided by friends and colleagues in Russia, suggest that they are by no means uncommon.

An early and highly explicit statement condemning those who contract HIV/AIDS as "social deviants" who deserve their fate appeared in 1987 in the youth newspaper *Komsomolskaia pravda*. Sixteen medical school graduates sent a letter to Pokrovskii, expressing the hope that a cure for AIDS not be found:

> We graduates of a medical institute categorically are opposed to combating the 'new disease' AIDS! And we intend to do everything in our power to impede the search for ways to combat this noble [*blagorodnoi*] epidemic. We are certain that, after a brief time, AIDS will destroy all drug addicts, homosexuals and prostitutes . . . Long live AIDS![35]

In the first years after the virus appeared in the USSR, most doctors refused to treat such patients. Even a 25 percent supplement to their salaries was not enough to compensate for the added risk.[36] At first, patients were kept in special cubicles and were forbidden to leave the hospital's premises. Only after medical personnel learned that protective gloves and masks would protect them were patients permitted to attend movies or to go shopping.[37] But the fact that so many men and women in the medical field embrace homophobic views makes it more difficult for them to help patients who are HIV-positive. No courses dealing specifically with the disease are offered in medical schools, although in some areas, local physicians, medical associations, hospitals, or foreign experts put together lectures on the topic.

If "experts" are loathe to deal with sexual matters, it is not surprising that ordinary citizens find it even more difficult. For example, one can meet Russians who believe (like their counterparts in other nations) that the disease can be spread through handshakes, swimming pools, pocket money, shop counters, restaurant dishes, or by mosquitoes and other blood-sucking insects. In addition, one can find frequent reports in the press of a new phenomenon—"AIDS phobia," the fear of being infected with the HIV virus.[38] In 1987, Gennadii Gerasimov, the official spokesman of the USSR Ministry of Foreign Affairs, suggested that "maybe [AIDS] can be regarded as the scourge of God against the doubtful morals of our world."[39] Today, too, a Finnish journalist has pointed out, "there are still people who throw out their children when they hear about their being HIV-positive.... Those [who are] infected are considered addicts and rejects."[40]

Inadequate Funding for Treatment

As the 1990s wore on, the state provided less and less money to the health care sector. Today, even though WHO recommends that countries devote at least 5 percent of their gross domestic product (GDP) to basic health care, Russia spends only 2.2 percent. The health ministry has calculated that by the year 2000, it will cost at least $5.6 billion a year to treat the nation's HIV/AIDS patients. At the present time, the entire federal health budget is $10 billion, and an increase in allocations is unlikely. Furthermore, the health ministry generally receives less than half the money budgeted for its

AIDS program, and oftentimes it receives no money at all to carry out educational or preventive programs.[41] Ignorance, denial, and shortsightedness conspire to keep anti-AIDS budgets small. Indeed, Pokrovskii has alleged that "a kind of informal group of those opposed to fighting AIDS has been created," one that actively disseminates its point of view among the leadership." These doctors, he went on, believe that "the threat of AIDS is seriously exaggerated."[42]

Russia lacks the medical facilities, physicians, and drugs needed either to treat or to prevent the disease. In the United States, it took years of public education programs and billions of dollars in research before the number of HIV cases finally stabilized. In Russia, as a scientist has pointed out, "It's as if we're standing on the beach watching a giant wave coming right at us. We know it, we see it and we can do almost nothing about it. We're just going to get swept away."[43]

What Is to Be Done?

What is being done to counteract such ignorance and prejudice?

Laws and Regulations

Various laws, decrees, and regulations designed to limit the further spread of HIV/AIDS have been promulgated by federal and local authorities. The first of these measures was adopted in 1987; it was followed by others, the most recent of which was passed in 1995. These measures include regulations aimed at controlling entry into the country (providing obligatory tests for certain tourists, students, and other visitors), requiring Russian citizens to undergo medical examinations if public health agencies believe they are infected with the virus, establishing criminal liability for anyone who "knowingly puts another person at risk of infection or infects another person with HIV," and providing (at least on paper) for confidentiality in the doctor-patient relationship when a diagnosis of HIV or AIDS is established.

On 14 August 1987, the Politburo of the Communist Party approved "additional measures aimed at preventing an outbreak of AIDS in our country,"[44] and on August 25 of that year, the Supreme Soviet passed a law, "On the Prevention of Infection with the AIDS Virus." The latter included the following provisions:[45]

(a) It made any carrier of the virus who had sexual contact with another person liable for a five-year prison term—whether or not the virus was transmitted from the former to the latter individual.

(b) It made "the infection of another person with AIDS by a person aware of having AIDS" punishable by up to eight years in prison.

(c) It threatened Soviet citizens, as well as foreigners who resided in the Soviet Union or who intended to visit for three months or more, with the prospect of compulsory testing.

(d) It authorized the police to detain any individual suspected of harboring the virus and taking him or her (by force if necessary) for testing.

In April 1990, a "Law on the Prevention of the Illness AIDS" was passed, followed later that year by additional "Rules for Medical Examination for the Detection of the Human Immunodeficiency Virus (AIDS)." (The latter came into effect in January 1991.) These documents called for testing on a large scale; the penalties were identical to those first set down in 1987.[46] In addition, the legislation passed in 1990, like the 1987 law and the 1989 regulations, identified certain groups whose members were to be tested "if there were grounds to suspect" that they were HIV-positive. Other categories were added to the list, however, e.g., homosexuals, bisexuals, and Soviet citizens returning from extended trips abroad to areas where AIDS was rife. But the new rules were far more detailed, listing the following categories of people who were required to undergo AIDS testing:

a. Donors of blood and other substances, at each donation.

b. USSR citizens returning from visits abroad lasting longer than three months.

c. Foreigners arriving in the USSR, within ten days of their arrival, unless they had a recognized certificate testifying that they had the appropriate antibodies.

d. Students arriving in the USSR, within 10 days of their arrival, and thereafter once a year.

e. Soviet and foreign citizens who had had sexual contact with AIDS sufferers (to be examined once every six months for a year).

f. Children of HIV-positive mothers, at birth, at six months, and at one year of age.

g. Pregnant women, at the time of registration as pregnant and again within 30 weeks of pregnancy.

h. Medical personnel working with the AIDS virus, once a year.

i. Drug addicts, homosexuals, bisexuals, prostitutes, and vagrants, twice a year. Prisoners from these groups, upon entry into, and upon departure from, prison.

j. Diplomats, the regulations stipulated, "may be examined only with their consent."

The 1990 law also promised complete confidentiality of diagnosis, that the health and other rights of patients would be protected, that doctors and other medical personnel would be held legally responsible for the safety of those being tested, and that compensation would be provided if an individual nonetheless became infected while being tested. Not surprisingly, however, it proved impossible to reconcile the promise of confidentiality with the requirement that individuals suspected of being HIV-positive undergo testing.

The 1995 law stipulated that foreigners and stateless persons—except individuals with diplomatic immunity—would be given visas only if they provided certificates "proving" that they were HIV-negative, if they planned to visit Russia for more than a month.[47] Anyone who refused to be screened or who tested positive when he/she arrived in Russia was to be deported. How much of a difference, if any, such laws have made is difficult to ascertain.

Fashioning a "National Program" to Combat AIDS

During the Soviet period, Russia had no broad national program to define and coordinate the battle against AIDS, an arrangement that resulted in fragmentation and duplication, and that seriously impeded the scientific community's prospects for success. But in March 1992, shortly after the collapse of the communist regime, one was created.[48] This program was supposed to educate Russians about the risk of HIV/ AIDS, but it was designed to last only three years and, though extended for a year, expired just as the number of AIDS cases was beginning its exponential increase in 1996.[49]

Mass Testing or "Screening" of the Population

Rather than wasting money examining healthy people, Pokrovskii has argued, "it would make better sense to spend [the funds] on prevention."[50] Devoting so much attention to testing (or "screening," as it is known in Russia) means denying resources to preventive efforts. According to Onishchenko, "we spend almost our entire budget testing risk groups for HIV infection every year, and there is nothing left over for scientific research or public education campaigning. It's like trying to fight an invading army without weapons or defensive walls."[51]

Every year new groups are selected for screening—homosexuals, drug abusers, people with venereal diseases, the homeless, promiscuous persons, etc. But more often than not, members of these groups are not registered by either the health or interior ministry, nor are they likely to come in voluntarily for a checkup. They "screen themselves out," in a manner of speaking. Over a period of seven years, starting in 1987, the government screened approximately half the population of the USSR, 140 million in all, discovering a total of only 774 HIV-positive people. This whole approach, with its emphasis on quantitative indicators, is Soviet, rather than scientific.[52]

More important, AIDS has a so-called "silent stage" or a period of "zero-conversion," when a person is already HIV-positive, but his/her immune system has not produced a sufficient quantity of antibodies for a blood test to reveal the presence of the virus. The duration of this zero-conversion stage varies widely, but it sometimes involves years. Obviously, this makes the government's fixation on screening all the more questionable.

Treatment

Approaches to treatment vary widely, depending on time and place, as well as on the financial resources available to the patient. Still, almost anyone who seeks medical aid will confront poorly equipped hospitals and, frequently, staff who are unaware of the latest advances in AIDS care. Most Russian hospitals are unable to afford the new drugs now available in the United States; in particular, protease inhibitors must be obtained at Western clinics or, in rare cases, are brought in by (or for) patients who are rich.

Even if the level of treatment available were first-rate, though, doctors would be stymied by the lack of up-to-date equipment. Thus, blood samples often have to be sent to far-away cities to be analyzed, a process that may take several weeks.[53] Medical instruments need to be boiled for several hours, but at the offices of some private doctors and dentists, as well as at most hospitals, it is not uncommon for staff to neglect to sterilize instruments or use fresh ones for each patient. In the case of complex medical devices such as endoscopes, hemodialysis equipment or artificial kidneys, which come in direct contact with bodily fluids, thermal treatment does no good whatsoever, so the devices themselves are potential carriers of infectious diseases.[54]

The medication most commonly employed for infected men and women is Russian-made (and thus of indifferent quality) AZT (azidotimidine), which was first produced by Soviet pharmaceutical plants in 1987. But many afflicted individuals, either out of ignorance or too depressed to care, do not bother with medication.[55] The conclusion is inescapable: money spent for treatment could, and should, be put to better use as part of a public-education campaign. In 1997, Nikolai Gerasimenko, chair of the Duma's Health Care Committee, declared that "prevention is much cheaper than treatment, and if we do not spend money on education about AIDS, people will continue to die."[56] Unfortunately, it will not be possible to obtain the necessary funds for this in the near future.

Shortages of Medical Equipment and Pharmaceutical Products

Treatment has been made more difficult by widespread shortages of drugs and medical equipment. At the same time, deteriorating public health institutions are less and less able to cope with the upsurge in the number of HIV/AIDS cases. "We seemed to be insulated for so long, and thought that maybe Russia was an exception to global trends," Narkevich said in 1997. "Now we are facing the flood with almost no defenses."[57]

Throughout the entire period during which HIV/AIDS has been present in Russia, a lack of hard currency and the leadership's priorities have made it exceedingly difficult to obtain sufficient quantities of the pharmaceuticals with which patients could be treated. While supplies of AZT are adequate, there is a shortage of drugs

such as Pentamidine and Ganciclovir, employed in the United States
to treat various "opportunistic" infections.

As regards the lack of disposable syringes and needles, physicians and nurses generally have responded by reusing conventional
syringes, a practice that was common in the West until only a few
decades ago, and that still could offer proper protection today. In
Russia, however, the syringes often are simply "stored" in a bath of
disinfectant solution—without, however, having been placed in boil-
ing water or an autoclave. Not only do few hospitals have adequate
supplies of disposable hypodermics; many also experience shortages
of nondisposables. In Western countries, single-use hypodermics
have been almost universally employed for two decades. In both the
USSR and post-Soviet Russia, though, disposable equipment often
disappears or is reused, practices guaranteed to place patients, as
well as their physicians and nurses, at risk.[58] In fact, the alcohol that
is supposed to sterilize nondisposable equipment routinely was or is
in short supply, partly because people prefer to drink it.[59]

Whether or not there was (or is) a shortage of condoms is
largely a matter of definition. During the 1980s, Soviet manufac-
turers produced 220 million annually, i.e., three per year for every
male, including little boys and old men.[60] But the "shortage" of
condoms was offset by low demand, which meant that there really
was no shortage at all. In 1992, demand was estimated at 1.2 billion, while only 226 million were produced. But condoms could
usually be found in stores, evidence that the population preferred
not to use them.[61] Today, even more than was true in communist
times, domestic production and foreign imports of condoms are
sufficient to assure the practice of safe sex. But availability is not
the same thing as use: most Russian men and their partners stay
away from condoms.

Maintaining the Purity of the Blood Supply

Another problem concerns inadequacies in the system of supply-
ing blood. Of particular concern are shortages of needles, plastic
containers, and other equipment, inadequate and outdated storage facilities, poorly trained technicians, and an alarming indifference to the need for proper screening of blood donors. In Soviet
times, because of the scarcity of diagnostic kits, blood from 10–15
different individuals would first be pooled, and a sample from

each pool would then be tested for the AIDS virus. This approach made it possible to save money by not having to purchase large numbers of diagnostic kits. "It was also clearly stupid," Jerome Groopman has observed. Because of dilution, the level of antibody in a given sample would have to be 10–15 times the minimum level to be detected.[62]

In May 1995, Moscow health care officials admitted that "the most serious blunders" were taking place in the capital's hospitals. The head of the municipal health department spoke of "a disheartening complacency" among officials with regard to the threat of HIV infection.[63] Two years later, the Moscow Public Health Committee issued a directive prohibiting all medical institutions from purchasing donor blood on their own, and today, the supply of all blood to hospitals is in the hands of the city blood-transfusion station (known in Russian as the OSPK). The main problem, according to the Moscow OSPK's chief physician, is underground trafficking in donor blood—which, he said, "has grown to menacing proportions recently." Moreover, according to a journalist, "until recently, dubious types of people have been hanging around official donor stations and outbidding them for donors. These people paid twice what the city station pays for the standard 450 milliliters [about a pint]." After such transactions, the blood can be delivered to any city hospital without undergoing proper testing.[64]

Why is there underground trafficking in blood? According to the chief physician at the Moscow OSPK, in 1993 the city needed 1.2 million blood donations a year but received only 100,000. Today, the situation is worse. In addition, it used to be that 30 percent of the donors were paid and 70 percent were volunteer; now the opposite relationship prevails. Among the explanations for this change is people's fear of becoming infected with the AIDS virus when they give blood.[65] As a result, Russian hospitals, especially those in Moscow and St. Petersburg, experience a chronic shortage of blood. Stocks at some hospitals are as low as one-fifth of desired levels, and the relatives of patients scheduled for surgery are routinely asked to provide blood. According to a report in a British medical journal, "It has become so bad that medical staff often have no alternative but to give their own blood to patients."[66]

Among the few OSPKs that have taken steps to improve the purity of blood and enhance the safety of its procedures is the Smolensk Province Blood Transfusion Station. Its facilities have undergone modernization, and it has purchased state-of-the-art technology, e.g., improved freezers, heat generators, and plasmapheresis apparatus, which it uses to ensure quality control during transfusions. This protects patients against posttransfusion complications.[67] Blood is procured, processed, checked, and stored in accordance with the most up-to-date procedures. It is tested in the AIDS laboratory for HIV antibodies, hepatitis C, and other dangerous impurities. Furthermore, the center has gone over to a system whereby blood components are stored in composite plastic containers (as required by international standards) 70 percent of the time, rather than mainly in glass packaging, as had been the case until 1998. The new Smolensk OSPK also has created a computer data bank on all donors from the city; this makes it possible to avoid the problems caused by donors with chronic infectious diseases or those belonging to high-risk groups, including individuals infected with HIV. The data bank, in other words, permits the authorities to weed out "undesirables."[68] But Smolensk is exceptional in this regard.

Needle-Exchange Programs

While officials in most parts of the country lack the resources to deal with the relationship between IV drug use and HIV/AIDS (as well as other infectious diseases), several cities have tried to curb the spread of the virus by offering disposable syringes and needles free of charge, in exchange for used ones. The first such effort was launched in 1996 by the European Union's TACIS program (Technical Assistance for the Commonwealth of Independent States). Run by a Christian charity that works with addicts, and operating out of a bus parked at a St. Petersburg market, it handles 300 people a day.[69]

A second, more substantial needle-exchange project was introduced in the city of Yaroslavl, not far from Moscow, in 1997. Administered by the Russian nongovernmental organization Friends Help Friends, it receives money, advice, and supplies from the Soros Foundation.[70] Other needle-exchange programs exist, but almost all of them are funded by outside agencies such as Doctors Without Borders and UNAIDS. Many, perhaps most, Russian specialists on substance abuse are skeptical of such efforts, arguing that instead of fighting the spread of disease, they encourage drug use.[71]

Sex Education and Discussions of "Safe Sex"

Virtually without exception, the media during the Soviet period—and to a lesser degree even now—were reluctant to confront issues of human sexuality. In 1987, Pokrovskii complained about the "fear" and "shame" the media had shown when they tried to deal with the question of how to prevent the disease. "For some reason," he said, "French television is able to say unabashedly, 'Madames, messieurs: use condoms!' But with us, the word causes us to have a fit."[72] At the same time, schools offered no systematic sex education programs. The materials that were used—literary, psychological, biological, and/or legislative—focused on the animal and plant kingdoms, rather than on human sexuality. Their tone was almost always moralistic; whether in courses on hygiene or (at a later date) marriage and the family, they condemned "those who were viewed as promiscuous (prostitutes, deviant teenagers, etc.), arguing that they deserved what they got."[73]

In virtually all public opinion polls taken since 1989, a substantial majority of the adult population—ranging from 60 percent to 90 percent, depending upon age and social background—strongly supported school sex education, with only 3 percent to 20 percent against it. But in Russian families, intergenerational taboos on discussions of sexuality are very strong. According to one survey, only 13 percent of parents have ever talked with their children about sexual matters, and the mass media provide precious little scientific information about STDs in general or HIV/AIDS in particular. This widespread reluctance by both adults and teenagers to learn more about human sexuality derives largely from the Victorian, almost puritanical, attitudes that traditionally have characterized Russian culture.[74]

Other studies, confined to the sexual behaviors and attitudes of urban teenagers, have revealed the following: in 1993, 25 percent of 16-year-old girls and 38 percent of boys had had intercourse; in 1995 the figures were 33 percent and 55 percent, respectively. Among 17-year-olds, the respective changes were from 46 percent to 52 percent (females) and from 49 percent to 57 percent (males). As Russia's most prominent specialist on sexual matters, Igor Kon, has pointed out, the absolute figures are comparable to those found in the United States and Western Europe, but in Russia the change has come about rapidly—probably too rapidly for the youngsters, their parents, and the school system.[75]

Russia's first serious attempt to introduce sex education classes for teenagers began only in 1996, with a modest pilot project directed at grades 7–9 in a handful of schools. But the teachers were hardly ready to help. As Tatiana Pestich, who managed the program for the Ministry of Education, complained in 1996, "The teachers we have now were brought up in the old atmosphere and are part of the problem rather than the solution."[76]

For years, educators attributed the failure to introduce sex education in Russian schools to a campaign organized by communists, extreme nationalists, the Russian Orthodox Church, and outspoken members of "pro-life" organizations. "One of their main targets is the Russian Planned Parenthood Association," Kon asserted in 1997. The organization is denounced by Christian fundamentalists as "a 'satanic institution' which propagates abortion and depopulation."[77] Other critics allege that sex education programs "warp children's minds" and "pervert minors." The work of the Vologda Center for Medical and Psychological Assistance and Family Planning, for example, has been accused of propagating homosexual values and "poeticizing lesbianism." The center's efforts to ensure that young people practice safe sex is seen by some as instruction on the virtues of "masturbation, anal, oral and vaginal sex, homosexuality, sodomy, lesbianism and bestiality." The program, one critic has asserted, "instills in young minds a cult of 'sex' in all its varied forms, including . . . sexual perversions and transgressions."[78]

Sex education programs are not aimed only at children. In June 1997, the Russian government, together with the French group Doctors Without Borders, introduced a mass advertising campaign in Moscow to help combat the spread of AIDS.[79] The TV advertisements consisted of 30-second messages featuring a procession of handsome young Russians "pushing the message home against a dizzying backdrop of Moscow and a steady techno beat." Television stations ran it as a public service. In addition, 45 Moscow buses carried the message, and it was also posted at 16 metro exits and on four metro lines. Finally, 100,000 leaflets and cards were distributed free of charge on streets throughout the city, and the slogan "Safe Sex—My Choice" was placed on billboards and appeared in magazines and newspapers. One of the advertisements featured a young man announcing, "For me, safe sex is as natural as washing and brushing my teeth in the morning."

In response to criticisms from the church, the Communist Party and ordinary citizens, the Moscow city government decided to discontinue the effort at the end of 1997.[80] The television network TV-Center, which was controlled by the municipal government, also ceased to air commercials promoting safe sex. At a November 1997 roundtable discussion of the campaign, many members of the State Duma expressed concern over its purpose and content. One of them said it violated both the Russian constitution and Russian law, while another argued that the project was designed by Western "experts" to lower birthrates in Russia. Others contended that the program would only corrupt teenagers and encourage them to have sex—precisely because it contained a section on "safe sex" and made condoms available to students.[81]

The Role of Nongovernmental Organizations (NGOs)

Because of official indifference and laxity, the main responsibility for dealing with the crisis has fallen to various NGOs. Some of these groups were set up and are being run by Russians, e. g., churches, the Red Cross and Red Crescent Society, doctors' and nurses' associations, and other bodies. But most are offshoots of Western (especially American) organizations, including a number that continue to receive financial support from abroad. They provide medications for HIV/AIDS patients, donate electronic equipment to anti-AIDS groups, create e-mail links with experts and concerned citizens in the West, publish literature and disseminate it among HIV/AIDS patients and their doctors, establish libraries with AIDS-related literature, translate scientific and other educational materials into Russian, set up "hotlines" (the first of which appeared in Moscow in 1990), "walk-in" centers, and anti-AIDS clubs, and distribute condoms to sexually active men.

There is even a newspaper, *SPID-INFO* (AIDS-INFO),[82] with a circulation of 3.7 million copies. When it first appeared, it provided sex education, along with information about human physiology, drugs, homosexuality, and prostitution, with a view to encouraging safe sex and curbing the spread of AIDS. Unfortunately, as time has gone by, its editors have shifted away from the prevention of disease; today, the newspaper publishes racy discussions of sexual infidelity, offers "information" (along with product advertisements) on how to enhance one's sexual pleasure, and provides photographs of scantily attired young women.

The most effective of these organizations, AIDS Infoshare, was founded to provide both ordinary Russians and specialists with the information they need to curb the spread of STDs and HIV/AIDS.[83] Among other things, the group offers: (1) an information service through its library and special publications, (2) training through seminars and workshops on human rights and public health, organizational and project management, computer skills, etc., and (3) consulting on information storage and retrieval, project management, medical diagnosis and treatment, etc. AIDS Infoshare also issues a Russian-language quarterly, which describes publications available to Russian organizations, offers a free mail-order service, and distributes a newsletter for HIV-positive people and their caretakers that deals with medical, social, and psychological issues. Its principal projects include:

- "Health and Human Rights in Russia," which develops guidelines to help the Ministry of Health and the Duma prepare legislation. There is also an educational component, which consists primarily of workshops, translated materials, and a newsletter.
- Infoexchange, which focuses on STD/HIV/AIDS prevention among women, helping Russian organizations carry out activities in their regions, providing computer equipment and training in computer and project management skills, offering small grants (up to $3,000), and putting people in touch with appropriate American or European counterparts.
- SPIDNET, an electronic mail network, funded by USAID, that disseminates information in Russia on HIV/AIDS.
- AIDS Infoshare Library, the first library in Russia specifically devoted to HIV/AIDS and STDs, consisting of books, articles, essays, videos, and brochures. Over 200 pages of material are translated into Russian and distributed each month at the request of specific users.
- Database/Resource Guide, which created an electronic database concerning individuals and institutions working in the fields of HIV/AIDS prevention, education,

care, policy making and research. This information has
been put together in a Russian-language resource guide
and is scheduled to be published in English.

The Red Cross and Red Crescent Societies have also become involved in combating HIV/AIDS. In 1989, a group of physicians,
nurses, feldshers (paramedics), and representatives of the Red Cross
in the Chuvash Republic put together leaflets, posters, and articles
in the local press, and arranged lectures and discussions on the subject of AIDS.[84] The Moscow City Committee of the Red Cross Society visits schools, distributes literature free of charge and arranges
"information-education skits."[85] Other branches of the Red Cross
and Red Crescent Society have similar programs in dozens of cities
around the country.

Table 7.1 provides some background on other national or local
NGOs active in this sphere. In addition to the activities described in
the table, these organizations are involved in other consciousness-
raising efforts very much like those seen in the United States. For example, in the summer of 1996 and then again in the summer of
1997, several NGOs in Nizhnii Novgorod took advantage of the
city's Hot Air Balloon Festival. Anti-AIDS activists distributed pam-
phlets about the risks of HIV/AIDS and drug abuse and gave away
free condoms.[86] In the spring of 1994, the homosexual advocacy
group *Krylia* helped to organize a ceremony, lighting candles on
May 22, the Memorial Day for Those Who Have Died of AIDS. A
similar group, the Tchaikovsky Fund, carries out educational work,
primarily among young men who are gay, urging them to practice
safe sex. Members of the foundation also visit local hospitals, which
provide AIDS patients with psychological and financial support.[87]

Concluding Remarks

Most communities lack the funds to conduct preventive work or
help those who are infected; medical personnel, administrators, and
legislators feel awkward talking about sex; and the notion of
"screening" looks, at least at first glance, as though it is ideally
suited to protecting public health, welfare, and morality. For all of
these reasons, few government officials invest either time or effort
in preventing the virus from spreading. This situation is especially

Table 7.1 National or Local NGOs Involved in the Fight against AIDS in Russia

The Russian Names Foundation	Friends and relatives of AIDS victims have created a giant blanket from their clothes, photographs, and names, distribute literature, and have created a support group for HIV-infected women.
Moscow's Social and Psychological Support Center	People who have come in contact with HIV infection are helped by a social worker, a lawyer, and a psychologist.
"A Future Without AIDS"	A Nizhnii Novgorod group seeks to raise public consciousness about the disease and has set up various programs to help individuals who are HIV-positive or who have the disease itself.
The Anti-AIDS Foundation	The foundation publishes a journal, *Chelovek i zdorove (Man and Health),* and finances AIDS prevention programs.
AESOP	AESOP criticizes mandatory HIV testing, has introduced sex education in several schools, and publishes a journal, *AESOP's Fables,* which includes material on sexual health, the prevention of HIV/AIDS, family planning, and combating discrimination against gays and AIDS victims.
The Agency for Social Information	ASI publishes a newsletter on health and other social issues.
Vy i my	"You and We," a support group, helps its members find jobs, obtain legal assistance, and learn more about safe sex, partly through its anonymous AIDS hotline.
Russian AIDS Relief	Another support group, Russian AIDS Relief, distributes food, clothing, and medication to people affected by HIV/AIDS.

(continues)

Table 7.1 *(continued)*

M & M	Man to Man is an organization that promotes safe sex among gay men.
The Russian Association of Gays, Lesbians, and Bisexuals	Also known as *Krylia,* or "Wings."
Sokol	"Falcon" is a youth organization that distributes literature and encourages students to call the confidential telephone line of the Nizhnii Novgorod AIDS center.
The Triangle Center	The International Gay and Lesbian Human Rights Commission.

unfortunate because Russian and Soviet "traditions" could be put to use. Behaviors and expectations that have been molded by centuries of hierarchy, discipline, etc., could be exploited by public health agencies to combat HIV/AIDS. That is, a well-designed program of prevention, if supported by adequate funds, medical supplies, literature, and advice, could be effective precisely because of Russia's historical experience.

But if Russians can hope for the best outcome, they still must prepare for the worst. History and culture, as well as current political and economic realities, have conspired to make the HIV/AIDS threat a clear and present danger to the very survival of the nation. Barring a (highly unlikely) massive transfer of human and financial resources from the West, the people of Russia will watch with mounting horror as the epidemic continues to spread. What is imperative, though, is for the government to acknowledge the crisis, mobilize its scientific resources, collaborate with Western experts, and develop some sort of education campaign.

The population's decades-long experience with Soviet propaganda—the constant campaigns to eradicate such "social evils" as religion, alcoholism, crime, and poor work habits—makes any attempt to change their attitudes and behaviors problematic. But the gravity of the situation facing the country's leaders and people requires a massive public-private alliance to re-fashion Russians'

approach to the horror confronting them. This must include public
service announcements, safe-sex instruction in schools, clergy who
will devote themselves to their church's social mission, and support
and understanding for NGO activism. The only alternative is self-
induced genocide.

NOTES

1. The following data are drawn from the Joint United Nations Pro-
    gram on HIV/AIDS (UNAIDS) and the World Health Organization
    (WHO), *AIDS Epidemic Update: December 1998* (Geneva and New
    York: 1999), as well as UNAIDS and WHO, *Report on the Global
    HIV/AIDS Epidemic: June 1998* (Geneva and New York: 1998).
2. *Meditsinskaia gazeta,* 27 November 1998.
3. *Moskovskiy Komsomolets,* 28 July 1999.
4. Reuters, cited in *RFE/RL Newsline* 3, no. 129, part I (2 July 1999).
5. *RFE/RL Newsline* 2, no. 109, part I (9 June 1998) and Reuters,
    "Drug-taking Threatens Russian AIDS Explosion," cited in *John-
    son's Russia List,* no. 2211 (9 June 1998).
6. Derived from *Kommersant,* no. 21 (16 February 1999).
7. Cited in *The Hindustan Times,* 2 June 1997. See also *Newsweek,* 14
    April 1997.
8. InterPress Service (Moscow), 28 November 1997.
9. The figures for Moscow come from *Moskovskii Komsomolets,* 28
    July 1999. Data for other areas were reported in *Sovetskaia Rossiia,*
    13 September 1997, *Argumenty i fakty,* no. 39 (September 1997),
    and ITAR-TASS, 12 November 1998.
10. See, e.g., *Literaturnaia gazeta,* 13 November 1985 and 19 Novem-
    ber 1986.
11. *Sotsialisticheskaia industriia,* 6 December 1986.
12. The following discussion relies chiefly on *Trud,* 26 January 1989;
    Moscow News, 18 and 23 February 1989; *Izvestiia,* 23 February and
    6 May 1989; *Komsomolskaia pravda,* 28 January and 6 May 1989;
    Literaturnaia gazeta, 15 March 1989; and *Selskaia zhizn,* 18 April
    1989. See also *The Sunday Times* [London], 21 May 1989, and
    "Children Infect Mothers in AIDS Outbreak at Soviet Hospital,"
    Nature 337, no. 6207 (9 February 1989): 493.
13. *Izvestiia,* 17 February 1989.
14. *Komsomolskaia pravda,* 24 May 1990. See also *Ogonëk,* no. 26 (27
    June 1989): 30.
15. *Izvestiia,* 23 June 1989.

16. UNAIDS and World Health Organization, *Epidemiological Fact Sheet on HIV/AIDS and Sexually Transmitted Diseases: Russian Federation* (Geneva and New York: 1998).

17. *St. Petersburg Times,* 1–7 December 1997. See also the chapter by John M. Kramer in this volume.

18. *Segodnia,* 26 May 1999.

19. *Voprosy narkologii,* no. 3 (July-September 1996): 4–7.

20. For an early criticism of the view that HIV in Russia was spread primarily through sexual contacts, and a suggestion that the real problem was multiuse, inadequately sterilized hypodermics, see John R. Seale and Zhores A. Medvedev, "Origin and Transmission of AIDS: Multi-use Hypodermics and the Threat to the Soviet Union: Discussion Paper," *Journal of the Royal Society of Medicine* 80 (May 1987): 201–204.

21. *Helsingin Sanomat* (Helsinki), 3 August 1997, in FBIS-WEU-97–40 (28 August 1997).

22. *Newsday,* 2 November 1997.

23. *Los Angeles Times,* 11 July 1997.

24. *New York Times,* 18 May 1997.

25. *Kommersant,* no. 21 (February 1999).

26. *Hindustan Times,* 24 November 1996.

27. *Report on the USSR* 2, no. 24 (1993).

28. *Newsweek,* 14 April 1997.

29. ITAR-TASS, 14 October 1997, and *Sovetskaia Rossiia,* 13 September 1997.

30. Reuters, 14 October 1997.

31. NTV, 5 October 1997, in FBIS-SOV-97–279. See also *Komsomolskaia pravda,* 2–5 December 1994.

32. *RFE/RL NEWSLINE,* 29 October 1997.

33. UN Population Fund, *The State of the World's Population,* 1998.

34. *Voprosy narkologii,* no. 3 (July-September 1996): 4–7; *Kommersant-Daily,* 27 February 1997; and *Meditsinskii kurier,* no. 1 (1997).

35. *Komsomolskaia pravda,* 1 August 1987. The term *blagorodnoi* was, of course, being used ironically.

36. *Pravda,* 30 April 1989.

37. *Argumenty i fakty,* no. 45 (1991).

38. *Severnyi Kavkaz,* 18 December 1995, in FBIS-TEN-96–002 (4 March 1996).

39. *The Guardian,* 18 November 1994.

40. *Helsingin Sanomat* (Helsinki), 3 August 1997, in FBIS-WEU-97–40 (28 August 1997).

41. *New York Times,* 18 May 1997.

42. *Meditsinskaia gazeta,* 27 November 1998.

43. *Newsweek,* 14 April 1997.
44. *Pravda,* 14 August 1987.
45. See *Izvestiia,* 26 August 1987.
46. *Izvestiia,* 11 May 1990 and *Meditsinskaia gazeta,* 14 December 1990.
47. *Rossiiskaia gazeta,* 12 April 1995.
48. *Meditsinskaia gazeta,* 27 November 1998.
49. See the remarks of Gennadii Onishchenko on 8 June 1998, in *RFE/RL Newsline,* 2, no. 109, part I (9 June 1998).
50. *Meditsinskaia gazeta,* 30 November 1994.
51. *Hindustan Times,* 22 April 1998, cited in *Johnson's Russia List,* no. 2161 (22 April 1998). See also *Meditsinskaia gazeta,* 30 November 1994.
52. This paragraph and the one that follows are derived from *New Scientist,* 4 February 1989, 30, and *Segodnia,* 24 July 1996.
53. *Helsingin Sanomat* (Helsinki), 3 August 1997, in FBIS-WEU-97–40 (28 August 1997).
54. *Segodnia,* 24 July 1996.
55. *Newsweek,* 14 April 1997.
56. *Molod Ukrayiny,* 7 August 1997, in FBIS-SOV-92–253 (10 September 1997).
57. *The Hindustan Times,* 2 June 1997.
58. *Molod Ukrayiny* (Kiev), 1 December 1990, translated in JPRS-TEP-92–007 (24 April 1992): 22–23.
59. Jerome Groopman, "Red Scare," *The New Republic* 200, no. 3874 (17 April 1989): 26.
60. *Pravda,* 21 February 1989.
61. *Nezavisimaia gazeta,* 24 March 1992.
62. Groopman, "Red Scare."
63. *Segodnia,* 20 May 1995.
64. *Moskovskii komsomolets,* 5 July 1997.
65. *Moskovskii komsomolets,* 5 July 1997; *Pravda,* 21 May 1993; and *Meditsinskaia gazeta,* 16 December 1998.
66. *British Medical Journal* 309 (8 October 1994): 899–900.
67. The following discussion is derived from *Meditsinskaia gazeta,* 16 December 1998.
68. *Meditsinskaia gazeta,* 16 December 1998.
69. *St. Petersburg Times,* 1–7 December 1997.
70. *Izvestiia,* 7 December 1996.
71. *Newsweek,* 14 April 1997.
72. *Komsomolskaia pravda,* 1 August 1987.
73. Christopher Williams, *AIDS in Post-Communist Russia and its Successor States* (Brookfield, VT: Ashgate Publishing Co., 1995), 87.

74. This discussion relies on *Kuranty*, 21 February 1992.
75. InterPress Service, "Health-Russia: Drugs Spark HIV Infection Explosion in Russia," 28 November 1997.
76. *Hindustan Times*, 24 November 1996.
77. BBC World Service, 4 and 7 April 1997.
78. *Rossiiskaia gazeta*, 10 June 1999.
79. This discussion is drawn from *St. Petersburg Times*, 30 June–6 July 1997, and personal observations.
80. *Segodnia*, 24 December 1997.
81. *Segodnia*, 24 December 1997, and *ASI Bulletin*, no. 46 (14–21 November 1997).
82. *SPID*, pronounced "speed," is the Russian acronym for Acquired Immune Deficiency Syndrome or AIDS (*sindrom priobretennogo immunisticheskogo defitsita*).
83. The following discussion relies on *ASI Bulletin*, no. 28 (137) (11–17 July 1997).
84. *Zdravookhranenie Rosskiiskoi Federatsii*, no. 11 (1991): 24–26.
85. *Trud*, 27 November 1991.
86. *ASI Bulletin*, no. 22 (131) (30 May–5 June 1997).
87. *ASI Bulletin*, no. 35 (144) (29 August–4 September 1997).

CHAPTER 8

The Disabled in Russia in the 1990s

Ethel Dunn

RELATIVELY LITTLE IS KNOWN ABOUT THE DISABLED in Russia, although more information is available now than when it was thought that talking about the disabled or showing pictures of them was as taboo as talking about train wrecks or natural disasters. The situation began to change in the early 1990s as mass-circulation newspapers began to publish photo and other types of stories about the disabled, but discussions of problems the disabled faced were still rare, except in the pages of *Sotsial'noe obespechenie,* a journal supported by the Russian Ministry of Social Protection. More recently, some information appears fairly regularly in the popular press. *Ogonëk,* a mass-circulation magazine, has in the last few years published a number of sympathetic depictions of the disabled,[1] including a discussion of terminally ill cancer patients.[2] *Izvestiia* reported as news in 1998 that in Artem, a city in the maritime region, several dozen blind people and children were picketing and living in tents in front of the city's administrative offices, to protest the fact that their dormitory, built in 1957, has neither lights, nor plumbing, nor water.[3] There are quite a few stories dealing with participation by the disabled in various sports, with the theme generally that such participation returns the individual to life.[4]

Attitudes toward the Disabled

It is estimated that 30 percent of the disabled never leave their homes or apartments,[5] only 45.8 percent of the disabled have a necessary minimum of clothing, and only 40 percent have TVs and radios.[6] Some attempts have been made to provide disabled schoolchildren with the same experiences as their able-bodied peers—a graduation ball in St. Petersburg, for instance, followed by a boat ride down the Neva—sponsored by local businessmen.[7] However, sheer lack of contact with the disabled elicits negative attitudes from the able-bodied about whether the disabled should be integrated into society. A survey of attitudes in Vologda, Moscow, Chelyabinsk and Ufa in 1991 found that women and severely disabled people most frequently sensed a disdainful attitude toward them. Young people and workers in the field of social protection had the most negative views, with 64 percent of the youth saying that they didn't want a disabled person as a relative, nor as a colleague (44 percent), as a boss (52 percent), or as a representative of the organs of power (48 percent).[8]

Negative attitudes toward the disabled, particularly on the part of the young, still trouble veterans of World War II, one of whom wrote to *Izvestiia* to report that one well-built young man looked at a World War II veteran who was trying to get ahead of him in a line at a clinic (as he had a right to do) and said, "Are you still crawling around?" The veteran also notes the failure on the part of young people in subways to give up seats set aside for the disabled, the elderly, and passengers with children. He attributes this to a lack of culture and of a firm sense of morality.[9]

The Prevalence of Disability

How many disabled are there in Russia? Statistics on the total number of disabled are not plentiful, and when available are contradictory, but at least the definition of what constitutes a disability now approximates the one in general use internationally: any condition that inhibits the individual from performing the usual activities of daily living, undermines health, or prevents the person from studying, working, or communicating.[10] Until recently, the disabled and the elderly were combined in statistical tables as a single category of persons receiving pensions,[11] and until recently disabled children did not get pensions, because the right to a pension was based on a person's work history. Some rural residents also did not qualify for pensions, because the *kolkhozy* evolved their own pension system (when and if they could afford it). It seems that Russian public health officials know how many disabled people there are only by counting those who have pensions,[12] and that responsibility for the disabled is spread among several agencies, giving rise to contradictory figures. A handbook of medical statistics[13] lists 5,100,700 disabled on the rolls of the Ministry of Social Protection in 1993, an increase of 326,700 since 1992.[14]

At an international conference on rehabilitation practice held in Moscow, A. I. Osadchikh, formerly deputy minister of social protection and presently deputy minister of labor and social development, reportedly stated in 1997: "In Russia according to the official statistics there are about four million disabled. These are people who receive pensions for disability. If however we include all (some disabled receive pensions on other grounds) this figure probably rises to eight million." Osadchikh reported that as of 1 January 1997 there were 7,284,000 disabled on the rolls of the social-protection agencies. He also remarked that about a million persons are added to the rolls yearly, more than 50 percent of them of working age.[15] A 1998 statistical handbook gives a figure of 9,110,100 disabled under the Ministry of Social Protection, based solely on the number of people receiving a pension.[16] Osadchikh himself was quoted in 1995 as saying that not less than 30 million people needed the products of a rehabilitation industry that barely existed in Russia at the time.[17]

Russian commentators themselves say that it is difficult to have exact figures on the disabled, largely because the criteria for establishing disability are not fixed, and the practice of the certifying body, the Medical-Social Expert Bureau, which has replaced the older Physician-Labor Expert Commission (VTEK) as of 1996, slows down the process of giving pensions.[18] For example, a woman wrote to *Sel'skaia zhizn'* that she lost her left hand in childhood, but her pension came to her as the result of the death of her father when she was 15, and of her mother at 16. She was given a Group III (able to work) disability rating and after completing her studies at an institute, she went to work, still receiving the original pension for loss of a breadwinner (at age 29). The local department of social protection, which accused her of hiding the fact that she was working, made her go through the certification process once more, in order to receive a Group III disability pension, since legally she was too old for a pension based on loss of a breadwinner. She asked whether this new rating deprives her of certain benefits, because Ul'ianovsk

Oblast, where she lives, does not give Group III disabled certain housing and consumer benefits to which they are entitled by law.[19]

Benefits for the Disabled

However illegal practices like the ones described above may be, they may be forced upon the local agencies for lack of funds. In Samara Oblast, the benefits of monetary compensation for transport and treatment at sanatoria are paid from the local budget.[20] The government of the Russian Federation appears to be shifting more and more of the welfare budget to regional agencies. Rehabilitation services also are not funded from the federal budget,[21] and this fact has definitely hindered the integration of the disabled into Russian society, though at the rehabilitation conference referred to above, A. I. Osadchik tried to put a brave face on the matter. In 1997, he said: "[W]e have a branching network of appropriate rehabilitation facilities. We have more than 1600 Medical-Social Expert Bureaus,[22] 12 boarding-school-tekhnikums for the disabled, seven higher educational institutions and more than 30 professional-technical schools for disabled. There are sanatoria in which pensioners and disabled are receiving rehabilitation and over 70 firms producing prostheses and orthopedic equipment. . . . The basic problem is to unite them all under one administration or one structure, which . . . could be called the state rehabilitation industry service."[23] A modest start has been made, with rehabilitation and technical centers in Novosibirsk, St. Petersburg, and Petrozavodsk. In the Republic of Karelia, three territorial centers have been opened as well, in Pitkyaranta, Segezha, and Kem.[24]

Can organizations of the disabled do what the state cannot? The largest organized group of disabled is the All-Russia Society for the Disabled (ARSD), formed in 1988, with 2.4 million members. By way of comparison, the All-Russia Society for the Blind, according to *Ogonëk*,[25] has about 300,000 persons with visual disabilities. More than three-quarters of them are older than 50. The Moscow city branch of the ARSD claims that there are a million disabled people in Moscow, 220,000 of whom are members of the ARSD, according to their official newspaper *Nadezhda,* but the overwhelming majority of the disabled must somehow fend for themselves or organize into small independent groups. For example, an association for epileptics, Mutual Aid, has just been formed in Moscow.[26]

The city of Moscow in 1994 gave a fair amount of aid to almost one third of its population, including a million schoolchildren, 700,000 poor pensioners living alone, 570,000 disabled, 110,000 children from large families, and 18,500 families with disabled children.[27] Free dinners were provided to 40,000 people, and 67,000 elderly and disabled who needed home care were served by 537 departments for social assistance.[28] In 1992, according to Ella Pamfilova, then minister of social protection, Russia-wide there were 7,800 such departments, serving 724,000 persons, as well as 321 territorial centers. By 1993, the head of the service reported that 952,200 elderly and disabled needed such assistance.[29] By way of comparison, on January 1, 1994, the Kursk Oblast Department of Social Protection had on its rolls 397,000 people who received pensions or grants of aid, including 47,300 pensioners, 30,000 disabled, 21,300 families with children, 16,300 refugees from various war zones, and the homeless. Repair of 1500 apartments occupied by elderly pensioners living alone and by the disabled was among a fairly long list of activities undertaken from regional and local resources.[30]

Special Categories of Disabled Persons

War Veterans

Disabled veterans of World War II in Russia numbered 659,200 in 1989, but their numbers increase as those veterans who survived the war without crippling injuries (2,660,000 in 1994, and another 13 million who are recognized as having worked in the rear of the army) age and acquire multiple disabilities.[31] There is also a very prominent group of veterans who fought in the Afghan War—the so-called Afghantsy. A statistical handbook lists 372,700 in the USSR as of 1989, with 167,700 in Russia. Three percent of the total (11,181) are disabled, almost half of them with Group I and Group II (severely disabled and usually considered at present unable to work) disabilities.[32] In 1989, some 2,000 of them were in need of prostheses.[33] According to an interview with the chairman of the Union of Afghan Veterans published in *Literaturnaia gazeta,* they were so well supplied with wheelchairs from foreign donors that they gave some to World War II veterans and people disabled from childhood. Two of the functioning prosthetics shops in Moscow and St. Petersburg were set up by the veterans, as were two-year training courses abroad. Veterans have also contributed equipment to various hospitals to aid in rehabilitation. When asked where the money came from, the chairman said that in 1993, their 184 regional organizations had 2,500 enterprises bringing in money.[34] The ARSD during the same period had 78 regional member organizations, 4,429 district and city member organizations, and over 19,000 local ones, and, according to a World Institute on Disability report, about 1,300 enterprises.

The Afghantsy are a privileged group compared to thousands of soldiers in the Russian army today who became disabled during their tour of duty and who do not qualify for pensions,[35] and to veterans in rural areas who, because of their location, have reduced access to jobs and medical care. *Ogonëk*[36] published a letter from a man living in a village in Voronezh Oblast who was called up for army service in September 1958, was hospitalized in October with "a bouquet of illnesses," but who nonetheless served until November 1960, when he received leg wounds in the course of duty. By March 1961, he was released from the hospital to rejoin his unit. Now, 34 years later, his health has been undermined, but he apparently cannot turn to the Ministry of Defense, or any other ministry, for help.

The Homeless

Prisoners released from confinement are a neglected but large proportion of the disabled. In 1992, 203,000 prisoners were released, 11 percent (22,330) of whom were aged, or Groups I and II disabled. There were only 4,000 places in homes for such people, and local inhabitants are not above picketing against the building of new facilities.[37] More than 60 percent of the homeless are former prisoners.[38] *Izvestiia,* with a banner headline warning of the threat of mass epidemics, reported that in 1993, according to official figures, there were 150,000 homeless in Moscow alone, most of them diseased and louse-ridden. Of these, 87,000 in Moscow are former prisoners, with another 57,000 unable to find housing or work in the Moscow area. For Russia as a whole, the figure rises to about 1,500,000.[39] *Ogonëk* notes that the source used as official is the local police count of those detained for lack of a residence permit or registration at a residence, and by this count in 1998, there were between 100,000 and 350,000 homeless in Moscow, with perhaps as many as five million throughout Russia.[40] Judging by the pictures accompanying these stories, many homeless are also disabled. The threat of epidemics seems real enough: in Russia as a whole, the rate of illness with tuberculosis is 70 per 100,000; in the Northern Caucasus, 200, and in prisons 3,395 per 100,000.[41] In addition, strains of tuberculosis are developing that are resistant to drugs.[42]

The ranks of the homeless and potentially homeless have also been swollen by Russians and people of other nationalities coming from the "near abroad" (the Baltic area, Central Asia, Kazakstan, and the Causasus and Transcaucasus), most of whom are leaving very unstable areas with little more than what they can carry. *Sel'skaia zhizn'* reports that the Swiss Red Cross was willing to build a Social Center for the Unprotected in the refugee center "Novosel," in Kaluga Oblast, which would have served pensioners and the disabled from all the "hot spots" of the former Soviet Union, but the oblast administration declined the offer, saying that it knew better than the Swiss what was needed.[43]

Children

The number of disabled children has been growing steadily in recent years. In 1996 state statistics on the number of disabled children under the age of 15 became available for the first time: there are 462,300, 43.4 percent of whom are in the 10–14 age group. Almost 40,000 of them need constant care (there are 4,311 totally blind, 27,515 with hearing difficulties, and 3,449 with amputated limbs). More than a third of the total number suffer from diseases of the nervous system and sensory organs (including almost half with cerebral palsy); 19.7 percent suffer from psychic disorders, and more than 70 percent of this group have some form of mental retardation.[44] Children with Down's syndrome are frequently abandoned by their parents and considered by most Russian doctors to be ineducable, and therefore most boarding schools give the children very little, even in terms of socialization. A Russian Association for Down's Syndrome had begun by 1995 to distribute literature,[45] but information has been slow to filter out to the provinces.

A study done in Nizhnii Novgorod (a city in a region where reforms were achieving some results) revealed that from 1993 to 1996 the number of disabled children grew by a factor of 1.4 and stands at 12.4 per 1,000 children. A special study of 148 families was done, comparing those families with those of preschool children who are not disabled. In the group with disabled children, 29.7 percent of the mothers (10.1 percent in the control group) gave birth at relatively late ages (after 30). Most of the families (54.7 percent and 49.3 percent respectively) had only one child; those with a disabled child feared having another. Even so, 11.1 percent of families had a second child with developmental deviations. In 19.6 percent of families with disabled children, conflicts arose because of difficulties in raising a disabled child, and every ninth family had problems with alcohol. Only 29 percent of the families were optimistic that the child would come out all right. More than a third of these parents worked with the children only periodically. Disabled children were seldom outdoors, either because the children had difficulty walking, or the parents didn't have time. Only 39.1 percent of the disabled children were undergoing rehabilitation, and 12.1 percent of the families treated the children at home, citing the child's health and mistrust of doctors as reasons. Apparently some parents are unaware of their options, because 9.5 percent of the children receive no treatment at all.[46]

The attitudes and behavior of parents whose disabled child is at least ambulatory are somewhat different. A study of 203 families of children with cranio-facial pathologies in Ekaterinburg revealed that the presence of such a child had a less disastrous effect on family relationships, that 88 percent made the rehabilitation of the affected child their main goal, that 46 percent blamed the ecological situation for the child's disability, or the mother's poor working conditions (20 percent), or past parental illnesses (21 percent), or poor medical care (15 percent). Although 68 percent of these families planned no more children, 46 percent already had two, 15 percent had three, and 6 percent had four or more.[47]

Education of the Disabled

It seems clear that the majority of disabled people in Russia are poor because they frequently subsist on their pensions alone, live in substandard housing, and have less education than other classes of Russians, although it really cannot be said that these facts are the result of discrimination. The problem once more is that of attitudes. A case in point: Igor Markov is a resident of the House of the Disabled in Moscow. He has cerebral palsy and walks on crutches, and cannot use the subway. His mother sent him at birth to a boarding school where he was potentially able to attend a normal school, but the school was across a street, and the director of the boarding school would not designate a nurse to help him with the journey. So he got basic reading, writing, and arithmetic, and a second diagnosis of "oligophrenia" (mental retardation). For many years, he was shunted around boarding schools for retarded children and passed through more than a dozen psychiatric evaluations, during which he was told, "You are first of all disabled, and a person only second. No one will ever accept you in a normal fashion." Igor, during his stay in one boarding facility, wrote a letter to then-General Secretary (of the CPSU) Andropov and got his psychiatric evaluation removed. For the next 12 years he began trying to change his fate. He took classes by correspondence in the M. Torres Institute of Foreign Languages in the Spanish division, and translated some Spanish poetry. Then he became attracted to the history of philosophy and took courses in the Russian Open University by correspondence. He came up against the problem of how to attend the university every day for a month for testing, which he couldn't do, and the university told him that sessions now needed to be paid for, and furthermore, he didn't qualify. He heard of a school for advertising art in Moscow, but the new curator of the school told him that as a disabled person, he didn't need the schooling, the diploma cost $3,000, and he, as a moron, was completely unsuited for study. Then Igor thought that he should try to get his secondary schooling and apply to higher educational institutions on his merits. At last he found School No. 199 for External Studies, whose director said, "Of course we will help him." Now at age 31 he has finished the tenth grade, is studying in the eleventh, and is very happy.[48]

T. A. Dobrovol'skaia and N. B. Shabalina, in a 1991 survey of 1,321 persons with varying degrees of loss of working capacity in Moscow, Chelyabinsk, and Ufa and the surrounding oblasts, found that more people had incomplete secondary education than higher education. Being disabled, they say, diminishes the chances for getting an education, but even so, among people disabled from childhood, 12.6 percent had attended institutions of higher education.[49]

Until very recently, few disabled students were enrolled in higher educational institutions, probably because of problems with accessibility. For example, *Uchitel'skaia gazeta* reported that in 1991 there were only 648 disabled students in 514 higher educational institutions.[50] *Ogonëk* says that less than 1,000 members of the Society of the Blind (a group said to have the resources to aid its members) were studying in 1995 at higher educational institutions or technical schools.[51] In July 1991, a special boarding school and institute was set up for the motor-disabled in Moscow. Its five departments include information science and applied mathematics, foreign languages, economics, editing and publishing, and law—a welcome change from the usual shoemaking, watch repair, and tatting. In St. Petersburg there is a Center for the Professional Rehabilitation of the Disabled, so far the only one in the country, at which 250 students are studying business basics, with a view to acquiring various skills such as lab techniques and computer repair. The administrators of the school hope that with such skills the presence of a disability will not be as limiting.[52]

Whether or not the disabled attend regular schools depends on their ability to walk (since most buildings are not wheelchair accessible) and to use their hands. Disabled children have the right to an education, which is supposed to be provided at home if the child cannot be placed in a special boarding school (such schools had and have long waiting lists). In practice, home schooling is probably limited because of teacher shortages.

Children who are considered educable are the responsibility of the Ministry of Education, and those who are judged "without prospects" are served by the Ministry of Social Protection. Children placed in special boarding schools must leave them at age 16 when their training ends. Usually an attempt is made to find them living space with relatives, but if no one can or will claim them (many children are abandoned at birth by their parents), the adolescents attempt to return to the school, or land on the streets. The Ministry of Social Protection also reports that in its experience, people classified as Group III disabled with psycho-neurological disorders, even when housing is found for them (usually in a communal apartment), are usually unable to cope and request readmission.[53] Sometimes an individual with very limited personal resources is moved to set up a group home, as in the case of Svetlana N. Protsenko, a retired translator, who now lives on a farm near Moscow most of the year, and who is aided by one of the private farmers.[54]

In recent years special schools using innovative techniques have been set up to rehabilitate disabled children. One of the most serious problems a disabled child faces is social isolation. Moscow School No. 1673, a state school and the first of its kind in Russia, integrates disabled and able-bodied children, but it initially encountered resistance from parents who did not want their children stigmatized by attendance at a school for disabled children. It was staffed by people without pedagogical training and did not have all the money it needed for its programs (which included free meals, support for parents' groups, medical services, and home schooling for those who need it).[55] Most facilities for disabled children, whether from staff shortages or lack of funds, are pretty grim places. A mother with an epileptic child reports seeing in a home for disabled children how children without hands lap up their food like kittens, because there is no one to help feed them. The school for retarded children in the village of Pervomaiskoe, the Altai, shows that when Russian educators try a progressive approach, they do very well. The school is organized into family groups, with each having a separate apartment. In this way the children are given individual attention, and allowed to work on the land and with a small horse.[56]

Employment of the Disabled

How many disabled people are employed? Under the Soviet system, by law, two percent of the work places were to be set aside for the disabled, but even this (by European standards) low percentage was frequently violated as factory managers struggled to meet the output plan set centrally for their enterprises. "During the transition to new economic relationships," as Ella Pamfilova described the present regime in Russia, the number of disabled employed continued to decline, from 727,400 in 1991 to 702,300 in 1992.[57] The head of the Russian Federal Employment Service reported that in 1993, 82,690 pensioners came looking for work, including 26,572 disabled. The service was able to aid in the placement of 14,470, half of them disabled.[58] The small soviet in Tiumen' (Siberia) decided in February 1993 to reduce by half the taxes on profits from those enterprises where 25–40 percent of the workers are disabled or pensioners.[59] By 1998, the law stated that not less than 3 percent of job slots at enterprises with 30 or more workers (including private enterprises) were to be set aside for the disabled, and not less than 1 percent for young people. In places like Astrakhan Oblast, certain tax advantages are extended to enterprises that will exceed these percentages, and enterprises that fail to meet the quota are fined.[60]

According to an interview in 1993 with the deputy minister of social protection, L. P. Khrapilina, who is a trained rehabilitation specialist, the work the disabled do only enhances their sense of hopelessness. There has been at least one case in which there were two brigades of disabled workers: one knit socks and the other unwound them so that the first one would have work. When asked whether it wouldn't make more sense to sell the stockings, she answered, of course, but then you'd have to organize getting raw material and selling the finished product, and the businessmen made their computations and figured "that it was more economical simply to imitate work. And they were able to think of themselves as philanthropists because the disabled people received wages."[61]

Many professionals in Russia whose job it is to help the disabled hoped that organizations for the disabled would provide the social services, education, and employment that state services fail or are unable to provide. This approach is sometimes criticized as an attempt to create "reservations," segregating the disabled in isolated communities. Organizations of the disabled originally looked forward to the return of more than 8,000 production units (artels) and 100 professional training schools expropriated by the state during the Khrushchev era, leaving many disabled workers without any means of subsistence.[62] The return of these enterprises would mainly have benefited the Society of the Deaf and the Society of the Blind, which have existed since the 1920s, but there was a catch: the return would take place only with the agreement of the present workers in the enterprises. Only in Nizhnii Novgorod Oblast have "practically all" the enterprises been returned.[63] *Ogonëk* reported that only 50,000 of the 300,000 members of the Society of the Blind are working at trade schools or in agriculture.[64] In an article appropriately flagged as good news, *Sotsial'noe obespechenie* reported that the Ufa factory for metal and plastic wares had opened a center for using waste products to make briquettes, dress hangers, plastic wrap, and compost boxes. An agreement was reached with the Bashkir Society of Disabled to hire the disabled, including Group I.[65]

In 1994 Vladimir Kaznacheev, a reporter for *Nadezhda*, indicated that about 21,000 workers were employed in enterprises owned by the All-Russia Society for the Disabled, but the figures he cited show that most of them are very small. The Moscow city ARSD, for example, has 34 enterprises, with 225 disabled workers. The mayor's office has not turned over a single enterprise to them. There are 24 enterprises in Moscow Oblast that employ disabled workers. In one city, Khimki, in 1994, there was a plastics factory whose director refused to upgrade his equipment because it would throw many people out of work. This attitude is still a fairly common one, which clearly exhibits a sense of responsibility on the part of directors to provide a social safety net. The district had 7,000 disabled, 803 classified as Group III—able to work—but only 533 of them were working.[66] At least some regional cities extend tax advantages to enterprises that will hire the disabled, but the number of disabled people working continues to fall, at least among Group III disabled. Employment among Group II disabled had risen somewhat, thanks to the efforts of local departments of employment.[67]

The Impact of the Yeltsin Reforms

The benefits to which disabled people were entitled under the Soviet system for the most part survived into the Yeltsin era but are being slowly eroded by the failure to fund social and public health services at the necessary level. Formerly free medicines are no longer free,[68] and the disabled complain that often a cheaper and less effective medication is substituted for a higher-priced one. Many medicines are too expensive for most pensioners. In Moscow, at one pharmacy, Tamoxifen sells for 349 rubles a package; a person with a Group II disability (including people with cancer) gets a pension of 400 rubles a month. Many Moscow pharmacies apparently are not receiving the subsidies that would allow them to dispense the medicines free.[69] This may be one reason why the average life expectancy of the disabled is 3.7 years less than for other Russians.[70] Veterans, families with many children, disadvantaged elderly, and the disabled sometimes are able to shop at stores for food at discounted prices, but diabetics have difficulty finding suitable food at any price.[71] An auditor with the rank of minister in the accounting office of the Russian Federation, in a 1998 interview, put the blame for the food situation squarely on the Russian government, saying that "30 percent of the population lacks the means to acquire food at a minimal physiological level of consumption," and he likened the situation to that of Leningrad during the blockade in World War II.[72] Another source sets calorie consumption at 2,000–2,200 calories per day in a country where hard physical labor is still the norm, and bread, potatoes, and pasta are the main items in the food basket. Little meat, dairy products, fish, fruits, or vegetables are consumed.[73]

Other benefits that have stretched small pensions are being threatened by the capitalist climate in Russia. For example, the phone company in Rybinsk charged a disabled veteran twice for service, when by law he was entitled to a 50 percent discount on the telephone in his home.[74] The specially equipped car to which veterans and disabled people are entitled is not only in short supply, but acquiring it is a process entangled in bureaucratic regulations, and the vehicle is poorly made.[75]

According to a spokesman from the general procurator's office, in 1994 there was almost no law or instruction relating to the disabled or those in need of social protection that had not been violated. For instance, children in St. Petersburg and Samara have been denied pensions, allegedly because they already were living at full state expense. People eligible for telephone installations have been denied them, supposedly for lack of equipment, and some offices have also refused to install telephones free. The right to free or reduced-rate bus and train travel suffers from inflation, but in some places agencies have refused to reimburse even the very small pre-inflation fees. People who should have their expenses for gasoline and repairs for their cars covered find that these amounts too are either refused or were insufficient. Only about half of the trips to sanatoria authorized by the Ministry of Social Protection have been honored.[76]

Political Activity

The involvement of the disabled in the present-day political situation in Russia is uneven. According to *Ogonëk*[77] there are 200 deputies at local levels who are members of the Society of the Blind.

During the discussion about the adoption of the Law on Social Protection of the Disabled in the State Duma, Oleg N. Smolin, a blind deputy representing the city of Omsk, spoke in the Council of the Federation in favor of the law's adoption. Smolin had also worked on laws guaranteeing rights for the disabled in the Supreme Soviet, before the collapse of the Soviet regime. There may be other deputies at the federal level who are disabled, but the question is whether they identify themselves as disabled. In 1993, a party fraction that the ARSD had helped to form, *Dostoinstvo i Miloserdie,* received enough qualifying votes (5 percent) to win seats in the Duma, but failed to do so in the 1995 elections.

According to a sociological study sponsored by the ARSD, headed by E. Okhotskii and A. Kolesnikov in 1993, the activity of the electorate represented by the disabled is significantly lower than the rest of Russia's electorate. If the pre-election activity for all social groups was predicted to be close to the 60 percent level, among the disabled, it reached only a quarter. In addition, almost a third of the disabled, according to the experts, did not support the forthcoming elections, considering them only a formality, and not particularly democratic. Twenty-eight percent were indifferent to them or neutral, and an additional 14 percent had no definite position. According to the World Institute for Disability, however,

> The data adduced by no means show that the disabled are a politically passive part of the population. The research results show that only a third of the members of the Society of Disabled Persons take no part at all in the socio-political life of the country. According to 54 percent of the experts, the main part of the disabled to one or another degree participates in various socio-political and economic activities. According to another 22 percent of the experts, the Society is extremely active in deciding all the vitally important problems of the regions.[78]

Certainly political involvement by disabled groups and organizations is essential, because even they are not immune to the problems of crime and corruption currently plaguing Russia. The Afghantsy are rather more involved in politics than other disabled groups, and perhaps to pacify them, Yeltsin issued a decree in 1991 creating a Russia fund for veterans of the Afghanistan War, which, according to *Izvestiia,*[79] had over a billion rubles, tax free.[80]

Future Prospects

Summing up, it is difficult to know how to improve the situation of the disabled in Russia. Humanitarian aid is only a short-term solution, however necessary. The World Institute on Disability, which has received a number of grants from USAID and IREX, decided to concentrate on institution building and advocacy in its dealings with the All-Russia Society for the Disabled, and if one believes that Russian disabled people need to be taught how to help themselves, WID started on the right course. However, given that WID operates on the thesis that the disabled the world over have the same culture, it is not clear how much they have helped the Russians. The Wheeled Mobility Center at San Francisco State University carried out a three-year project in Novosibirsk centered on setting up factories to produce inexpensive wheelchairs with local materials, but the center realized that it had to mobilize disabled people not only by giving them wheelchairs but by helping them to think of ways to interact with local authorities. Unfortunately, disabled activists in Novosibirsk are struggling on alone, and may have to continue to do so for many years. It is too simplistic to say that the government does not place the disabled very high on its list of priorities, nor can the Russian government be forced to reorder those priorities. Given the devastating and ongoing impact of the August 1998 financial crisis, it is difficult to imagine new government flows of resources in this direction. Whatever steps are taken, they must be grounded in knowledge of the context in which the disabled live their lives.

NOTES

1. For instance, *Ogonёk* has run an article about a blind couple (no. 34 [1995]: 56–57), an article about a 56-year-old woman in a wheelchair disabled as the result of being in a war zone in World War II (no. 30 [1995]: 51–52), children disabled by Down's syndrome (no. 9 [1997]: 40–43; no. 39 [1997]: 37), a performance by six actors with Down's syndrome based on Biblical themes (no. 38 [1998]: 38–41), and motor-disabled children (no. 8 [1996]: 46–48). There are supposed to be about ten million children in this latter category, including 120,000 in Moscow alone.
2. *Ogonёk*, no. 29 (1998): 38–45. The hospice described provides outpatient services to 1,000 people.

3. *Izvestiia*, 20 August 1998, 2.
4. See *Izvestiia*, 28 October 1993, 8. Whole books are devoted to the topic, celebrating individual wheelchair athletes. See, for example, Dmitri Shparo and Irina Grigor'eva, *Repetitsiia s anshlagom: rasskaz o supermarafone v invalidnykh koliaskakh Moskva, Kiev, Krivoi Rog* (Moscow, 1992), published in an astonishing 50,000 copies, with photographs.
5. *Golos,* no. 4 (1993): 3. This statistic may come out of a state report on the situation of the disabled.
6. *Sotsial'noe obespechenie,* no. 7 (1998): 30.
7. *Izvestiia,* 2 June 1994, 1.
8. T. A. Dobrovol'skaia and N. B. Shabalina, "Sotsial'no-psikhologicheskie osobennosti vzaimootnoshenii invalidov i zdorovykh," *Sotsiologicheskie issledovaniia* no. 1 (1993): 62–67.
9. *Izvestiia,* 21 August 1998, 5.
10. *Sotsial'noe obespechenie,* no. 10 (1996): 4.
11. This may be because most of the disabled are elderly. In a study of Moscow Oblast mentioned in *Sotsial'noe obespechenie* (no. 9 [1996]: 4, 8), 66.5 percent of the disabled were over 56 years of age (see also *Sotsial'noe obespechenie,* no. 8 (1998): 23). In an earlier statement, then-Minister of Social Protection Ella Pamfilova reported that many elderly people have been applying for disability benefits, thereby significantly increasing the number of newly disabled (75.7 per 10,000 in 1992). See *Sotsial'noe obespechenie,* no. 8 (1993): 4–5.
12. L. L. Grishina, a professor at the Central Institute of Examination of Labor and Organization of the Work of the Disabled (TsIETIN) under the Ministry of Social Protection, reported that there were 8.2 million disabled in 1991 (5.5 percent of the population). In 1992, the figure grew to 8.4 million (5.7 percent of the population), 70 percent classified as Group I or Group II; 17 percent were young people (1.5 million) and 60 percent were elderly (5 million). See *Sotsial'noe obespechenie,* no. 5 (1994): 19. Under the Soviet system Groups I and II (severely disabled and at present usually considered unable to work) did work when positions could be found for them. For more details, see Stephen P. Dunn and Ethel Dunn, "Everyday Life of the Disabled in the USSR," in *The Disabled in the Soviet Union,* eds. McCagg and Siegelbaum (Pittsburgh: University of Pittsburgh Press, 1989), 227–228.
13. *Meditsinskoe obsluzhivanie naseleniia Rossiiskoi Federatsii v 1993 godu* (Moscow: 1994), 123–134.
14. *Sotsial'noe obespechenie,* no. 3 (1995): 4.
15. *Sotsial'noe obespechenie,* no. 4 (1998): 30.

16. *Sotsial'noe obespechenie,* no. 7 (1998): 18.
17. *Sotsial'noe obespechenie,* no. 3 (1995): 4.
18. *Sotsial'noe obespechenie,* no. 9 (1996): 4, 8.
19. *Sel'skaia zhizn',* 9 July 1998, 13.
20. *Sel'skaia zhizn',* 9 July 1998, 13.
21. *Sotsial'noe obespechenie,* no. 7 (1998): 19.
22. *Sotsial'noe obespechenie,* no. 9 (1996): 8; no. 11 (1996): 36–37, 39.
23. *Sotsial'noe obespechenie,* no. 12 (1997): 6.
24. *Sotsial'noe obespechenie,* no. 9(1998): 27.
25. *Ogonëk,* no. 17 (April 1995): 28–29.
26. *Uchitel'skaia gazeta,* 20 August 1998, 9.
27. *Sotsial'noe obespechenie,* no. 3 (1995): 5.
28. *Sotsial'noe obespechenie,* no. 3 (1995): 5.
29. *Sotsial'noe obespechenie,* no. 8 (1994): 26. In 1992, elderly persons applying for disability benefits significantly increased the number of newly disabled (75.7 per 10,000). See *Sotsial'noe obespechenie,* no. 8 (1993): 4–5.
30. *Sotsial'noe obespechenie,* no. 9–10 (1994): 15.
31. *Sotsial'noe obespechenie,* no. 3 (1995): 2.
32. *Okhrana zdoroviia v SSSR* (Moscow: 1990), 163.
33. *The Station Relay,* 4 (1988–1989), 93. The number of shops producing prostheses appears to have remained at 66, according to A.I. Osadchikh. See *Sotsial'noe obespechenie,* no. 3 (1995): 4.
34. *Literaturnaia gazeta,* 8 September 1993,15.
35. *Sel'skaia nov',* no. 3 (1994): 7–9.
36. *Ogonëk,* no. 52 (December 1994): 13.
37. *Sotsial'noe obespechenie,* no. 9 (1993): 13–14.
38. *Sotsial'noe obespechenie,* no. 6 (1994): 15.
39. *Izvestiia* 8 September 1993, 7; 19 August 1993, 8.
40. *Ogonëk,* no. 16 (1998): 21.
41. *Sel'skaia zhizn',* 29 July 1998, 3.
42. E-mail posting from *promed@usa.healthnet.org* on 16 September 1998.
43. *Sel'skaia zhizn',* 22 August 1998, 3
44. *Zdravookhranenie Rossissskoi Federatsii,* no. 4 (1996): 16.
45. *Literaturnaia gazeta,* 19 July 1995, 12.
46. M. A. Pozdniakova, et al., "Mediko-sotsial'naia kharakteristika osobennostei uslovii i obraza zhizni detei-invalidov," *Zdravookhranenie Rossissskoi Federatsii,* no. 4 (1998): 46–48.
47. *Ogonëk,* no. 4 (1996): 52–54.
48. *Literaturnaia gazeta,* 23 September 1998, 14.
49. T. A. Dobrovol'skaia and N. B. Shabalina, "Invalidy: diskriminiruyemoe menshestvo?," *Sotsiologicheskie issledovaniia,* no. 5 (1992): 104.

50. Uchitel'skaia gazeta 9, no. 37 (1991): 7.
51. *Ogonëk*, no. 17 (April 1995): 28.
52. *Ogonëk*, no. 11 (March 1998): 9.
53. *Sotsial'noe obespechenie*, no. 9 (1993): 7.
54. *Sel'skaia nov'*, no. 6 (1994): 24–35.
55. *Sotsial'noe obespechenie*, no. 7 (1994): 9.
56. *Uchitel'skaia gazeta*, no. 27–29 (6 July 1993): 10.
57. *Sotsial'noe obespechenie*, no. 8 (1993): 6.
58. *Sotsial'noe obespechenie*, no. 8 (1994): 26.
59. *Izvestiia*, 23 February 1993, 1.
60. *Ogonëk*, no. 11 (March 1998): 9.
61. *Golos*, no. 4 (1993): 6.
62. *Nadezhda*, May 1995.
63. *Nadezhda*, no. 9 (July 1993).
64. *Ogonëk*, no. 17 (1995): 28.
65. *Sotsial'noe obespechenie*, no. 9 (1993): 30.
66. *Sotsial'noe obespechenie*, no. 11–12 (1994): 15.
67. *Sotsial'noe obespechenie*, no. 7 (1998): 3.
68. *Izvestiia*, 23 July 1998, 4.
69. *Izvestiia*, 20 October 1998, 1. The problem is a long-standing one. In 1993, the minister of health said in an interview with *Izvestiia* (3 September 1993, 5) that an attempt was being made to control the price of medicines, and to assure an adequate supply of the most necessary ones. It was a losing battle.
70. *Sotsial'noe obespechenie*, no. 7 (1998): 18.
71. *Izvestiia*, 28 June 1994, 4; *Saratovskie vesti*, 16 March 1996; even insulin is in short supply.
72. *Literaturnaia gazeta*, 8 April 1998, 5.
73. *Sel'skaia zhizn'*, 16 August 1998, 1, 3.
74. *Izvestiia*, 24 July 1998, 8.
75. *Izvestiia*, 31 July 1998, 8.
76. *Chelovek i zakon*, no. 7 (1994): 57–60.
77. *Ogonëk*, no. 17 (April 1995): 28.
78. Author's translation for the World Institute on Disability, unpublished.
79. *Izvestiia*, 8 November 1994, 2.
80. *Sotsial'naia zashchita invalidov* (Moscow: 1994), 114–115.

PART II

Social Issues

CHAPTER 9

The "New" Sexism:
Images of Russian Women
during the Transition

Valerie Sperling

FOR ALL OF THE CHAOS THAT HAS OVERTAKEN RUSSIAN politics and society in the last decade, perhaps the most profound change has been
the introduction of glasnost and the decline in the censorship of
public speech and action. As a result of these new freedoms, at the
end of the 1980s women in Russia were able to start speaking out
publicly about discrimination, about the gendered division of labor,
about the paucity of women in high political positions, and so forth.
Women's organizations began to form independent of state control,
national-level women's movement conferences were held starting in
the early 1990s, women's newspapers and other publications
emerged, and the women's movement, non-existent in the mid-
1980s, is now growing apace. Estimates of the number of women's
groups in Russia today range from 400 to 4,000.

But this veritable explosion of women's organizations was occurring against the background of another explosion enabled by the
newfound freedom of speech, namely an explosion of overt sexism.

This took various forms, some of which were old, and others quite new. One of the most visible manifestations of sexism and the objectification of women was the rapid proliferation of printed pornography—which had been prohibited until recently. This formerly forbidden fruit became a commonplace presence in the public realm. Pornographic materials were sold in underground street crossings (*perekhody*), dubbed "*porno-khody*," and wallet-sized pictures of naked women became a staple on the dashboards of many taxicabs. One of the most incompatible sights in the new Russia, particularly in Moscow, was that of elderly women standing on busy sidewalks, doing a brisk business in the sale of plastic shopping bags, nearly all of which sported a partially naked, voluptuous woman, against the background of a variety of Western corporate symbols. The spread of pornographic images in a country where, for decades, laws forbade it, was seen by some women as downright oppressive. Others regarded it as simply a phase, a natural reaction against (or liberation from) the asceticism of communism. Either way, it sent a clear message that one of women's roles in the new Russia was that of sexual object.

Sexual objectification of women was also the message expressed in the veritable epidemic of beauty contests that began in the late 1980s and that glorified various body parts: "Miss Bust, Miss Legs, Miss Ass, and so forth."[1] The Soviet bloc's beauty contest craze took off in 1988, with flight attendants taking the lead: one popular magazine reported on the "Miss Airspace" (*vozdushnyi okean*) contest, held in Budapest, with contestants from five East Bloc countries. A Russian woman won, and was crowned "Miss 10,000 Meters" (cruising altitude for airplanes).[2] Marina Liborakina, a Russian feminist critiquing such phenomena, pointed out that these contests became popular at the same time as free elections began for Russia's Supreme Soviet. Liborakina noted with irony that as women's representation in politics plummeted, these contests became their own version of "democracy for women."[3] The beauty contests were part of a clear trend toward the commercialization and objectification of women's bodies in Russia, soon to expand to advertising, with the advent of an emerging market economy in the early 1990s.[4]

While I would not argue that pornographic and consumerist images of women created an obligatory new identity for women in Russia during the economic and political transition period, I would suggest that the proliferation of these images had an effect on women, and on women's self-image, not to mention on the ideas and stereotypes that both men and women develop about women's capacities and proper social roles.[5] In the remainder of this chapter, I will address the phenomenon of the "new" sexism in Russia, first in the political sphere, second in the economic sphere, and third in the social sphere, focusing on the media. I will argue that a long-standing pattern of discrimination against women on the basis of sex forms the background to Russian women's present-day socio-cultural status, and that although discrimination on the basis of sex has always existed in Soviet Russia, such discrimination became increasingly overt with the advent of glasnost (especially in the form of biological reductionism) and perestroika (in the form of labor discrimination). During the transition period, women and women's movement activists have contended with a "newly" overt sexism, pornographic images of women, a patriarchal-nationalist upsurge that espouses the return of women to the home, and a renewed stress on women's "natural predestination" as wives and mothers. The image of women in Russian society is shaped in part by the overt messages about women's proper roles expressed by public officials, in social structures, in daily interactions, and in the mainstream media. I will conclude the chapter with some thoughts about the effects of sexist social attitudes and discourse about the proper role of women on the women's movement itself.

The "New" Sexism in the Political Sphere

Aside from the newfound freedom of speech that Gorbachev brought to Soviet women's lives, the political transition in Russia has been detrimental to women's status. The percentage of women in high politics has declined from the albeit quota-based levels of the Soviet era, and it has remained low, to the extent that in 1999 there was only one woman in the upper house of Russia's legislature, and only 46 in the lower house, the Duma (out of 450 deputies). The women's party that had emerged to win 8 percent of the vote in December 1993 did not break the 5 percent barrier in 1995; in part as a result of this loss, the percentage of women in the Duma fell from 13 percent in 1993 to 10 percent in 1995.

Women politicians in both the legislative and executive branches of Russia's political system have complained of sexist and disdainful attitudes from their male counterparts. For example, Alevtina Fedulova, then a leading member of the Women of Russia (WOR) political bloc in the Duma, claimed in an interview shortly after the 1993 elections that the Women of Russia deputies "feel comfortable, so far," although she added, "As before, people can still be heard saying, 'Give the girl the floor!', and in the corridors, men say to me, 'Alevtina, no other woman gets talked about more than you do.' We understand that it'll be difficult for us. After all, we're the first."[6]

Fedulova's sentiment was echoed in 1995 by Ekaterina Lakhova, chair of the WOR faction, in an interview, where she stated directly that "male deputies don't accept us as politicians on an equal basis (*kak ravnopravnykh politikov*)."[7]

It is not only WOR deputies who have noticed the prejudicial slant of male parliamentarians on the subject of female politicians. Irina Khakamada, a popular deputy with a liberal political stance, complained that "women in government constantly have to prove that they are not fools," and explained that she had split from Boris Fedorov [who had formed the December 12 faction with her] due to his "boorish" attitude, which apparently emerged when she criticized his leadership capacity. Rather than debating with her, he dismissed her opinion, saying, "What does it matter what you say, you exotic woman!"[8]

Yet this overt sexism in the political sphere is not new. According to eyewitnesses, attitudes toward women in the parliament have remained somewhat consistent since the institution of Russia's Supreme Soviet. Asked in 1991 whether it was hard for women deputies to operate there, Ekaterina Lakhova acknowledged that, out of the 1,000 deputies in the Supreme Soviet, there were only 50 women, and that of them, only three were chosen to work on committees. Women deputies felt a lack of respect. Said Lakhova, "We thought we would come in and quickly carry out our election platforms. But here, they look at us (*vosprinimaiut*) just as they do in the provinces. Men see us as women, but not as deputies. You're explaining something to him about infant mortality, and he says that it doesn't become you to talk about such serious things, that you have to be a woman."[9]

According to Galina Sillaste, a public opinion researcher and women's movement activist, in sessions of the Supreme Soviet, the devaluation of women's role in Soviet society was visible, evidenced by the "disrespectful attitude towards women who speak from the tribune."[10] Galina Starovoitova, a deputy to Russia's Supreme Soviet who was assassinated in 1998, confirmed this. At a 1995 feminist conference in St. Petersburg, she recalled an illustrative incident:

> Once, when the well-known democrat Bella Denisenko—a professor, the deputy Minister of Health—took the floor to put the issue of medical insurance on the agenda, speaker [Ruslan] Khasbulatov interrupted her. And when the people in the hall demanded to let her finish talking, he turned the microphone back on and rudely said, "Well, what else did you want to say?" At that, Denisenko, upset, answered, "But you hit me below the belt, now I'll just gather my thoughts and conclude." Ruslan Khasbulatov reacted immediately, saying, "I've got nothing to do with what's below your belt." And he turned off the microphone again.[11]

Nor is sexism a problem limited to the legislative branch. The executive branch too has been indicted by women who have achieved ministerial status. Ella Pamfilova, as of November 1993 the only female minister in the Russian Federation (her position as minister of social protection was later taken by Liudmila Beslepkina), answering a question about what it was like to work in an entirely male environment and whether she was able to influence the male ministers in a positive way, responded, "It depends. Sometimes I manage to get somewhere with them, but more often, not. Men often don't accept women in politics—or in other spheres. And that's not always fair (*verno*)."[12] The lack of respect for her positions and her concomitant lack of influence may have been a factor contributing to Pamfilova's resignation in February 1994.[13]

In part, such disrespectful attitudes toward women on the part of state officials and legislators are a reflection of societal perceptions about women's proper role in Russian (and/or late Soviet) society. Virulently negative attitudes toward Gorbachev's wife, Raisa Maximovna, the first wife of a Communist Party general secretary to play an extensive public role, are illustrative of the staunchly patriarchal atmosphere. Indeed, the perception that women's roles during the transition period ought to be limited to domestic ones held true even with regard to women who succeeded in entering the very highest echelons of power as politicians. Galina Semenova, former editor of the women's magazine *Krestianka,* in a talk she gave at a meeting of Moscow's feminist discussion club (Klub F-1), related several stories about her brief experience as a Politburo member toward the end of the Gorbachev period, which tellingly reveal societal attitudes toward women in politics:

> I went to the salon located [near the Kremlin] and explained that I was a new Politburo member, and wanted my hair cut. The hairdresser told me she could do it between 2 and 3 PM. I said, "Excuse me, but I need an appointment before work!" The hairdresser said, "Well, before WORK, I have to cut the wives' hair." Meaning—the hair of the wives of Politburo members.[14]

Survey research suggests that the public's view reflects the idea that women and politics do not mix. A survey cited in a speech by Alevtina Fedulova in 1995 claimed that 65 percent of men and 35 percent of women "would under no circumstances support a woman for office in the legislature."[15] The societal message that women have no place in politics, particularly as politicians, is clear.

The "New" Sexism in the Economic Sphere

In the economic sphere, the transition has had extremely important and negative effects on women. Unemployment appeared in the early 1990s, along with privatization, and women quickly became disproportionately unemployed—making up as much as 90 percent of the unemployed in some cities. Part of the reason for this was that with the state no longer subsidizing factories, employers had little incentive to retain women, who were thought to be potentially more costly employees, due to the fact that women were entitled to maternity leave and other benefits and privileges associated with motherhood. Another reason was that certain industries that were female-dominated, like the textile industry, were particularly hard hit by the transition period, and their production levels fell dramatically, along with demand for employees. Social welfare spending was cut, and, in part as a result of structural adjustment programs, child-care centers closed down—5,000 closed in 1993 alone.[16] This threw many women into a position where they had to either quit their jobs and face economic hardship, or find some other means of taking care of their children—not necessarily an easy task, especially because the new, privately run day care centers were prohibitively expensive for most of the population.

Rather than recognizing this turmoil as being somehow detrimental to women, and to the Russian economy's productivity overall (many of the women who lost their jobs were specialists with a higher education), the Russian government chose to propagate an argument made popular during the Brezhnev era—namely, that women's place was in the home, and that women's unemployment was not, in fact, disastrous, but rather natural. Such attitudes were endorsed by the labor ministry itself. For example, in 1993, then–Labor Minister Gennadii Melikian was quoted as saying, "There is no point in creating jobs for women, when there aren't enough jobs for men."[17] The subtext of Melikian's argument was the widespread notion that women should be at home, raising the children, rather than working outside the home for a salary. Such role stereotypes persist, despite the fact that under current economic conditions, most families require two salaries in order to meet the minimum living standards.

These role stereotypes are also reinforced with statistical data. One monograph, published in 1994, argued that the level of women employed in the economy (*obshchestvennoe proizvodstvo*) had "exceeded the normal level, having an adverse effect on production, as well as on the family, fertility, and children." The authors stated that the level of women's employment was more than twice as high as that in "developed" countries, where women did not exceed one-third of the workforce. They drew special attention to the inefficiency of women's labor, especially those women who had young children: these women fail to fulfill their "duties," both at work and at home. Thus, freeing women in part from their employment in the economy, stated the authors, "cannot be evaluated as a singularly negative idea."[18]

This image of women as being primarily mothers lies behind other manifestations of sexism in the economic realm, but again, some of these are not of recent vintage. For example, women's labor in certain professions is prohibited, and has been so since the Soviet era. Women are barred from 460 occupations by government decree, because these jobs are deemed dangerous to a woman's reproductive health. Sometimes these regulations seem ludicrous. Because underground work is forbidden to women, they may not work as metro train drivers—although they are permitted to sweep the floors in metro stations. And although women are not allowed to work as pilots, they are permitted to work as flight attendants.

Sex-role stereotypes are reinforced continually, among children as well as adults. For instance, in 1994, a two-volume encyclopedia was published, called "Encyclopedia for Boys" and "Encyclopedia for Girls." Aside from chapters on health and beauty, the girls' volume was exclusively concerned with domestic labor, from taking spots out of clothes to special ways to prevent bread from spoiling. The boys' volume, in sharp contrast, contained chapters ranging from apartment repairs ("Your home is your fortress"), to hand-combat skills, to methods for starting one's own business.[19] These encyclopedias were distributed in one of my interviewees' daughter's first grade class, and were widely available in local bookstores. The girls' proper sphere was clearly delineated, beginning and ending within the home, whereas the boys' sphere extended throughout the socio-economic arena. This stands in sharp contrast to the Soviet regime's official rhetoric, which proclaimed that Soviet women and men were equal in all ways, with similar responsibilities and identical opportunities in the labor sphere, and even in contrast to the new Russian constitution of 1993, which recognized that men and women have equal rights and should have equal opportunities to realize them.[20] Judging from official statements and occupational segregation, however, the constitution is not as influential as the prevailing set of role stereotypes.

Moreover, today's labor market reflects a new type of sexism regarding women's roles and employment opportunities. In addition to the prevailing image of women as mothers, a newer image of women—as sexual objects in the labor force—has begun to spread. Job advertisements, for instance, openly exhibit discrimination on the basis of both sex and age. According to feminist journalist Nadia Azhgikhina, classified ads seeking exclusively male applicants to fill positions as accountants and lawyers in new private businesses are commonplace.[21] "For hire" advertisements in Russian papers sometimes read more like personal ads than want ads. It is not unheard of to encounter advertisements that state, "seeking attractive woman, with European features, under 35, and without hang-ups." The latter phrase is even abbreviated, as b/k (*bez kompleksov*), and signifies either sex work or that the woman in question should be willing to put up with sexual demands by bosses, clients, and so on—an institutionalized form of sexual harassment. Activist Elvira Novikova, speaking at a seminar on the image of women in the media in March 1992, noted several such examples from want ads:

> Look at this announcement from the journal *Rovesnik* (no. 2), from this year. The firm "Superelectro" is announcing a superprize. The winner (*pobeditel'nitsa*) will work at Superelectro offices and get a salary of 2,500 rubles. They're asking the competitors to submit a full-body photograph of themselves, preferably in a bathing suit, "so as not to hide your super-attractiveness." [They ask for] her height, bust measurement, and so on. Just what is that young woman going to be doing at work?[22]

Novikova also described a cartoon in a popular humor magazine, *Krokodil:* "In the first frame, a woman is being prevented from going into her boss' office; she's asked, 'Why aren't you dressed properly?' In the next frame, you see this woman almost totally naked; now the response is, 'Well that's more like it!' (*Vot eto drugoe delo!*)."

Images like these are being inscribed in want ads, cartoons, and other media that both reflect and promote given societal attitudes. In such guises, women's roles in the private sector of the economy are being restricted, reflecting and reinforcing a specific societal attitude about women's proper place.

Images of Women in the Media

Images of women as sex objects and as beings best restricted to the domestic sphere have found a major outlet in the mass media. Several women activists in Russia have argued that, at the outset of perestroika, an unofficial campaign began to "facilitate women's return to their natural predestination," a campaign that intensified as the transition toward a market began, and that reinforced Russian women's limited socio-cultural status.[23] This "return to the kitchen" campaign was promoted in the mainstream press, accompanied by warnings about the dangers wrought by women's emancipation. Feminist philosopher Olga Voronina described the trend:

The pages of newspapers and journals were covered with articles on the "women's" theme, though they only printed the opinions of fans of patriarchal values. Even the *Domostroi* [a sixteenth-century Russian guide to household management], in which, as is well-known, beatings were considered the favored means of educating one's wife and children, started being propagandized as a monument to national culture. The point of the overwhelming mass of publications was one—everything was the fault of women and their emancipation. [Valentin] Rasputin [a well-known writer], for example, affirmed that "emancipation is a moral mutation, the moral degradation of the weaker sex." It was increasingly emphasized that today's women suffered from over-emancipation and its costs.[24]

The idea of separate spheres and roles for men and women was also reinforced during the transition period by representatives of the Russian Orthodox Church. Church adherents argued that accepting women into the priesthood was "a perversion of the norm, not the establishment of equality," and, while claiming to describe "reality," instead prescribed separate spheres of life and activity for women and men, based ostensibly on women's and men's essential natures:

> Let's leave aside the . . . fact that in each man there's something female, and in each woman there's something male, and let's stick to the main thing: a man is more aggressive, more active, more curious, more risk-taking; his creativity is a constant search for innovation. Women create continuity, peace, reliability. Man creates, woman reproduces.[25]

Newspapers and Television

The point may be further illustrated with specific examples of images of women in the media during the last few years. As the spectrum of available media sources has spread, so has the range of these images. The emergence of glossy, expensive women's magazines, such as *Cosmopolitan* (in Russian), for instance, spreads a familiar picture of well-dressed, anorexic models. The content of *Cosmopolitan* may not be entirely offensive in the Russian context, since the editors have chosen to publish rather needed information about sexual technique, female orgasm, and even lesbianism—formerly taboo subjects. Other magazines contain familiar and laudatory images of Russia's female celebrities; some (including *Rabot-nitsa,* since the early 1990s) portray activists in Russia's fledgling women's movement in a positive light, as women working to counter discrimination (particularly economic discrimination).

But examples of media reinforcement of sexist images of women abound. Marina Liborakina, an activist with several Moscow-based women's organizations, argues, for example, that the above-noted "return to the kitchen" campaign took on a mass character, in the media, advertisements, television shows, and women's journals, accompanied by a "blaming mechanism" for women who resisted it—such women were doing harm to men. Liborakina writes, "In this context, a woman's desire to have a well-paid, skilled occupation is seen as egoism: not only does she want to work, she wants to steal this work away from her husband, her brother, her father...."[26] The preferred image for women was that of a happy wife and housekeeper, "creatively (!) actualizing herself by mastering a variety of pretty, shiny, convenient [household] items."[27] The resemblance to the image of the ideal housewife of the post–World War II era in the United States described by Betty Friedan is striking.[28]

A related media trend allowed for women to have careers, but stressed the importance of maintaining one's femininity. A representative article from *Moskvichka* (now a weekly Moscow-based woman's newspaper with a circulation of 175,000, tabloid-size, usually 16 pages, with more of a stress on human interest stories than on high politics), in 1995, called "Businesslike, but Even Still, a Woman," began with a long list of all the things that men don't like about career women: "Most men do not like it when the woman they love earns more than they do . . . even fewer men like it when a woman gets home from work later than her husband, who is tired from work." The article concludes by reassuring women that it is possible to succeed in business without making it "a family tragedy," as long as one recalls that in men's eyes, "you are first and foremost a wife and mother, and only thereafter the head of a firm."[29] In a similar vein, *Moskvichka* published an article about Duma deputy Aleksandra Ochirova under the headline, "A Woman-Deputy, Who Remains a Woman, All the Same." The first question posed by the interviewer, emphasizing the fact that *Moskvichka* was a *women's* publication, was about the appearance of female Duma deputies—their "ability to dress." The remainder of the interview focused on the issue of clothing (both for male and female deputies), and fashion crimes, such as trying to wear a deputy's button [*znachok*] on a "frivolous dress, a romantic lacy blouse," and so on.[30]

This is not to suggest that there are no media portrayals of successful and happy career women. *Sveta,* for example, in 1992, published an article about three female entrepreneurs, strongly critiquing the idea that the words "woman" and "business" could not go together. On the other hand, the article was printed alongside an advertisement for a firm that specialized in helping women attain an "ideal" figure (the dimensions given were 90–60–90 centimeters), featuring a naked woman, photographed seated, from behind.[31]

The housewifization of women, and the transformation of women's bodies into "objects of consumption," extended to television advertisements, where women began to appear in seductive poses, seeming to exist in order to serve men and please the (heterosexual) male eye.[32] Also, TV advertisements very often showed women with children, in a domestic setting.[33] And sometimes, women in advertisements were portrayed as childlike beings who could not survive in the new Russia without the guidance of knowledgeable men. Marina Liborakina described such an advertisement for a firm called Telemarket:

> An energetic young man is explaining the worthiness of the [Telemarket] system to a pretty but obtuse young woman. When he asks her, "Well, now do you understand?" she, in tears, responds, "uh-uh," and then the emblem of the Telemarket company appears on the screen. A masculine voice resounds: "For those who understand!"[34]

Television shows, as well as advertisements spotlighting the image of helpless women who must rely on men to get along under the new conditions of a market economy, echo the division of labor and social roles described above in the 1994 children's encyclopedia. One game show on ORT (the state television station), sponsored by SPID-INFO, in 1996, called "Love at First Sight" (similar to the "Dating Game"), featured three young men and three young women who enunciated statements that seemed to be generated by an automated role-stereotyping device: for example, one female contestant argued that "a man should support the family," while a male contestant stated unequivocally that "a woman should be a housewife (*domokhoziaika*)." The female contestants even willingly reduced themselves to role-stereotypes, with one contestant telling the host that she had "picked Sergei [her date] because he said he wants an attractive housewife, and I'm attractive, and I cook really well!" The role of television in spreading fads, fashions, and attitudes should not be underestimated.

This selected presentation of evidence from the media and from Russian researchers' own work suggests that, over the course of the economic and political transition in Russia, a hegemonic discourse on the part of the state has been at work, reinforcing traditional sex roles, stressing women's primary role as reproducers of the nation, and unofficially also granting women a new role as objects for sexual consumption. Although it is difficult to gauge cultural responses to this discourse, we might hypothesize that the effect of such rhetoric may be to depress the likelihood that any women's movement message about uprooting sex-role stereotypes would get a widespread and sympathetic hearing. It is, however, also possible that the blatantly patriarchal rhetoric itself may have inspired transformation of consciousness and awareness of sexist oppression in some women.

Conclusion: Images and Reality

The images of women that we see on television or in ministerial pronouncements—as happy domestic servants and sex objects who play very restricted roles in the public sphere—do not reflect the reality of women's lives in Russia today. Although it is commonly asserted that men run everything from politics to the emerging market economy, it is women that we see everywhere in action, striving to keep their families afloat during an extremely unstable period. And the images we bring with us from visits to Russia are sometimes not so much sexist as they are sobering. It is not for fun that aging women, the proverbial *babushki,* stand in front of the Novyi Arbat supermarket in Moscow selling plastic bags with pornographic images on them to passersby. This is perhaps the latest version of a phenomenon that began in the early 1990s, when the gauntlets of women began to appear, lining the sidewalks near Moscow's main farmers' markets, selling a variety of goods, from dishes and glassware to old clothes to matches. Indeed, Russia's female street merchants of the

1990s have metaphorically joined the ranks of Soviet (and Russian) women employed as broom-bearing street-sweepers—all endeavoring to scrape a living off of Moscow's dirty sidewalks.

Yet women in contemporary Russia are also challenging the images and realities of Russia's "new" sexism. Women's movement activists are tirelessly struggling to improve their status, and that of other women, by lobbying state officials, starting women's employment training groups, women's business clubs, women's advocacy groups, rape crisis centers, domestic violence hotlines, and so on. No doubt one of the effects of sexist discourse and images has been to instill distorted and restrictive pictures of women's roles and abilities in the minds of the population, and to make it even more difficult for women to become conscious of their own oppression, or to believe that it would be possible to change societal attitudes about women in a nonsexist direction. However, another of the effects has been to awaken some women to the need to struggle against these images, and to insist on their right to create different images of women: as citizens with equal rights and equal opportunities to enjoy them; as independent actors on the Russian political and economic stage; and as creators of their own, varied images of themselves.

NOTES

Some material in this chapter is excerpted from the author's *Organizing Women in Contemporary Russia* (New York: Cambridge University Press, 1999), reprinted with the permission of Cambridge University Press.

1. Marina Liborakina, *Obretenie sily: rossiiskii opyt* (Moskva: CheRo, 1996), 78.
2. See *Ogonëk*, no. 14 (April 1988).
3. Marina Liborakina, *Obretenie sily,*78. Free elections to Russia's legislature did not take place until 1990.
4. It was also in 1988 that *Ogonëk* printed an article about cosmetic surgery in Russia (see *Ogonëk*, no. 10 (March 1988)). I am grateful to Christoph Neidhart for the references to *Ogonëk*.
5. Some women have reacted with outrage to the spread of pornography in Russia. The St. Petersburg Center for Gender Issues, for example, initiated a suit against Russian Playboy magazine, after it published a series of "misogynist" painted images of famous Russian

women (Catherine the Great, topless; mathematician Sofia Ko-valevskaya, masturbating, and others). See "PCGI protest against Playboy," conference "women.east-west" <women-east-west@igc.apc.org>, 11 July 1996.

6. "Mnenia zhenshchin-politikov o politicheskoi situatsii v rossii," in *Zhenskii diskussionyi klub,* Interlegal, January 1994 (citing articles in *Moskovskaia pravda* and *Moskovskii komsolets*).

7. WOR, *Informatsionnyi bulleten',* no. 2 (1995): 34.

8. Khakamada is half-Japanese, which may explain Fedorov's use of "exotic"—or it may have reflected his sense that women in politics generally are "exotic." See Penny Morvant, "Bearing the Double Burden in Russia," *Transition,* 8 September 1995, 9, quoting *Moskovskaia pravda,* 21 June 1995, 16. In advance of the December 1995 elections, Khakamada formed a new bloc called *Obshoe delo* (Common Cause), hoping in part to draw voters from Women of Russia's constituency. Khakamada successfully re-entered the Duma from a single-mandate district.

9. "Nashe interv'iu," *Zhenskoe dvizhenie v SSSR* (later, *Women's Discussion Club*), no. 2 (January–March 1991).

10. Galina Sillaste, "Any state is strengthened by women's prudence," *Moskvichka,* no. 2 (1991): 3.

11. Galina Starovoitova, "Kakovo byt' zhenshchine-politiku v rossii segodnia," (stenogramma vystupleniia), in *Feministstkaia teoriia i praktika: vostok–zapad: Konferentsiia 9.6–12.6.95* (Sankt-Peterburg, 1996), 36.

12. "Ia videla reform obshchestva s iznanki,". *Moskvichka,* no. 34 (November 1993): 1, 3.

13. Interestingly enough, Beslepkina was quoted in 1991, when she was deputy minister of the State Committee on Labor and Social Issues, reporting a conversation in which she overheard her colleagues insisting that a woman could never be the chair of the committee: "No, a woman can't be, can't be and that's that," her colleague said. (See Sheila Puffer, "Women Managers in the Former USSR: A case of 'Too Much Equality'?" in *Competitive Frontiers,* Nancy Adler and Daena Izraeli, eds., 282, citing V. Kopeiko, "Destruction of a Stereotype, or a Monologue of a Woman about the Woman," *Soviet Woman* 1 [1991]: 5.) Despite her male colleagues' skepticism, Beslepkina did become the head of the Ministry of Social Protection.

14. Galina Semenova, speaking at Klub F-1, 20 March 1996.

15. See "Zhenshchiny v politike, politika dlia zhenshchin," *Moskvichka* (WOR Bulletin #5), no. 22–23 (June 1995).

16. The trend continued in 1994. See Ekaterina Lakhova, "Vcherashnie shchi liubite? Zakhodite zavtra," *Izvestiia,* 19 April 1995, 4.

17. Anastasia Posadskaia, "Demokratiia minus zhenshchina—ne demokratiia," *Ogonëk*, no. 38 (1993): 9.

18. N. V. Zvereva and E. S. Vazhenova, *Nekotorye demograficheskie aspekty regional'nykh rynkov truda v Rossii* (Moscow: 1994), 43–45. This booklet was distributed to those attending a women's conference in November 1994 in Moscow, called "Labor, Employment, Unemployment."

19. *Entsiklopedia dlia devochek, Entsiklopedia dlia mal'chikov* (St. Petersburg, 1994).

20. Despite such guarantees, under Soviet rule and continuing up to the present, there existed a list of occupations forbidden to women. These included night work, work underground, and a variety of jobs deemed too dangerous to women's reproductive capacity and health. Despite these regulations, however, women were and continue to be disproportionately employed in heavy manual labor and in hazardous occupations.

21. See "A Movement is Born," *The Bulletin of Atomic Scientists* (July/August 1995): 49.

22. "Obraz zhenshchiny v sredstvakh massovoi informatsii," *Zhenskii diskussionnyi klub* (March 1992): 5.

23. The most highly placed official statement of this campaign was made by Gorbachev, who wrote of the need to establish conditions that would facilitate returning Soviet women to their "purely womanly mission"—in other words, the private sphere of household and family—in his 1987 book, *Perestroika: New Thinking for Our Country and the World,* 116–117.

24. Olga Voronina, "Zhenshchina i sotsializm: opyt feministkogo analiza," in *Feminizm: vostok, zapad, rosiia,* ed. M. T. Stepaniants (Moskva: Nauka, 1993), 206.

25. Iakov Korotov, "Liubov' ne ishchet svoego: ni muzhskogo, ni zhenskogo," *Segodnia,* 18 March 1995, 5. On the same page, *Segodnia* published an interview with an orthodox priest condemning abortion, as well as a pro-choice article, "Vox Feminae," whose author took a representative of the church to task for condemning contraception.

26. Marina Liborakina, *Obretenie sily: rossiiskii opyt* (Moskva: CheRo, 1996), 50.

27. Liborakina, *Obretenie sily,* 51.

28. See, for example, Betty Friedan, "The Way We Were—1949," in *The Ethnic Moment: The Search for Equality in the American Experience,* ed. Philip L. Fetzer (Armonk, NY: M. E. Sharpe, 1997), 53–67.

29. "Delovaia i pri etom—zhenshchina," *Moskvichka,* no. 9–10 (1995):16.

30. "Oprava k statusu—sharm i iziashchestvo," *Moskvichka,* no. 4 (1995): 10.

31. Irina Korchagina, "Gruppovoi portret biznes-ledi na fone otechestvennogo predprinimatel'stva," *Sveta* (September 1992): 7–10.

32. Among the first discussions and critiques of the objectification of women in Russia was Olga Lipovskaia, "Woman as an 'object of consumption'," *Moskvichka,* no. 8 (1991): 7.

33. This trend is not unfamiliar to the observer of U.S. commercial television, where most of the advertisements for household products feature women actors, along with voice-overs by men, whose authoritative presence ostensibly reassures the consumer that a product is reliable.

34. Liborakina, *Obretenie sily,* 79.

CHAPTER 10

New World of Work: Employment, Unemployment, and Adaptation

Walter D. Connor

WHEN THE TIME COMES TO WRITE THE FIRST ECONOMIC HISTORY of post-Soviet Russia, it is probable that, given sufficient perspective, the whole period from 1 January 1992 until the summer of 1998 will be treated as a single period—or at most two periods—wherein the working population of the Russian Federation, as earners, consumers, and providers for their dependents, underwent a harsh and wrenching, but not altogether negative, period of adjustment to new economic conditions. This transitional period, it will be argued, came to an end with the devaluation of the ruble, the effective default on most of its external debt, and the consequent collapse of Russia's precarious position in the world economy. At home, the crash of the ruble and consequent rapid inflation experienced by a population more and more dependent on imports threatened the measure of comfort and security—thin as it was—that *some* Russians (not just the "new Russian" super-rich) had achieved, and heralded further distress for the larger numbers who had experienced mainly economic disadvantage since the end of 1991.

This chapter focuses primarily on issues of employment, wages, unemployment, and labor militancy in that 1992–1998 period—matters on which, by now, we have some perspective—and offers in conclusion some thoughts on the near- and middle-term implications of the chaos unleashed in the summer of 1998.

Employment: Persistence and Change

The immediate historical context to the present situation in the post-communist Russian Federation lies in the mature, late-Soviet years. It is a heritage of full, or "overfull," employment, driven by the Soviet economy's commitment to imposing the obligation to work on all, and its tendencies to generate construction projects, new plants, and consequently new workplaces needing hands, in the pursuit of a crudely conceived quantitative economic "growth" that began with Stalin's first five year plan. In the later Brezhnev years, the planning process took rather little account of the limits of manpower supply, thus creating chronic labor "shortages" in an economy where unemployment was "unknown"—a fact of which Soviet propaganda never tired of reminding both the capitalist and third worlds.

Employment was particularly full and shortages acute in the Russian Federation's predecessor, the RSFSR, and in the other better-developed republics in the European parts of the USSR. There, relatively low fertility rates over time meant aging populations and, combined with health problems, made for an excess of people exiting the labor force, in death or retirement, over younger people entering. As students of USSR population and labor force dynamics noted, the Soviet Union of the late 1970s and 1980s faced, in fact, a situation wherein the *net* increase in population and labor force size, modest as it was likely to be, would come almost totally from the higher-fertility republics of the Caucasus and Central Asia, rather than from the core European industrial areas.[1]

With the bulk of the Soviet land area and more than half its population, the RSFSR/Russian Federation contained the majority of the Soviet workforce. Figures for 1980–1993 (including the self-employed—a category virtually nonexistent before the late 1980s) indicate an average in the lower 70 million–plus, with moderate growth in total numbers employed from 1980 to 1990 (many of pensionable age went on working), and no massive fall-off in the numbers as the USSR came to an end, but only a modest contraction, all the more modest given the fall in actual production in the terminal year of 1991 (see table 10.1).

Overall, employment throughout these years remained heavily tilted toward the traditionally favored industrial sector, with largish numbers in agriculture as well testifying to the persistent backwardness and inefficiency of that sector. Thus, in 1980—the depths of

Table 10.1   Employment, RSFSR/Russian Federation, 1980–1993
(millions)

1980	1985	1990	1991	1992	1993
73.3	74.9	75.3	73.8	72.0	71.0

Source: Russian Economic Trends, no. 2 (1994): 101.

Brezhnevian stagnation—fully 47.5 percent of the 73.3 million employed were in industry (32.5 percent) or agriculture (15.0 percent). By 1993, this had changed relatively little: 29.3 percent were in industry, 13.5 percent in the farm sector, for a still-high 42.8 percent of the employed. Even modest changes of this sort, and allowing for retirements on pension, involve millions and are thus not to be lightly dismissed. But what was most striking in the early transition was that these declines in industrial employment—roughly down a million persons each in 1992 from 1991, and in 1993 from 1992— barely hinted at the massive falls in industrial output. These reportedly amounted to 18 percent from 1991 to 1992, and a further 16 percent in 1993 over 1992's reduced base. Thus, large numbers of workers, by world standards never very productive to begin with, were early in Russia's transition to the market still "working" but producing even less than heretofore. The legacy of classic Soviet over- and mis-industrialization was a heavy one, and a landscape without massed ranks daily entering and exiting the familiar backdrop of concrete, steel, and smokestacks was hard to imagine. As a contemporary comment put it, "clearly enterprises are loath to reduce employment."[2]

That "reluctance," and alternative explanations for worker retention, will be addressed later. Meanwhile, we need to make a few more points on other aspects of change from 1992 to 1998. First, gross changes in total employment figures become more impressive after 1993, as they begin to show more clearly the turmoil and adjustment accompanying privatization and other changes. By the end of 1997—on the eve of the crisis year of 1998—the employment figures had trended steadily lower (see table 10.2)

Second, while overall employment fell by 6.9 percent in the period 1992–1995, structural readjustments—reallocation between sectors—were more impressive. Over that time, employment in

Table 10.2　Employment, Russian Federation, 1994–1997 (millions)

1980	1990	1991	1993
68.5	66.4	66.0	65.3

Source: Russian Economic Trends, no. 1 (1998): 28.

(mainly state-sector) industry declined by fully 19.2 percent, in construction by 6.7, and by 21.4 percent in transport and communications. Agriculture remained mired in a deadlock over the issue of ownership, underemployment, and unrecorded subsistence activity and only "shed" small numbers. Smaller sectors, underdeveloped or absent in the Soviet period, grew. From 1992 to 1995, trade and catering increased by 16.1 percent, commercial services by 13.8, "credit, finance and insurance" (still small in absolute numbers but virtually nonexistent before) by 40 percent, a residual "other" category by 38.1, and—more ominously—"public administration" by 13.3 percent.[3]

Third, it should be noted that these figures "track" most accurately the state and newly privatized former state sectors: they are weighted toward larger enterprises and organizations, where data gathering has been more comprehensive. Over the period to 1995, they capture less well the outflows of those leaving employment in such enterprises in industry, construction, transport, and retail trade/catering, to find new and typically better-paid work in the same sectors, but in smaller enterprises newly formed and private from the outset. In the one year 1994–95, the numbers employed in small firms (under 20 employees) grew from 6.8 to 8.8 million, or by over 29 percent.[4]

These changes, in turn, partially reflect the massive revolution of the privatization of the major components of an overwhelmingly *state* economy that got underway in 1993. Following on the earlier growth of individual proprietorships, the founding of new private businesses, and smaller-scale privatizations of small retail outlets, restaurants, and the like, this amounted to reallocating workers and employees who actually stayed in the same workplaces from a declining "state" to a new "private" sector, as medium- and large-scale state enterprises first took on "corporate" form, with the state holding 100 percent of the shares, and were then privatized according to two major procedural variants, both of which left sitting work forces—but more importantly, managers—with large-to-majority equity stakes in the new entities.

Thus, by the second quarter of 1995, fully 47 percent of all employed were in the private sector (either originally private enterprises, or ex-state ones in which the state now held at most a minority interest). One year later, the statistical reversal of the state's longtime role as the employer and paymaster of all had been achieved: 59 percent of Russia's employed worked in the private sector, and the self-employed had grown to slightly over 10 percent of all employed.[5] For all the blight, corruption, pains, and messy execution of the state's withdrawal from ownership, the deals that favored managers over rank-and-file workers in the allocation of shares, thus converting power to property for many,[6] and the failure of most ex-state enterprises to behave like the textbook model of the profit-maximizing, market-seeking entrepreneurial firm, these numbers reflect a hitherto near-inconceivable break with the legacy of 60-plus years of the Soviet-model economy: the leviathan had been laid to rest.

In 1996 and 1997, the economy exhibited a fair amount of flex, the low unemployment earlier in the period trending upward (see below) but not yet assuming massive proportions, and the shrinkage of total employment figures moderating. Goskomstat reported a fall in employment levels of 0.5 percent in 1996, vs. the sharper drop of 2.5 percent in 1994's shake-out. In large and medium enterprises, more than 11 million workers quit or were laid off—24 percent of those employed in such places, and among them fully 27 percent of those in large and medium industrial enterprises. But versus the 11 million exits, there were 9 million hires: the outflow was largely "voluntary" rather than a matter of forced redundancy that would create factual or state-registered unemployment.[7] Notable by mid-1997 were Goskomstat estimates that both employment and unemployment had fallen since the end of 1996—the former from 65.9 million in December 1996 to 65.3 million at the end of July 1997, the latter estimated actual unemployed, not the much smaller numbers registered as such with the Federal Employment Service (FES), from 6.8 to 6.7 million in the same period. Though these figures are essentially estimates drawn by extrapolation from parameters established by earlier surveys, and therefore somewhat questionable, the general impression they convey is that the overall labor force, the "economically active" population, was contracting somewhat (retirements, emigration, deaths), while some of the recorded shrinkage also reflected people exiting recorded employment to work, unreported, unrecorded, and untaxed, "off the books."

Though wage/salary inequalities are not the concern of this chapter, it should at least be noted in passing that these employment dynamics have been taking place against a background of massively increased inter-branch and -sector differentials in average pay levels. The old relatively "flat" pattern of the Soviet period has given way to a pattern of very steep differentials, and thus more inequality. For example, among industrial branches, the fuel-energy complex was traditionally favored; but if in 1990 its workers earned 1.7 times the all-industry average, by 1995 this had increased to 2.7.[8] Light industries like textiles and footwear, low-paid in Soviet times, have come to suffer even more from rising input costs, flagging demand, and competition from imports: textile workers in the mid 1990s were earning on the average only about one-eighth of workers in the energy giant Gazprom.[9]

The "good news" about Russia's rough transition is that money *can* now buy everything—reversing the old Soviet patterns of chronic shortage, rubles do convert into goods. The bad news, of course, is that the lack of rubles suffered by so many low-paid persons is, in the face of market-set prices, more painful. Russia has its "new poor," and obviously they are a much larger population than the newly rich, or merely "comfortable."

The full reality of the Russian employment picture is elusive, and likely to remain so for some time. Shifts out of the large, formerly state-owned heavy industrial and other enterprises and into similar work in smaller private plants have been a major development; also, many of the mobile have tended to move toward work in the service sector so underdeveloped in the Soviet period (in 1991, services accounted for only 39 percent of Russia's GDP, versus 59 percent in West Germany, and 61 percent in Mexico).[10] Some such moves are recorded in data on intersectoral flows, but others are probably cloaked in the numbers that simply record a switch from employee to "self-employed." Services have grown as a share of GDP—by 1993 roughly equal with goods production, services accounted for 50 percent of GDP by 1996 versus 41.2 for goods production, and in the second quarter of 1998, services were 54.3 percent of GDP versus 38.4 for goods production.[11] But it needs to be noted also that this growing "advantage" has as much to do with huge declines in goods production as with a massive revolution in services, or any huge intersectoral shifts. As it turns out, in all the transition economies, but especially in Russia, the "restructuring" that shifts labor out of declining sectors into ones that are the growth points of modern economies is a difficult and lengthy process.[12]

The brutal reality, overall, is that—as we shall see further below—the old Soviet Union's syndrome of permanent labor shortages created by the obsession with quantitative growth, and the "planning process" that expressed it, has been reversed in Russia's chaotic "market" economy. Given the reduced levels of activity, especially in the sectors that provided much of the "overfull" employment, Russia is now a country with a painful labor surplus.

Unemployment

While no one would call Russia's economic transition anything less than wrenching, the feared massive unemployment, as we noted earlier, did not emerge in the early post-Soviet times. Through the massive inflation of 1992–93, factories did not close, workers were not flung into the street—even though the decline in actual output, as noted earlier, was massive. Partly, this was a matter of enterprise behavior: factories still state-owned in 1992–93 were no longer run by the state, since the old branch-ministry structure was gone. But supplier and consumer plants continued "as before," receiving, producing, and shipping as they could, running up massive payment arrears—the typical plant was a large-scale creditor of its nonpaying customers, a debtor to its suppliers—and then pressuring a reluctant but vulnerable government to issue the subsidies that allowed the books to be wiped clean, the workers paid, and "social explosion" averted. The labor market "flexibility" characteristic of the East European market transitions, especially Poland's—the "shedding" of what had become excess labor as enterprises found themselves under the harder budget constraints of the new market—was not part of the Russian picture of the earlier 1990s.

The reasons are many: first, however, a caveat. Early on, some of the statistics on falling production required cautious interpretation. As a new tax regime emerged, reporting incentives for enterprise managers changed. Schooled throughout the Soviet period to *over*-report the physical volume of production, since managers' and workers' bonuses—a very significant part of the monthly pay-packet—depended on 100 percent-plus target fulfillment, managers now found themselves with an incentive—high taxes imposed on income derived from production—to *under*-report output and income. Consequently, some falls in plant output were not real, and would not, under normal circumstances, in fact imply a shedding of excess workers.[13]

But most of the fall in output—at least among large enterprises that are still the major employers—is only too real, and growing worse as time goes on. Despite intermittent expectations—and announcements—of a final "bottoming out," and an imminent return to GDP growth, it has not happened. According to one set of calculations, the last year of the USSR (1991) saw the Russian Federation's GDP fall by a massive 12.9 percent from the 1990 level (itself hardly a banner year). The newly independent Russia's GDP, according to one set of official statistics, fell in 1992 by a further 18.5 percent vs. 1991, and endured in 1993 a decline of 12.0 percent on the 1992 figure.[14] These grim figures were assembled in 1994, and may in retrospect tend toward the high side. But alternative series covering more years look, on the whole, no less grim: a World Bank series, covering 1991–1996, tracks the year-on-year percentage decline in GDP in constant market prices, and adds as well the worse falls of "manufacturing and construction"—those "goods-producing" activities that were so central to the old Soviet economy, and that have been under the greatest pressure as Russia has sought to find its way in the world economy (see table 10.3).

All such figures are approximate, to be sure: measurement and definitional problems make it hard to capture many economic activities, including much that does make a positive contribution to GDP. But they are probably good indicators of the falling output in most of the sectors that employed the bulk of the labor force, and thus represent the core of the Soviet economic legacy.

The economic contraction continued, obviously, into, and in a likely exacerbated fashion through, 1998. A series of GDP figures calculated by the Russian state statistical office (Goskomstat) early in 1998, with 1995 GDP taken as 100, estimated 1996's GDP as 96.5, and 1997's as 97.3 percent of the 1996 figure.[15] Russia's economy never managed to "bottom out," prior to the crisis year.

Table 10.3 Yearly Percentage Decline, GDP and Manufacturing/
Construction Levels, 1991–1996

	1991	1992	1993	1994	1995	1996
GDP	–5.0	–14.5	–8.7	–12.6	–4.3	–6.0
Manufacturing/ construction	–7.0	–21.0	–13.6	–20.0	–5.3	–5.0

Source: Statistical Handbook, 1996: States of the Former USSR (Washington, D.C.: The World Bank, 1996), vol. 21, 386.

Economic numbers like these generally have profound implications for "human" numbers: production collapses equal mass joblessness—a depression. (We are looking at numbers that add up to around a 50 percent decline in GDP from the 1989–90 period to around 1996: U.S. GNP, during the whole of the Great Depression, fell by about 30 percent.)

It needs to be understood as well that what distinguishes Russia is not a sharp fall in output right after the old regime ends, but that Russia's decline in GNP has continued, while East Central Europe's has not. One set of calculations highlights the differences: over the whole period 1989–1996, GDP grew in Poland by "only" 4 percent—but this was accomplished, after a sharp fall, by a 23 percent cumulative growth rate from 1993–1996.[16] In Hungary, a less stellar performer, GDP fell 13 percent over the whole period, but was recovering with a 5 percent rise from 1993 to 1996. Russia's 1989–1996 contraction was 49 percent—but most ominous, the 1993–96 figure was a minus 25 percent.

And even in an atypical Russia, unemployment, after the earlier "lag," has grown as output and GDP have fallen. Table 10.4 indicates the trends of two important indicators from 1992 through early (second-quarter) 1998.

These figures track two things: the growth of "real" unemployment, as defined by the International Labor Office, and the increase in the ranks of "registered" unemployed, i.e., the numbers of those who have registered with Russia's Federal Employment Service as jobless. The latter are much smaller than the former; the former are high enough to be painful, yet they are still low for an economy suffering a GDP contraction as severe (measurement problems aside) as

Table 10.4 Unemployment, Russian Federation, 1992–1998 (percent of labor force)

	1992	1993	1994	1995	1996	1997	1998
"Actual" (ILO definition)	4.8	5.3	7.1	8.3	9.2	10.9	11.5
FES-registered	0.8	1.0	1.7	2.8	3.5	3.1	2.6

Source: 1992: *Russian Economic Trends,* no. 4 (1997): 81; 1993–95: *Russian Economic Trends,* no. 1 (1998): 28; 1996–98: *Russian Economic Trends,* no. 3 (1998): 50.

Russia's today. Explaining both figures requires that we give attention to two kinds of forces in operation: (1) those that work on enterprise management—since privatization, a category also signifying predominant ownership interests—to encourage or facilitate the retention rather than the dismissal of "excess" labor; and (2) those that operate on workers positively to provide an incentive to remain on the plant's books, however poor the conditions, and negatively to deter them from registering with the FES as unemployed.

The massive problem of wage arrears, noted earlier in this chapter, offers a key to understanding managerial willingness to retain workers whose productivity may be zero. An unpaid labor force is a cheap one indeed to "maintain," even if its numbers are large. This is a striking characteristic, indeed a bizarre one, of the Russian economy that has no equivalent in East Central Europe. In many sectors of the economy, neither individually nor collectively have workers and employees the "clout" to compel bosses to pay them on time, or in some cases at all. Nor has government, national or regional, been particularly energetic at compelling managers, through administrative or legal measures, to pay workers the wages due them. Managers frequently plead nonpayment from their own customers, and a consequent lack of rubles in the wage fund, as the reason for wage arrears. Sometimes this is true, but as often as not, managers simply find other more directly profitable uses for the funds they owe their workers. The latter can do little about this, given the primitive and corrupt state of arbitration mechanisms and enforcement procedures.

Thus, average wage and salary figures published in official statistical sources measure "wages due, rather than what was actually paid."[17] But, were wages generally to be paid on time, throughout the economy, the wage bill would still represent a relatively small portion of the average plant's costs, compared to that in more developed market economies. Most Russian workers, even if paid their full wages on time, would still be cheap: management thus has less reason for the downsizing that has become such a hallmark of adaptation to globalization in many industries in the industrialized West.[18]

A kind of managerial "paternalism" was, early on in the transition, cited as a factor in labor force retention as well: a mix of simple habit and practice left over from the full-employment Soviet economy and its total lack of incentives to "economize" on labor at the plant level, and an "ethical" element that dictated managerial obligations to "take care" of their workers, formed again under the aegis of the Soviet system in which the efficiency of workers per se was not a major calculation, and "profit" a formal, essentially state-determined concept as well. Today, years further into the transition, there is little reason to credit any "paternalism" for the moderation of unemployment numbers. Those numbers are rising, and the growth of arrears, of low-pay/no-pay, belies any notion that we are still dealing with some kind of paternalistic inertia.[19]

There are other reasons, beyond their cheapness, for retaining workers. During privatization, managers and their inner circles typically acquired sizable equity, and have since bought more from the cash-poor workers who received shares. But workers still have some shares, and some managers have found a large population of "inside" shareholders on the plant floor a useful ally in fending off pressures from outside shareholders or hostile-takeover threats that might lead to changes in management. Workers will often vote as management directs, to retain their jobs, and because they see no reason to expect better treatment on the whole from the unknown outsiders who launch takeover bids. Tax incentives are working here as well: even honest managers who do pay wages in full and on time find it in many cases economically rational to retain lower-paid, less-skilled and -productive workers (among the first to be let go in economies that place a premium on employment flexibility). Such people depress the plant's average wage/salary figures, allowing it to avoid stiff excess-wage taxes.

Finally, "firing"—the unilateral management-initiated separation of a worker from his/her job—obligates the factory to pay a lump-sum severance of three months' wages. This is "expensive," especially if such a worker has scarcely been paid for months before the separation. Authorities also seem more responsive to complaints from fired workers about not receiving this severance pay than they are to wholesale protests about wage arrears.

So much for management. But what, one may ask, is there that prompts workers to remain where they are neither needed nor paid on time, nor even exalted in rhetoric and poster art as in the Soviet past?

The plant—the provider, in the Soviet period, of much beyond (and more important than) wages—of housing, medical services, child care, leisure facilities, etc.—still remains the point of access to such benefits for many workers. These in-kind services, free or subsidized, may be indifferent in quality and uncertain in delivery, but this was true as well in late Soviet times. Leaving a factory where one is paid poorly, late, or not at all for some time, one that has placed the worker on short-time or an indefinite unpaid furlough, will typically deprive that worker of the right to these things as well: sufficient reason for many who lack alternative employment opportunities to stay on the books. New "owners" might want to divest their enterprises of these costly noneconomic functions, but this is a complicated matter, because of the simple force of inertia, pressures from local governments who otherwise would have to take on many of these plant functions, and the fact that in the USSR, as opposed to Eastern Europe, factories took on even more of these functions, making the costs of "restructuring" all the greater.[20]

Further, plants that may be deplorable in their record of paying wages on time, and/or actually unable to collect on their receivables and thus cash-strapped, often do provide material compensation in addition to housing and other services. A factory may carry a large part of its labor force on the "furloughed" list and thus not be paying wages, but allow those same workers to use tools and facilities for various income-producing activities of their own, in return for "rent" charges—both factory and worker income from such arrangements largely hidden from the tax man. And, just as much inter-enterprise exchange is handled in a form of "barter" (frustrating statisticians), so some workers are paid not in cash but in shares of their own product. Producers of goods from matches to clothing items wind up selling, in sidewalk markets, their own product and realizing their own wages as "profits" from retail sale. Plants operating in this fashion need not report wages paid, nor do workers report incomes so realized.

Beyond this, what is left of the residence-control (*propiska*) system of Soviet days complicates leaving areas of economic stagnation for the greener pastures of Moscow, St. Petersburg, or other places that are atypically dynamic performers in the economic transition. Job-related geographic mobility is also hampered by the lack of anything approaching a housing market that would allow a ready exchange of residences. There is no reason to expect solutions here soon, and thus every prospect that economic problems in a given region will persist, and not be corrected by outflows of excess labor toward areas with more and better jobs on offer, as in the United States. Staying put—in one's job, in one's residence—is thus for many the only real option.

Furthermore, the attractions of "exit," insofar as they imply the status of a "registered" jobless person on the FES rolls, are moderate to say the least. The compensation payments are low, whether as a percentage of the average wage, of cost-of-living minimums, or any other economic "target" a person might aim for: they are very different from long-term joblessness benefits in some Western welfare states (and even some East Central European ones). Retraining programs under the FES are underdeveloped to nonexistent. As sources of alternate employment, FES job rosters are unattractive. The jobs they typically list are, one assumes, little better in pay and conditions than the jobs people have left—early (1992–93) in the transition, new private-sector employers in many areas did not even bother to list their jobs with the FES.[21] Little of the large volume of voluntary job-leaving and -finding involves the FES at all: successful job-changers typically never appear in its register figures. Indeed, in Moscow, where unemployment has been—at least until the 1998 crisis—quite low, and the range of jobs on offer high-paying by national standards, most FES efforts involve, and most of its funds go to, the processing of older, less-skilled workers into early pensions rather than new jobs.[22]

Strikes and Militancy

Given the record of real post-1991 economic woe in Russia, and recurrent references to the risk of "social explosion" by politicians and analysts alike, there has surely always been some justification for anticipating massive labor unrest, tumultuous strike activity, and the like. Such, however, has not been the case. Labor militancy, like unemployment, has been a lesser phenomenon than might have been expected.

There have, of course, been plenty of actions—work stoppages, protests, marches within and beyond factory gates—denominated strikes. And in earlier post-Soviet times (1992–93), strikes were often about demanding wage raises to keep up with punishing inflation, or to coerce subsidies from a government that was still the reluctant owner of Russia's industrial base.[23] But more recently, though it would be quite erroneous to say that the number of labor actions has declined, there is about the record of labor militancy a strong intimation of "ritualism," of a kind of conventionalized choreography, a ballet of protest in which all the players have learned to execute familiar roles. It has been a success in expressing the pains people endure, but on the whole less effective in advancing the sorts of objectives that promote strikes in more "normal" economies. The numbers of strikes, and indices of participant numbers and man-days lost, are recorded in table 10.5 for 1993 through the first quarter of 1998.

While 1995 obviously marked a massive upsurge in strike activity, it is important to understand—though the data are not complete—that there are strikes, and strikes: the scale of labor actions differs markedly. The "explosion" of 1995 looks different when one takes account of two facts. Whereas the 514 strikes in 1994 averaged around 300 participants each, of the 8,967 that occurred in 1995, fully 8,101 took place in the latter half of the year, with 5,021 in the third quarter and 3,080 in the fourth quarter, and

Table 10.5   Russian Federation: Strike Activity, 1993–1998

	1993	1994	1995	1996	1997	1998*
Strikes (number)	265	514	8,967	8,278	17,007	394
Strikers (1,000)	120	155	489	664	887	37
Days lost (1,000)	237	755	1,367	4,009	6,001	270

Sources: Russian Economic Trends, no. 4 (1995): 95; no. 2 (1996): 110; no. 1 (1997): 131; no. 3 (1998): 51.
*first quarter

the average number of participants in these was, respectively, 37 and 45. Especially dramatic again, at first glance, is the upkick from "only" 8,278 strikes in 1996 to a dazzling 17,007 in 1997. But the figures on total numbers recorded as striking do not double, growing only—though still substantially—from 664,000 to 887,000. This yields a per-strike average participation of 52 people, only marginally higher than the latter half of 1996.

What do such figures reflect? Beyond general economic malaise, a rather peculiar picture. Outside of some special sectors like coal mining, transport, and a defense industry that has suffered mightily since the later Gorbachev years, it is not on the whole yesterday's "favored" proletarians, the work forces of "material production," who are, as a segment of society, downing their tools in frequent and loud protest. It is not blue-collar Russia that is in collective revolt: rather, the most strike-prone sectors have proven to be the two major "helping" professions—medical care and education.

Ever since the 1992 launching of the new Russian economy, teachers and medical care personnel have been prone to organized protest, but their numerical impact has grown as the number of strikes recorded has skyrocketed, as indicated above. Of those 8,278 1996 strikes, 7,396 were in education: the smaller scale of schools, vs. industrial plants, explains the small average number of participants per strike. And, in what turned out to be a massively turbulent first quarter of 1997, 92 percent of the strikes took place in the education sector—though they accounted for "only" a 71.6 percent share of the 3.42 million days lost, because of their tendency to involve fewer participants per recorded action than those that take place in industry.[24]

Why the militant teachers, doctors, nurses? Several reasons may be offered. First, low pay: vs. the average wage/salary levels (not necessarily, as we have seen, actually paid) in industry and most other major sectors, this "helping salariat" is badly disadvantaged today, much as it was in the Soviet period. Salaries are near the poverty line, and working conditions are degraded by a lack of equipment and facilities—including massive gaps in the supply of medicines to doctors. Thus they have much to complain about. The legacy of low Soviet emphasis on rewarding rank-and-file professional work "outside material production" is now exacerbated by post-Soviet budgetary problems that see governments seeking to save money on their own employees. Second, there is a sense of "worth" involved. While economists have suggested that, as a matter of economics, workers in value-subtracting areas of material production are truly excess labor and must be "shed" in any rational economic transformation,[25] few would suggest the same of those who work in health and education.

Finally, workers in education and medicine are direct claimants on government as their employer. Is the state—as opposed to private employers—expected to be more ethical, circumspect, "up-front" in dealings with its employees? Teachers and doctors have in a sense asserted this, and, one might say, "bet" on it, but with indifferent results. Their strikes have been about low pay levels and impossible working conditions—but they have also been about arrears in the payment of even those pittances. Governments, especially the regional and local ones that employ the bulk of educational and medical personnel, have been dilatory—though perhaps not quite so blatantly as the managers of many ex-state privatized enterprises—in squaring accounts with those to whom salaries are owed.

However, blue-collar industrial Russia has been proportionally less likely to lay hold of the strike weapon. Again, there are reasons. First, there is a certain amount of flex in the blue-collar world lacking in the white-collar helping professions. Many workers, as we know, shifted after 1991 to private-sector opportunities in the same branches (especially in construction and certain industries) where pay was higher and more regular, and thus motivation to strike lower. Second, of course, pay on the whole is better in many predominantly blue-collar "worker" sectors than the national average. While most have indeed suffered, as a category the classic "worker"—the manual operative in material production—has not been disproportionately victimized by post-Soviet economic policies.[26] Even where payment in kind (goods) may substitute for wages, the goods represent something workers can sell or barter to some advantage—more readily, on the whole, than teachers and doctors, at least outside major cities, can turn their services into money on the side.

Finally, the relative quiescence of that majority of blue-collar Russia that has enjoyed no particular advantage in the economy that has emerged since 1992 may also be traced to the circumstance that strikes, as such, do not and cannot advance their economic interests. Workers in formerly state, now privatized industrial enterprises are the ones who suffer mightily from wage arrears, short-time, unpaid furloughs, etc. But what will strikes avail them? Management does not "need" these workers; many managements, after all, do not depend on products and their sale to make their money. Workers are on the whole very cheap—the human meaning of "wage flexibility" so marked in Russia, but absent in East Central Europe. Workers, however, "need" their jobs, or rather their affiliation with the plant (for housing and other goods). They are "cheap to keep" from management's viewpoint, and, since there is a surplus of labor, not worth more. Strikes thus cannot compel management to be more honest, forthcoming, or generous—nor can they compel government to compel managers to do the right thing. Striking workers, again, can be fired—they have little, they may have complaints, but they *do* have something to lose. They are—sadly perhaps but appropriately—wary of being too militant.

These general conditions of worker/employee weakness, "fixed" as they are at least for a time in an economy whose brute reality is an excess of workers over "output," limit as well what trade unions can accomplish. While the current chapter affords neither space nor place for discussing the details of trade union dynamics in post-Soviet Russia, some brief comments may be offered.

With a few exceptions, the organizations aimed at the organization and mobilization of "labor" in defense of its own interests have played symbolic rather than substantive roles in the period since 1992. Theirs—especially the FNPR, the Federation of Independent Trade Unions of Russia, the lineal descendant of the old Soviet state-controlled trade union organization—has been a politics of gesture, of widely announced nationwide protests, or "days of action," that always promise larger numbers than in the end actually turn out.[27] More often than not, in the early 1990s, the target of such protests was not "employers" as such, but the government. Threats of "social explosion," demands for subsidies and other government bail-out help often came from a "united" front of unions and management. After privatization, the situation in many large plants did not change that much. Management and union in some cases still sought state subsidies, and management and union officialdom "got along" together comfortably, even as the latter accomplished little for the workers.

A whole literature on late-Soviet and post-Soviet labor unions, both of the (ex-)"official" and independent variety, cannot and need not be recapitulated here.[28] It need only be observed that, on the whole, it has been no easier for unions to identify any long-term economic objective (protests over wage arrears, and attempts to block the closing of loss-making, value-subtracting enterprises, aside) that can be pursued collectively with any great promise of success than it has been for workers acting "spontaneously" to do so. And, while the politics of trade unions—especially the FNPR complex of branch and regional unions—may be dramatic, populist, and redolent of "social justice" at the rhetorical level, no really effective linkages between trade unions and larger political forces have developed in the peculiar Russian politics of the 1990s. Natural "partners" to labor unions—political parties from the "hard" left to the social-democratic center-left—have in no case proven strong or durable organizations themselves.

Concluding Thoughts

The continuing effects of what has, and has not, been done in Russia's pursuit of the market since 1992, and of the crisis of 1998 that devalued the ruble, fed renewed inflation, and thus further impoverished so many, necessarily will play themselves out into the future. GDP fell in 1998—as it did in 1997, a year when more optimistic analysts expected the long-awaited turnaround. As 1998 turned into 1999, little to no progress had been made by Yeltsin's government in its dealings with the holders of Russia's external debt, and not much more with respect to wage arrears and other problems at home—save for the printing of yet more devalued rubles to partially "cover" what was owed on several fronts.

There is thus little reason, at the end of this chapter, to predict any radical reversal of the trends sketched out earlier. Given the deepening crisis, unemployment will surely increase. Given the differential effect of the crisis on different sectors of the economy, flows out of battered sectors into ones more promising, or into hard-to-measure modes of self-employment, will continue—though they will be hamstrung by all the factors that limit geographic/residential mobility within Russia. Trade unions, notably the FNPR, will continue to protest at the national level, will continue to call Yeltsin's government—and whatever succeeds it—to account, but will find that their rhetoric, outside of certain atypical sectors, leads to little concrete results in the face of the brute fact that Russia's potential working hands vastly exceed the combination of physical infrastructure, managerial talent, and finance that could find value-producing, profitable work for them all.

NOTES

1. Ann Goodman and Geoffrey Schleifer, "The Soviet Labor Market in the 1980s," *Soviet Economy in the 1980s: Problems and Prospects* (Washington, D.C.: Joint Economic Committee, Congress of the United States, 1982), vol. 2, 333. Had the USSR and the Soviet economy survived, the leadership would have faced the choice of trying the bring the new labor northwestward to the areas where it was needed, or constructing new industry in the south and southeast, where the surplus "bodies" were. Neither choice would have been easy, or even in the end feasible in those post-Stalin times. There was little propensity for Central Asians to migrate; major industrial relocation south and east was a prospect Herculean and unaffordable. In the event, of course, the USSR did not survive.
2. *Russian Economic Trends,* no. 1 (1994): 72.
3. *Russian Economic Trends,* no. 1 (1996): 99–100.
4. *Russian Economic Trends,* no. 1 (1996): 99–100.
5. *Russian Economic Trends,* no. 1 (1997): 129.
6. Alexander S. Bim, "Ownership and Control of Russian Enterprises and Strategies of Stockholders," *Communist Economies and Economic Transformation* 8, no. 4 (1996): 471–500; Igor Gurkov and Gary Asselbergs, "Ownership and Control in Russian Privatized Companies," *Communist Economies and Economic Transformation* 7, no. 2 (1995): 195–211.
7. *Russian Economic Trends,* no. 2 (1997): 89.
8. Anan'ev, "Novye protsessy v zaniatosti naseleniia v usloviiakh perekhoda k rynochnoi ekonomike," *Voprosy ekonomiki* 5 (1995): 39.
9. Richard Layard and John Parker, *The Coming Russian Boom: A Guide to New Markets and Politics* (New York: Free Press, 1996), 109, 301.
10. Anders Aslund, *How Russia Became a Market Economy* (Washington, D.C.: The Brookings Institution, 1995), 44.
11. *Russian Economic Trends,* no. 3 (1998): 44.
12. Richard Jackman, "Unemployment and Restructuring," in *Emerging from Communism: Lessons from Russia, China, and Eastern Europe,* eds. P. Boone, S. Gomulka, and R. Layard (Cambridge, MA: MIT Press, 1998), 129–136.

13.   This leaves aside, for the moment, any consideration of "value-subtracting," as opposed to "real," production: much Soviet-era production subtracted value in the sense that the combined "world market" price of the inputs (labor, raw materials, and fuel, especially the latter) was often much greater than the value of the item(s) produced. In the early post-Soviet period as well, enterprises, zombie-like, continued to produce, as they could, the "old" items for which no effective demand existed, since they could produce no other. They survived heavily on subsidies coerced from the government via threats of a "social explosion." These were value-subtracting, effectively bankrupt enterprises—and their workers—to be cut loose from Moscow's apron strings. Yeltsin's government, in 1992–93, was no longer the effective manager of the factories—but it was still their owner, and proved vulnerable to such manipulation, largely due to precisely a fear of the social consequences of large-scale unemployment.

14.   Aslund, *How Russia Became a Market Economy,* 277–279.

15.   *Russian Economic Trends,* no. 3 (1998): 44.

16.   Richard Layard, "Why So Much Pain? An Overview," in *Emerging from Communism,* 2.

17.   *Russian Economic Trends,* no. 2 (1997): 47.

18.   It is by now the conventional view that the more successful transition economies (Poland, Hungary) did a better job at "pricing" things from the outset than did Russia: in "Eastern Europe, inflation was contained because unemployment was allowed to rise from the very beginning. . . . This has not happened in Russia." (Olivier Blanchard, et al., *Post-Communist Reform: Pain and Progress* (Cambridge, MA: MIT Press, 1993). Thus, in Eastern Europe, the "flexibility" is in employment, in the labor market, and resulted in rapidly rising unemployment rates in the early phases of transition, whereas in Russia, the flexibility is in wage levels, and the likelihood of their (non-)payment: "workers have traded real wages for relative employment stability" (Simon Commmander and Ruslan Yemtsov, "Russian Unemployment: Its Magnitude, Characteristics, and Regional Dimensions," in *Poverty in Russia: Public Policy and Private Responses,* ed. J. Klugman [Washington, D.C.: The World Bank,1997], 134). Of course, broader economic policy also influenced behavior at the firm level, leaving Russian plants early on with little incentive to shed excess labor, and if anything strong incentives to keep workers aboard. "Contrary to Eastern European experience, Russian firms have not operated as if governed by a hard budget constraint. Indeed, employment rather than, say, output, seems to have been the main factor determining the size and distribution of

government subsidies" (Commander and Yemtsov, "Russian Unemployment"). Further on—i.e., as of 1996—the results of this difference could be seen in the starkest of numbers. Poland's GDP had grown 23 percent between 1993 and 1996, and in the latter year it still had an unemployment rate of 13 percent. Hungarian GDP grew five percent during the same period, and Hungary posted a 1996 unemployment rate of 11 percent. Russia, whose GDP had fallen by 25 percent 1993–1996, recorded only 11 percent unemployed in 1966 (Richard Layard and Andrea Richter, "Special Report: Labour Market Adjustment in Russia," *Russian Economic Trends* 3, no. 2 [1998], 2).

19. Anders Aslund, "The Politics of Economic Reform: Remaining Tasks," in *Russian Economic Reform at Risk,* ed. Anders Aslund (London and New York: Pinter, 1995), 198–200; Bim, "Ownership and Control," 490.

20. "Roundtable on 'Divestiture' of Social Services from State-Owned Economies," *Economics of Transition* 3, no. 2 (1995): 247–256; Vladimir Mikhalev, "Restructuring Social Assets: The Case of Health Care and Recreational Facilities in Two Russian Cities," in OECD, Centre for Cooperation with the Economies in Transition, *The Changing Social Benefits in Russian Enterprises* (Paris: OECD, 1996), 61–93; Simon Commander and Mark Schankerman, "Enterprise Restructuring and Social Benefits," *Economics of Transition* 5, no. 1 (1997): 1–24.

21. G. Standing and T. Chetverina, "Zagadki Rossiiskoi bezrabotitsii," *Voprosy ekonomiki,* no. 12 (1993): 86–93.

22. Dadashev, "Regional'nii rynok truda v Rossii: formirovanie i effektivnost' upravleniia," *Voprosy ekonomiki,* no. 5 (1995): 68.

23. Walter D. Connor, *Tattered Banners: Labor, Conflict, and Corporatism in Postcommunist Russia* (Boulder, CO: Westview, 1996).

24. *Russian Economic Trends,* no. 1 (1997): 131; *Russian Economic Trends,* no. 2 (1997): 92.

25. Andrei Illarionov, et al., "The Conditions of Life," in *Economic Transformation in Russia,* ed. Anders Aslund (New York: St. Martin's Press, 1994), 143–146.

26. Walter D. Connor, "Observations on the Status of Russia's Workers," *Post-Soviet Geography and Economics* 38, no. 9 (1997): 550–557.

27. Paul T. Christensen, "Why Russia Lacks a Labor Movement," *Transitions* 4, no. 7 (1997): 44–51.

28. Blair A. Ruble, *Soviet Trade Unions: Their Development in the 1970s* (New York: Cambridge University Press, 1981); Simon Clarke, et al., *The Workers' Movement in Russia* (Brookfield, VT:

Edward Elgar, 1995); Walter D. Connor, *The Accidental Proletariat: Workers, Politics and Crisis in Gorbachev's Russia* (Princeton, NJ: Princeton University Press, 1991); Connor, *Tattered Banners;* Linda J. Cook, *Labor and Liberalization: Trade Unions in the New Russia* (New York: Twentieth Century Fund Press, 1997).

CHAPTER 11

Internal Migration: A Civil Society Challenge

Justin Burke

Overview

ONE UNFORTUNATE THOUGH PERHAPS UNAVOIDABLE consequence of the Soviet Union's disintegration was massive population displacement. An estimated 9 million people felt compelled to flee their homes in the late 1980s and early 1990s, as the Soviet empire collapsed under the weight of its own sloth. The only internal population movement larger in scale in the post–World War II era occurred in India and Pakistan following the departure of the British. A major cause of upheaval across Eurasia was interethnic conflict arising out of the nationalist passions stirred by former Soviet President Mikhail Gorbachev's *perestroika* policies. A wide array of confrontations—including those in Abkhazia, Chechnya, Nagorno-Karabakh and Tajikistan—created millions of refugees and displaced persons. Meanwhile, millions of Russian speakers have also been on the move. Feeling unwelcome in many of the newly independent states—particularly in the Baltics and Central Asia—large numbers of Russian speakers, most of them ethnic Slavs, have been leaving the "near abroad" and returning to the Russian heartland. In addition, economic hardships are influencing migration trends.

Tragedy is evident not only in the wrenching dislocation associated with the Soviet state's implosion, but also in the inability of millions to move. An important, albeit hidden factor impacting internal migration is bureaucratic procedures that limit freedom of movement. The system of residency permits, known as *propiska*, remains in effect, either in law or in fact, in most of the former Soviet countries.[1] In the Russian Federation, for example, the constitutional court has issued decisions striking down *propiska* regulations. But local governments willfully flout judicial rulings and persist in their enforcement of *propiska* procedures, which are effectively designed to keep out newcomers.[2] Without residency permit restrictions, perhaps millions of people in the CIS would change locations, driven mainly by a desire to improve living standards.

For most refugees, displaced persons, and economic migrants, life in the post-Soviet era has meant enduring hardship. A lack of job opportunities, suitable housing, and educational facilities hinders the ability of migrants to remake their lives in new locations. Governmental responses to migration in the Commonwealth of Independent States have proved ineffective. Authorities cite a lack of resources as the main limitation on government migration-related programs. A framework for international community action to regulate population movement was established in 1996, arising out of the CIS conference on migration-related issues. However, progress toward implementation of the Program of Action has been hampered by the muted enthusiasm of many donor governments, especially European Union member states.[3]

Forced Migration

Forced migrants represent the failure of post-Soviet governments to properly manage the transition from a totalitarian model to a more market-oriented system. Soviet successor states encountered problems in accommodating displaced persons, and these troubles influenced political, economic and social developments. Hundreds of thousands of refugees and displaced persons remain in search of durable solutions, having become the largely forgotten flotsam of various interethnic conflicts.[4]

The Russian Federation was home to about 325,000 refugees and asylum seekers at the beginning of 1998, according to the 1998 World Refugee Survey, prepared by the U.S. Committee for Refugees.[5] Only 240 of the 325,000 refugees came from the "far abroad," or countries that were not part of the former Soviet Union. An additional 957,000 individuals in Russia had been granted "forced migrant" status, effectively recognized as internally displaced persons (IDPs), by the country's Federal Migration Service.[6]

There was a plethora of causes for forced migration within Russia during the post-Soviet period, the most serious being the Russian government's ill-fated attempt to repress Chechen separatists.[7] The Chechen war, which achieved little in terms of resolving the region's political status within the Russian Federation, created approximately 600,000 displaced persons. Over 200,000 of those displaced, the overwhelming majority of them ethnic Chechens, subsequently returned to their homes.[8] Yet tens of thousands of IDPs from Chechnya, mainly ethnic Russians, were struggling to reestablish themselves in other parts of the federation. Of the 1.19 million overall registered "refugees and forced migrants" in the Russian Federation in 1998, almost 154,000, or 13 percent, came from Chechnya, according to Russia's State Committee on Statistics. Another internal conflict that produced significant displacements occurred in the autonomous republic of North Ossetia, where Ingush and Ossetians clashed in 1992.[9]

Russia also has served as a reluctant host for those fleeing conflict in the "near abroad," as well as in former Soviet satellites. Moscow, understandably, has been the most desirable resettlement destination, but estimates vary widely as to the number of displaced persons in the capital. According to the 1998 World Refugee Survey, city officials claimed that there were upwards of 1.5 million unregistered residents in Moscow, while representatives of migration-related nongovernmental organizations put the figure at approximately 100,000. Afghanistan has been the largest source of migration from beyond the borders of the former Soviet Union, with tens of thousands of Afghans—many of them adherents of the ousted Najibullah puppet regime—living in Moscow.[10] The southern Russian territories of Stavropol and Krasnodar also hosted large numbers of refugees and displaced persons, who fled Chechnya, Abkhazia and other battle zones.

Other CIS states, especially in the Transcaucasus and Central Asia, were struggling in 1999 to resolve migration-related issues. Armenia and Azerbaijan, for example, experienced ongoing hardships associated with population displacements brought on by the war in the disputed enclave of Nagorno-Karabakh, which lies within Azerbaijan, but is controlled by ethnic Armenians. The neighboring states had not been able to reach a political settlement that would clear the way for the voluntary return of refugees and displaced persons. Armenia was hosting about 220,000 refugees, virtually all of them ethnic Armenians who fled Azerbaijan during the Karabakh conflict. Meanwhile, oil-rich Azerbaijan was home to over 240,000 refugees and displaced persons, of whom the large majority were ethnic Azeris.[11]

The third country in the Caucasus, Georgia, grappled with the task of accommodating roughly 275,000 IDPs, mostly victims of the separatist struggle in Abkhazia. Interethnic fighting in the autonomous republic of South Ossetia also contributed to internal displacement. A political settlement to the Abkhazian conflict remained elusive. Commitments between Georgian government officials and South Ossetian representatives, reached in 1997, paved the way for repatriation in the enclave. But in the ensuing two years, authorities had achieved little in the way of implementing agreements.[12]

In former Soviet Central Asia, Tajikistan experienced the most significant forced migration emergency, sparked by the country's 1992–93 civil war and its aftermath. Roughly 100,000 Tajiks fled to neighboring Afghanistan, and another 100,000, mostly members of the educated elite, went to other countries, including Russia and Uzbekistan. About 600,000 were internally displaced as a result of the fighting. A peace agreement in June 1997 led to a large-scale repatriation of Tajiks from Afghanistan. However, ongoing economic and political turmoil meant that returnees faced an uncertain future.[13]

A separate group of forced migrants comprise formerly deported peoples who were uprooted from their homelands by Stalin during the late 1930s and early 1940s and sent into internal exile. Most formerly deported peoples—including Crimean Tatars, Meskhetian Turks, Koreans, Chechens, Ingush and Volga Germans—were either accused or suspected of collaboration with the Soviet Union's enemies, and banished to remote areas of Central Asia. De-Stalinization led to the rehabilitation of all ethnic groups, except Tatars, Meskhetian Turks and Germans. The stigma associated with deportation remained with these three ethnic groups—whose combined numbers approached 1.7 million people—throughout the Soviet period.

Perestroika created the first repatriation opportunities for formerly deported peoples. An estimated 275,000 Tatars returned to their ancestral homeland in Ukraine's Crimean Peninsula between

1988 and 1998, while at the end of 1998, roughly another 225,000 Tatars were living elsewhere in the former Soviet Union, mainly in Uzbekistan. Repatriation was facilitated greatly by the Tatars' cohesiveness as a people, exemplified by the effective advocacy work carried out by Mejlis, the Tatars' representative organization. Tatars additionally enjoyed the tacit support of the Ukrainian government, which viewed Tatar resettlement as a means to dilute ethnic Russian influence in the Crimea. Ethnic Russians comprised upwards of 70 percent of the peninsula's population, and residents' divided loyalties hampered Kiev's ability to govern Crimea.

The peninsula has been a focal point of contention for most of the 1990s. Ukraine and Russia haggled over Crimea's territorial status, as well as ownership of the Black Sea Fleet. The Tatars' return added to the interethnic and economic tensions. At the same time, Ukraine's reluctance to grant automatic citizenship to returning formerly deported peoples generated discontent among Tatars. However, dissatisfaction had not boiled over into serious interethnic clashes, although conditions were such that conflict remained possible.[14]

Of all formerly deported peoples, Meskhetian Turks have experienced perhaps the most misfortune since their 1944 removal from their homeland in Georgia's border region with Turkey. A pogrom in Uzbekistan in 1989 forced the concentrated Meskhetian population there to flee. The 200,000-strong Meskhetian Turk nation fanned out across the former Soviet Union, with tens of thousands going to Azerbaijan. Other destinations included Kazakstan, Kyrgyzstan, and Russia's Krasnodar territory. Return efforts suffered from the lack of a cohesive advocacy organization that could mobilize the widely dispersed Meskhetian Turks. In addition, the Georgian government, already confronted with difficulties connected with caring for the large number of IDPs, vigorously resisted Meskhetian Turk repatriation initiatives. In 1999, only a handful of Meskhetian Turks were living in Georgia. Meanwhile, a steady stream of Meskhetians were emigrating to Turkey in search of better economic opportunities.[15]

The Soviet Union's collapse greatly benefited ethnic Germans. Under reunited Germany's Basic Law, citizenship was defined according to bloodlines (*jus sanguinis*), rather than birthplace (*jus soli*). Thus, ethnic Germans suddenly found themselves eligible for German citizenship and immediately availed themselves of the emigration opportunity. Of the approximately 1 million Germans in the

Central Asian republic of Kazakstan at the time of the Soviet collapse, for example, over 700,000 departed for the *Heimat*, or homeland, before legislative changes reduced the outflow.[16]

The Return of Russian Speakers

State-building processes have prompted dramatic shifts in the populations of several former Soviet republics. A significant migration trend associated with the emergence of newly independent states has been the departure of Russian speakers, mainly ethnic Slavs, from former Soviet republics in the Baltics, Caucasus, and Central Asia, and their resettlement in the Slavic heartland of Russia, Ukraine, and Belarus. On the surface, the return of Russian speakers was a matter of individual choice, yet there existed an undercurrent of coercion that linked the process to forced migration. The building of new state identities—especially in the spheres of culture and education—fueled discontent among Russian speakers, prompting allegations of state-sponsored discrimination in some of the newly independent states. On the other hand, indigenous national elites were generally critical of Russian speakers for resisting change.[17]

A major feature of Soviet rule during the post–World War II era was the suppression of indigenous cultures in the peripheral republics. Russian culture comprised the foundation of the Soviet identity. The Russian language served as the *lingua franca,* and ethnic Slavs were encouraged to resettle in the borderlands. In this respect, Soviet authorities were to a certain extent following in the colonial footsteps of Tsarist administrators of the Russian Empire. Russian speakers in the union republics created a core of skilled labor that helped industrialize and administer non-Slavic territories. Their presence also performed a useful function for Moscow in facilitating sovietization, especially in the Baltic states.[18]

Kremlin leaders never succeeded in forging a common Soviet identity. Among local elites, many intellectuals continued to harbor nationalist aspirations and longed for a revival opportunity. The Soviet Union's sudden and largely unanticipated demise thrust these local elites into power, providing them with the chance to test their agendas. A dramatic swing in the pendulum thus occurred, as the priorities of governing elites shifted away from Soviet practices. Many of the newly independent countries in 1991 were unprepared for statehood, lacking in both infrastructure and personnel. At the same time, the economic chaos that accompanied political upheaval created scarcities of jobs and social services, heightening interethnic tensions and fueling animosities.[19]

The pressures of state building pushed indigenous national elites in some, but not all, newly independent states to view Russian speakers as interlopers and competitors for political and economic power. Local political leaders in some instances pursued exclusionary policies, manipulating citizenship and language legislation to secure advantages for the indigenous population. As a result, large numbers of Russian speakers suddenly found themselves effectively reduced to second-class citizens. The trauma produced by the sudden change in status was profound. Rather than adapt to new realities, hundreds of thousands of Russian speakers in non-Slavic republics chose to leave, Russia being the destination of choice.

Not every former Soviet republic experienced significant tension between Russian speakers and the indigenous population. One example was Lithuania, which opted for an inclusive state-building model after the Baltic state regained independence in 1991. The relatively low percentage of ethnic Russians in Lithuania's population (about 10 percent) facilitated the extension of automatic citizenship to all legal residents in 1991. Even so, tens of thousands of Russian speakers in Lithuania returned to Russia between 1992 and 1997.

The countries that encountered significant Russian-speaker discontent, and out-migration, also tended to be the former Soviet republics with the largest Russian-speaking populations, in terms of percentage of the overall population. This was especially the case for Estonia, Latvia, and Kazakstan.[20]

Almost 50 years of sovietization dramatically altered the demographic balance of both Estonia and Latvia. Estonia's pre-war population comprised only about 23,000 ethnic Russians, or roughly 8 percent of the country's population. Estonians made up 88 percent of the population and other nationalities comprised the remainder. In Latvia, the ethnic breakdown was similar, with Latvians making up about 76 percent, Russians 11 percent and other nationalities approximately 13 percent of the population.

By the time the two countries regained independence in 1991, the percentages of the population of the indigenous nationalities had declined dramatically. Among Estonia's 1.5 million inhabitants in 1991, about 550,000, or roughly 37 percent, were Russian-speaking

Slavs. Estonians, meanwhile, comprised about 61 percent of the population. In Latvia, about 900,000 of the 2.56 million population, or 35 percent, were ethnic Russians. Latvians' share of the population dropped to 52 percent.[21]

In the immediate post-Soviet period, demographic factors influenced important decisions concerning citizenship and language policy in both Estonia and Latvia. Topping the agenda of the new political leaders was a desire to protect indigenous cultural traditions that had suffered from decades of Soviet degradation. Ultimately, the Estonian and Latvian governments opted to revive interwar citizenship laws. Russian speakers who had arrived after the war were in effect disenfranchised, and required to go through a naturalization process to obtain citizenship. A major requirement for naturalization was demonstrated indigenous language proficiency. Estonian and Latvian authorities also made proficiency in the respective local languages a condition for employment in the government sector.

Citizenship and language decisions spurred widespread discontent among Russian speakers. Only about 100,000 Russian speakers in Estonia, and roughly 200,000 in Latvia, qualified for automatic citizenship. Russian-speaking noncitizens demonstrated little desire to go through the naturalization process. Instead, the years immediately following the revival of citizenship laws saw tens of thousands of Russian speakers leave Estonia and Latvia. The outflow eased after 1995. Despite the outflow, however, both Estonia and Latvia retain a relatively high number of Russian-speaking noncitizens. Although Russian speakers continue to complain about what they describe as state-sponsored discrimination, they are at the same time reluctant to leave, readily admitting that economic conditions in the Baltic states are far more favorable than in Russia and other former Soviet countries.[22]

Kazakstan has experienced perhaps the most dramatic outflow of Russian speakers since 1991. Precise data have been difficult to obtain, but some estimates show that over 1.3 million Russian speakers left Kazakstan and returned to Russia from 1991 to 1998.

During the Soviet era, Kazakstan was one of the most ethnically diverse union republics. The last Soviet census, in 1989, showed ethnic Kazaks comprising 39.7 percent of the population, only slightly higher than the ethnic Russian share of 37.8 percent. Since then, the country's demographic balance has shifted significantly. Information compiled by Kazakstan's State Agency for Statistics and Analysis indicates that ethnic Kazaks will comprise about 52 percent of the population in 2000, while the ethnic Russian share will fall to about 27 percent.[23]

State-building policies are a major factor in the emigration of ethnic Russians and Russian speakers. In particular, the government's prohibition of dual citizenship leaves many ethnic Russians feeling uneasy. In addition, Russian speakers express concern over 1997 legislation that established Kazak as the state language, while permitting the use of Russian in official dealings. Access to employment in the state sector became contingent on the ability to speak, read, and write the Kazak language. Less than 10 percent of non-Kazaks, including Russians, are estimated to have sufficient command of Kazak to meet language requirements. The language legislation thus makes many feel unwelcome. President Nursultan Nazarbayev's government did not demonstrate great concern over the outflow of Russian speakers as a reaction to state-building policies.[24]

Overall, just over five million ethnic Russians and Russian speakers returned to Russia from the CIS and Baltic states between 1992 and 1997, the International Organization for Migration said in its 1998 report "Resettlement of Refugees and Forced Migrants in the Russian Federation." Kazakstan was the country of origin for about 27 percent of all returnees to Russia. Over 1.1 million, or 22 percent of returnees, arrived in Russia from Ukraine during the period. About 552,000 people left Uzbekistan and resettled in Russia between 1992 and 1997.[25]

Economic Migration

The collapse of the planned economy, and the failure to establish viable market mechanisms in its place, caused sizable population movements throughout the former Soviet Union. In Russia, the hardships associated with the post-Soviet transition period contributed to the depopulation of broad swaths of territory, especially northern regions along the Arctic Circle and, to a lesser extent, the Far East.

Never self-sufficient in food or energy, the Russian North and Far East depended on state subsidization for survival. Not only were subsidies drastically reduced after 1991, but the payment of wages to state-sector workers was delayed, often for months at a time. Particularly in the North, residents had fewer resources to fall back on. The uninviting tundra and arctic conditions were unsuitable for the cultivation of garden plots that could augment the meager diets of inhabitants.[26]

Soviet authorities had settled northern and northeastern regions, such as Vorkuta, Yakutia and Chukotka, out of a desire to exploit the area's natural resources, including coal, iron ore, and precious metals. At first, authorities relied primarily on prison labor in their colonization efforts. Later, hundreds of thousands of migrant workers were lured to the area by a variety of incentives, including relatively high wages. The influx continued into the late 1980s. For example, approximately 50,000 people resettled in the North in 1987, according to World Bank estimates. By 1989, however, the migration trend had swung into full reverse.

The outflow peaked in 1991, when 150,000 people departed, and in 1992, when 200,000 left the economically devastated area. The migration tempo slowed in subsequent years, but the desire to leave remained high. Many simply could no longer afford to move, as hyperinflation, combined with delays in the payment of wages, wiped out savings and left residents without the cash needed to migrate. Still, between 1992 and 1995, about 57,000 people, or just over 5 percent of the population, departed the diamond-rich autonomous republic of Yakutia, according to research data published by the Carnegie Moscow Center.[27]

Migration trends were not as pronounced in the Russian Far East—namely the Primorsky and Khabarovsk territories, as well as the Amur Region. Nevertheless, the area witnessed a gradual outflow of people in the post-Soviet era, as the regional population declined from a 1992 peak of about 5.32 million to roughly 4.9 million in 1995, according to Carnegie Moscow Center data. Khabarovsk experienced the largest outflow during the period, with a 14 percent decrease in the territory's population. As in the case of the northern regions, the decline in the Far East's population was primarily attributable to the collapse of the Soviet infrastructure. The Far East's economy depended heavily on subsidization for energy supplies and other basic necessities. The breakdown of old distribution networks, exacerbated by the Far East's relative isolation from the rest of the Russian Federation, produced socio-economic turmoil, which prompted people to leave.[28]

Restrictions on Freedom of Movement

The movement of people within the Russian Federation, as well as the CIS as a whole, might have been far greater were it not for the existence of bureaucratic practices that hampered freedom of movement. In the more than seven years since the collapse of the union, many former Soviet states had not fully dismantled the Soviet-era residency permit system embodied by the *propiska*. And even in countries where national authorities had moved to abolish or overhaul *propiska* regulations, regional and local officials often persisted in erecting barriers to the freedom of movement of citizens and legal residents.

The origin of contemporary *propiska* dilemmas can be traced back to 1932, when Stalin introduced the internal passport system in order to control internal population movements, specifically to restrict migration from rural areas to cities. A *propiska,* or residency permit, was stamped in an individual's internal passport. During the late Soviet era and in post-Soviet times, a valid *propiska* was required for an individual to obtain work legally in a given location, as well as gain access to essential social services, including health care and education. The *propiska* system also placed limitations on political rights. For example, those without a proper residency permit could not vote.

In Russia, the 1993 constitution provided for freedom of movement. A formal registration procedure, in theory, replaced the rigid residency permit system. However, implementation of the applicable legislation has been sporadic. The World Refugee Survey 1998 said that 30 of Russia's 89 regions and autonomous republics restricted migration in one way or another. Some regional and local administrations simply gerrymandered regulations to deny residency permits, while other regions relied on bureaucratic instruments to restrict freedom of movement, including the imposition of unreasonably high fees.[29]

In maintaining barriers to population movement, Russia and other CIS states were in violation of a number of international treaties and obligations, including the 1948 Universal Declaration of Human Rights. Article 13, paragraph 1, states unequivocally that "everyone has the right to freedom of movement and residence within the borders of each state." Article 29, paragraph 2, goes on to clarify: "In the exercise of rights and freedoms, everyone shall be subject only to such limitations as are determined by law solely for the purpose of securing due recognition and respect for the rights and freedoms of others and of meeting the just requirements of morality, public order and general welfare in a democratic society."

Those lacking proper residency registration, especially refugees and displaced persons, found themselves cut off from employment opportunities and essential services. In addition, they were targets of discrimination and police harassment. Russian police "systematically harass" those lacking valid residency documentation, according to the U.S. Committee for Refugees.[30]

Since 1995, Russia's constitutional court has repeatedly issued rulings upholding the principles of freedom of movement. For example, a February 1998, constitutional court ruling, coming in response to an appeal filed by officials from the Nizhny Novgorod region, struck down certain provisions in the Regulations of Permanent and Temporary Registration of Russian Citizens that hampered freedom of movement. The court specifically overturned provisions in the regulations that permitted local officials to imposes a six-month limit on the validity of temporary registration, and broadened eligibility for registration. Despite the bevy of unequivocal rulings against the continuation of *propiska* practices, regional and local officials, most notably those in Moscow, continued to ignore constitutional court rulings. The court, meanwhile, did not have the ability to compel compliance with its rulings.

Elsewhere in the former Soviet Union, some states—especially Estonia, Georgia, Latvia, Lithuania and Ukraine—have made genuine efforts to eliminate some or all *propiska* restrictions, according to a 1998 survey of *propiska* practices conducted by the Organization for Security and Cooperation in Europe. Other states—including Belarus and the Central Asian nations of Kazakstan, Kyrgyzstan, Turkmenistan and Uzbekistan—have preserved many of the major elements of the *propiska* regime.

The Response

By most accounts, the challenges arising out of population relocation have been met with an inadequate response on the part of both regional governments and the international community. Russia and other CIS states were ill-prepared and therefore overwhelmed by the migration processes that commenced even while the former Soviet Union lingered on its death bed. The legislative frameworks and mechanisms established to address migration issues have been woefully insufficient. Meanwhile, the international community's effort to foster better management of population movements has lagged, in part because of a lack of interest on the part of donor governments.

In Russia, the government established the Federal Migration Service (FMS) in July 1992 to address the immediate needs of refugees and displaced persons. In 1994, the adoption of a migration program provided the theoretical basis for FMS activity. Over time, the FMS established dozens of reception centers for not only forced migrants, but also repatriating Russian speakers and even economic migrants. Government officials estimated that it cost the equivalent of $17,000 to properly accommodate each new migrant. From the start, however, the FMS has been plagued by a shortage of funds and has been beset by bureaucratic inefficiency. In addition, the governmental response has suffered from the inadequate implementation of legislation.[31]

International organizations, including the Geneva-based International Organization for Migration (IOM), have raised questions about FMS methods for counting refugees and displaced persons, as well as the agency's registration practices. FMS data significantly underestimated the number of forced migrants in Russia, the IOM asserted in its 1998 report on the "Resettlement of Refugees and Forced Migrants in the Russian Federation." The IOM report added that 75 percent of migrants in Russia did not receive any aid whatsoever from the FMS. In addition, the U.S. Committee for Refugees described as "sluggish" the FMS response to the implementation of an international agenda for addressing migration issues in the CIS.[32]

The international community framework, the Program of Action, was adopted at the 1996 CIS conference on migration-related issues. Officials from over 45 states, including all the countries of the former Soviet Union, participated in the conference. Also attending were representatives from a variety of international organizations, including various United Nations bodies, the International Committee of the Red Cross, IOM and OSCE, as well as nongovernmental organization activists.

In its declaration, the Program of Action sought to "establish national migration systems and to develop appropriate policies and operational activities." It also tried to advance preventative action to address the causes of future potential displacements, and to strengthen international cooperation on the governmental and nongovernmental levels. "This strategy is grounded in universal human rights and internationally accepted principles relevant to the management of population movements, and to the prevention of situations leading to further massive, involuntary displacement," the Program of Action states.

The Program of Action created a framework for policy development and implementation, and formulated operational guidelines for emergency assistance, repatriation and resettlement of forced migrants, the return of formerly deported peoples and illegal migrants, and the integration of displaced persons. It also provided a basis for preventative action and international cooperation. UNHCR and IOM were charged with overseeing the implementation of program projects.

The lofty ideals contained in the program have gone unfulfilled for a variety of reasons, including governmental disarray and malfeasance in CIS states. Another factor contributing to implementation woes is a dearth of enthusiasm among donor governments, particularly European Union members. UNHCR and IOM funding appeals have met largely with indifference.[33]

By 1999, doubt surrounded the future of a coordinated international response to migration issues in the former Soviet Union. The mandate for the Program of Action is due to expire in 2000, and no clear blueprint for further comprehensive action exists. International community interest in addressing migration issues lags. CIS governments lack resources, and local nongovernmental organizations do not possess the capacity to address migration dilemmas.

Conclusion

Population movements, including forced migration and the repatriation of Russian speakers, already have produced widespread privation during the post-Soviet era. There are myriad indicators that migration-related issues will continue to present stern challenges to the newly independent states. How governments in the region respond will significantly impact the development of former Soviet states, especially Russia.

To a certain extent, migration decreased following the August 1998 economic crisis in Russia. The financial fallout hampered the ability of many to afford the costs inherent in moving. According to FMS estimates, the number of people arriving in Russia during the months immediately following the economic crisis was about three times lower than the number of arrivals in the months prior to the ruble's collapse.[34]

The economic crisis, however, did nothing to eliminate the underlying causes of forced migration or the repatriation of Russian speakers. Durable political settlements had not been achieved, as of early 1999, in a number of conflict zones, including Abkhazia, Chechnya, and Nagorno-Karabakh. In addition, new potential conflicts were simmering. Russia's autonomous republic of Dagestan was among the hot spots that could develop into a source of forced migration. "There are conditions that provide for the escalation of existing disputes," according to a report on political-economic conditions in Dagestan prepared in April 1998 by the Moscow-based Institute of Ethnology and Anthropology of the Russian Academy of Sciences. Regarding repatriation, exclusionary citizenship and language policies, acting in combination with the reluctance of some Russian speakers to adapt to new conditions, maintained migratory pressure.

Additional threats loom, especially potential ecological problems, which could prompt new population displacements. For example, the Itar-Tass wire service reported in January 1999 that a primary source of drinking water for the Western Siberian city of Perm contained 40 times the normal level of the toxic chemical phenol. There were potentially millions of people at risk of dislocation due to environmental hazards.[35]

So far, migration management in the former Soviet Union has been haphazard. The indicators in early 1999 did not provide reason for much hope for a marked improvement in the response over the near and medium term. Particularly for CIS states, the manner in which regional governments address migration challenges will provide a useful gauge of their transition into law-governed civil societies. The easier it becomes for forced migrants to find durable solutions, the stronger democratic values will be in the region. Likewise, the longer donor malaise grips the international community, thereby frustrating multilateral efforts to ease individual hardships, the greater the risk that CIS migration-related problems will proliferate.

NOTES

1. For in-depth information on *propiska* issues see a background paper, "Freedom of Movement: The Issue of Internal Registration," prepared in October 1998 by the Organization for Security and Cooperation's Office for Democratic Institutions and Human Rights (OSCE/ODIHR).

2. See "The Propiska Legacy: A Source of Woe in Russia," *The Forced Migration Monitor,* November 1997, 1, published by the Forced Migration Projects of the Open Society Institute.

3. Funding appeals by the United Nations High Commissioner for Refugees (UNHCR) and the International Organization for Migration (IOM) have fallen short of their goals. A joint appeal issued in 1997, for example, sought about $88 million for CIS programs, but garnered less than $25 million from donor governments. Also, see *FM Alert,* a weekly electronic bulletin published by the Forced Migration Projects at *www.soros.org/migrate.html.*

4. Refugees from the Caucasus region of Russia face especially difficult circumstances. For background in conditions in Chechnya see "Chechnya Struggles with Aftermath of Conflict," *The Forced Migration Monitor,* May 1999, 1.

5. See the *World Refugee Survey 1998,* published by the U.S. Committee for Refugees, 199.

6. *World Refugee Survey 1998,* 199.

7. For an extensive analysis of forced migration patterns in the Russian Federation, see "The Resettlement of 'Refugees and Forced Migrants' in the Russian Federation," published by the International Organization for Migration in 1998.

8. *World Refugee Survey 1998,* 203.

9. *World Refugee Survey 1998,* 202.

10. *World Refugee Survey 1998,* 200.

11. *World Refugee Survey 1998,* 158.

12. For background see "Forced Migration: Repatriation in Georgia," a special report published by the Forced Migration Projects of the Open Society Institute,1995.

13. For background see "Tajikistan: Refugee Reintegration and Conflict Prevention," a special report published by the Forced Migration Projects of the Open Society Institute, 1998.

14. For background see "Crimean Tatars: Repatriation and Conflict Prevention," a special report published by the Forced Migration Projects of the Open Society Institute, 1996. Also see "New Crimean Tatar Library Project," *The Forced Migration Monitor,* September 1998, 8.

15. For background see "Meskhetian Turks: Solutions and Human Security," a special report published by the Forced Migration Projects of the Open Society Institute, 1998.

16. For background on the exodus of ethnic Germans from Kazakstan see "Kazakstan: Forced Migration and Nation Building," a special report published by the Forced Migration Projects of the Open Society Institute, 1998.

17. Statistics on the annual migration inflow to the Russian Federation from CIS states can be found in "The Resettlement of 'Refugees and Forced Migrants' in the Russian Federation," published by the International Organization for Migration, 1998, 19.

18. For background on migration trends in Estonia and Latvia see "Estonia and Latvia: Citizenship, Language and Conflict Prevention," a special report published by the Forced Migration Projects of the Open Society Institute, 1997.

19. "Estonia and Latvia," 1997.

20. "Kazakstan: Forced Migration and Nation Building," 1998, 12–13.

21. See Paul Kolstoe, *Russians in the Former Soviet Republics* (Bloomington, IN: Indiana University Press, 1995), 108.

22. For background on Baltic demographic and citizenship issues see Jeff Chinn and Robert Kaiser, *Russians as the New Minority* (Boulder, CO: Westview Press, 1996), 97–116.

23. Makash Tatimov, advisor to Kazakstan's President Nursultan Nazarbayev and specialist in demography, interview by author, May 1997.

24. A more detailed discussion of the impact of Kazakstan's language policies on ethnic Russians can be found in "Kazakstan: Forced Migration and Nation Building," 1998, 66–74.

25. See the migration table on annual migration inflow to the Russian Federation from CIS states found in "The Resettlement of 'Refugees and Forced Migrants',"19.

26. "Forsaken in Russia's Arctic: 9 Million Stranded Workers," *The New York Times,* 6 January 1999, 1.

27. See Vladimir Portyakov, "Migratsionaya situatsiya na dal'nem vostokye," published by the Carnegie Moscow Center information at www.carnegie.ru.

28. Portyakov, "Migratsionaya situatsiya."

29. *World Refugee Survey 1998,* 200.

30. *World Refugee Survey 1998,* 200.

31. See Kim Tsagolov, Russia's deputy minister for nationality affairs and federal relations, writing in *The Forced Migration Monitor,* January 1998, 1.

32. See "The Resettlement of 'Refugees and Forced Migrants,'" 39.

33. See "The CIS Conference: Reflections on Lost Opportunities and Potential for New Directions," *The Forced Migration Monitor,* May 1998, 1.

34. See Valery Tishkov, Director of the Russian Academy of Science's Institute of Ethnology and Anthropology, writing in *The Forced Migration Monitor,* November 1998, 1.

35. "Perm Water Supply Polluted?" *RFE/RL Newsline* 3, no. 7, Part I, 12 January 1999.

CHAPTER 12

Russia's Aging Population

Victoria A. Velkoff
and Kevin Kinsella

AS COUNTRIES OF EASTERN EUROPE AND THE FORMER Soviet Union
make the transition from planned to market economies, issues of
employment, labor productivity, and financial restructuring tend to
dominate social discourse. With immediate, sometimes day-to-day
crises commanding the public spotlight, attention fades from less
obvious, longer-term processes involving demographic evolution
and changing national health profiles. The effects of these processes,
however, will have a substantial, tangible impact on how countries
define and develop their new socioeconomic agendas.

In Western Europe and North America, there has been an increasingly intense debate about the division of social resources in
an era marked by a major shift in relative numbers of older and
younger persons. The shifting balance of young and old affects the
implicit social contract between generations. Social protection systems that developed and functioned under one set of demographic
circumstances may need revamping or radical restructuring in
order to remain viable for current and future generations. Many
Western nations have been able to address the myriad issues related
to population aging in a stable political environment and a relatively prosperous economic climate. The majority of Russia's elderly lived their entire lives, until 1991, under Soviet rule. The
changing economic structure is foreign to them, and the social services that they expected from the Soviet regime are no longer available or no longer meet their needs today. One serious challenge for
Russia and neighboring countries is to promote the well-being of

their elderly citizens in the context of rapid and uncertain socio-economic change.

One out of every eight Russians (12.5 percent of the population) was aged 65 or older in 1998. By 2025, this proportion is expected to rise to 18 percent. While Russia is not the oldest of the newly independent states or the countries of Eastern Europe in terms of its percent elderly,[1] it has by far the largest absolute number of elderly people. The 18.4 million Russians aged 65 or above in 1998 are more than double the number of Ukraine's elderly, the second largest total in the region. Three million of Russia's elderly are in the oldest-old category—persons aged 80 and over. These large numbers of elderly and oldest-old pose challenges to Russian policy makers as they try to deal with the current economic transformation. This chapter will examine the demographic and socio-economic characteristics of Russia's elderly population at both the national and the subnational level.

The Process of Aging

In the simplest terms, population aging refers to an increasing proportion of older persons within an overall population age structure. In 1950, the share of Russia's population aged 65 and over was about 6 percent. This share had reached 10 percent by 1980 (United Nations, 1997), and is nearing 13 percent as we approach the millennium. By industrialized-country standards, Russia is not especially aged. Italy presently is the world's "oldest" major country, with 17.6 percent of its population among the ranks of the elderly. Most other Western European nations are near or above the 15 percent level. All such countries will experience a rise in their percent elderly over the next three decades.

Another way to think of population aging is to consider a society's median age, the age that divides a population into numerically equal parts of younger and older persons. Russia's median age in 1960 was 27 years, and in spite of a slight decline in the mid-1970s,[2] had risen to 36 years by 1998. We expect to see a further gradual rise to about 39 years between 2000 and 2020,[3] and then a more accelerated increase to 48 years by the middle of the 21st century. The concept of a nation in which half of all people are aged 50 or older is fairly radical in the 1990s, yet this is one likely scenario for Russia and other industrialized countries in the not-so-distant future. Beyond the fiscal and health ramifications of rising median ages lie the intriguing implications of a social fabric that will have a much different texture than is felt today.

History is clearly reflected in Russia's current age and sex structure (see figure 12.1), and past events will continue to influence the country's demographic future. Smaller-than-average cohorts were born during World War I and the subsequent civil war period 1917–1922. Many males in these small birth cohorts survived to become soldiers who were directly involved in combat during World War II. The Soviet Union suffered massive human losses during World War II; war-related deaths have been estimated at more than 20 million.[4] Because men were more likely than women to perish during the war, women currently constitute a disproportionate share of Russia's elderly population. While older women outnumber older men in most countries of the world, sex ratios at older ages in Russia are perhaps the most skewed in the world today. Among those aged 65 and older, there are only 45 men for every 100 women. At the oldest ages the imbalance is extreme, with 24 men aged 80 and over for every 100 women in this age group. In comparison, sex ratios for the United States are 70 for ages 65 and over and 49 for ages 80 and over. Even in Germany, which likewise felt the brunt of heavy war mortality, the corresponding figures are 60 and 36.

Although war mortality had a significant impact on Russia's population age structure, an even greater demographic impact associated with World War II was the sharp decrease in fertility during the war years, represented by the indentation in the population pyramid at and around age 55. This birth cohort was much smaller than the cohorts born before and after the war, and will influence the future aging of Russia's population. While elderly population size in most industrialized countries is projected to increase steadily over the coming years, Russia is an exception: the population aged 65 and older in 2010 is likely to be virtually the same size as it was in 1998. This stasis is a direct result of the small World War II birth cohort that will enter the ranks of the elderly between 2005 and 2010. After 2010, Russia's older population is projected to increase fairly rapidly, much as will be the case in the United States when the fabled post–World War II baby boom begins to reach age 65. By 2025, Russia will be home to more than 25 million people aged 65 and older, nearly 5 million of whom will be in the oldest-old age category.

Other historical events also have affected Russia's population age structure, the most prominent of which were Stalin's political and military purges and the famine of the early 1930s. The direct effects of the purges have largely disappeared from the age structure, but the famine had a much greater effect on infants and children who are now reaching older age. The higher mortality rates and lower fertility rates associated with the famine significantly reduced the size of cohorts born in 1933 and 1934.[5] One impact, as seen in the indentation at/around age 65 in figure 12.1, was to reduce the numbers of persons entering the ranks of the elderly in the latter 1990s. Another notable feature of figure 12.1 is the indentation around age 30. These smaller-than-average cohorts represent the children of the small World War II birth cohorts. These "echo cohorts" will affect the aging of the population in the same manner that the war will, though much less severely. In other words, the aging of the population will slow somewhat around the year 2030, when today's thirty-somethings begin to reach age 65. Finally, the narrow base of the population pyramid reflects the steep drop in fertility that has occurred in the 1990s. While Russian fertility generally has been below the natural replacement level of 2.1 lifetime births per woman since the early 1970s, the level has plummeted in recent years, from a total fertility rate[6] of 1.9 in 1990 to 1.3 in 1996, one of the lowest levels in the world. Sustained low levels of fertility eventually accelerate the pace of population aging by producing successively smaller birth cohorts, which increases the relative weight of adult age groups in a population age structure.

Figure 12.2 contrasts the projected size of different population subgroups in 2025 with their estimated size in 1998. It is clear that Russia's elderly, and especially the oldest old, will have the greatest percent increases during this period. The growth in Russia's elderly will be fueled by the aging of relatively large numbers of persons who today are in their late 30s and 40s. The corresponding bulge in figure 12.1 is evidence of a post–World War II increase in fertility. This increase in births appears more pronounced than in many Western European nations, but less so than in the United States, where the annual number of births nearly doubled between 1940 and 1961.[7] At the other end of the spectrum, there are likely to be far fewer persons under the age of 40 in 2025 than is the case at the end of the twentieth century. Such sharp differences in the growth of different age groups highlight the planning challenges that Russia and other countries in the region now or will soon face. The changing balance of children versus the oldest old has wide-ranging implications for educational outlays and the orientation of health services. Declining numbers of young adults portend an eventual decrease in labor force size at the same time that the population of pensionable age is expanding rapidly, with ominous fiscal ramifications. Continued low fertility will contribute to the decline in total population size that is already underway, perhaps giving rise to contentious political debates involving natalist policies (which were used successfully in the 1980s to increase numbers of births) and changes in immigration quotas.

The Importance of Changing Mortality

Although the effect of fertility decline usually is the driving force behind changing population age structures, current and future changes in mortality become increasingly important in societies with low rates of fertility and infant mortality. Countries have made enormous strides in extending life expectancy at birth since the beginning of the 1900s; in the first half of the century, many industrialized nations added 20 or more years to their average life expectancies.

Beginning in the 1950s, the sustained increase in life expectancy at birth in developed countries began to take different paths. Broadly speaking, female life expectancy continued to rise, while male gains slowed significantly or leveled off.[8] Deterioration of adult health in parts of Eastern Europe and the former Soviet Union resulted in declining male life expectancy at birth in the 1970s and 1980s. By the late 1980s, Russia, along with many of its regional neighbors, was experiencing a decrease in life expectancy at birth for both males *and* females. The decline was particularly severe for men, more than 7.5 years between 1988 and 1994.[9] The decrease in life expectancy was due primarily to increased mortality at older adult ages for both sexes, but the rise in mortality rates has been much larger for men. Increases in deaths from accidents, homicides, and suicides accounted for most of the increase in male mortality,[10] although elevated levels of circulatory-system mortality also played

Figure 12.1   The Population Structure of Russia: 1998

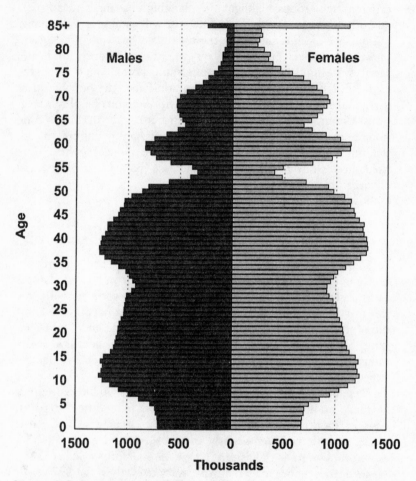

Source: U.S. Census Bureau, 1998.

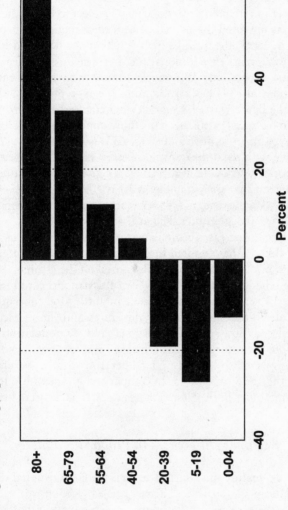

Figure 12.2   Age-Specific Population Change: 2025 Versus 1998

Percent change in the 2025 size of each age group relative to 1998.
Source: U.S. Census Bureau, 1998.

an important role. Population projections suggest that the recent mortality crisis will result in fewer adults reaching old age, thus mitigating to some extent the aging of Russia's population.[11]

Today's elderly themselves have not been immune to worsening mortality. The recent trend in life expectancy at age 65 (i.e., the average number of remaining years one might expect to live if one reaches age 65) has mirrored the overall pattern of changing life expectancy at birth. In 1991, the average man reaching age 65 could look forward to 12.2 years of additional life, but a man who turned 65 in 1994 could expect only 10.8 more years. A woman celebrating her 65th birthday in 1991 had an additional life expectancy of 16.0 years, whereas the figure was 14.8 years for her counterpart in 1994.[12]

The most recent available data show improvements in mortality, and life expectancy at birth and at age 65 is once again rising for both sexes. Even with the improvements, however, male life expectancy at birth remains very low in historical perspective. Official estimates for 1997[13] suggest that a Russian boy born in 1997 might be expected to live 61 years on average, two fewer years than the corresponding national average (63) that prevailed at the end of the 1950s.

The larger decrease in life expectancy for males versus females in recent decades has resulted in the widest known sex difference in life expectancy at birth in the world. Based on the estimated age-sex mortality schedule in 1998, a newborn Russian girl could expect to live a full 13 years longer than a male infant.[14] One consequence of large gender differentials in mortality rates and life expectancy is that the already-low sex ratio of Russia's elderly population will remain low in the future. In 2010, the sex ratio for those aged 65 and older is projected to be just 47 men per 100 women, barely different from the 1998 ratio of 45. In comparison, the sex ratio for those aged 65 and older in the United States in 2010 is projected to be 75.

Regional Differences in Proportion Elderly

One striking feature of aging in Russia is the large regional variation in population age structure. There are 89 administrative areas[15] within the country, and the proportion of population that is elderly in these areas varies substantially, particularly by urban/rural residence. The age structure of many rural areas is skewed in favor of older people.[16] For example, figure 12.3 displays the age and sex

Figure 12.3   Urban and Rural Population in Kursk Oblast: 1996

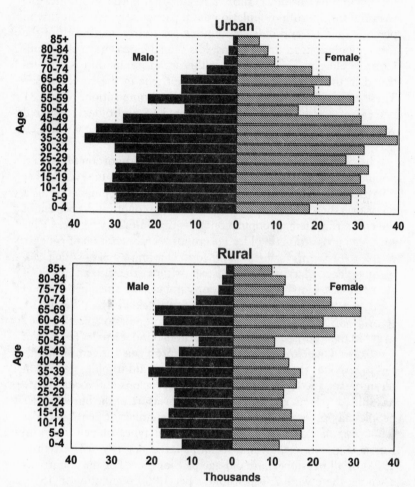

Source: U.S. Census Bureau, 1998.

distribution of urban versus rural populations in the Kursk Oblast, located in the Central Chernozem Region that borders Ukraine. The pyramid for the rural population has a particularly odd shape, with persons aged 65 and older accounting for nearly one-fourth of the total population. In urban areas, less than 12 percent of the population is elderly. The majority of the urban population is concentrated in the working ages, which is not true in the rural areas.[17] These pyramids also show disparities in sex composition. Nearly 31 percent of Kursk's rural females are aged 65 and older, compared with just 15 percent of rural males. The sex ratio for the rural elderly population is 41 men per 100 women.

Kursk is not the only oblast to have a large proportion of its rural population, particularly women, in older age groups. In several other oblasts, more than one-fourth of the rural female population is aged 65 or over. In seven oblasts, elderly women account for 30 percent of the entire rural female population. One reason that rural areas have such high proportions in older age groups is out-migration of younger people to urban areas in search of work. Out-migration of young people may leave older women and men without the direct support of their families. Harsh living conditions and lack of amenities in many rural areas pose additional difficulties for the elderly. In 1996, for instance, only 23 percent of Russia's rural population had running water in their homes, and only 3 percent had indoor toilet facilities.[18]

Skewed age structures may present problems for certain localities in terms of the provision of services and aid to older people. In recent years, the fiscal responsibility for pensions and medical care has shifted to local governments.[19] One measure of the burden older people may place on local finances is the number of pensioners per 1,000 population. While there are several types of pensioners in Russia (e.g., old-age, invalid, social), a large majority (77 percent in 1996) of all pensioners are old-age pensioners.[20] For the country as a whole, there were 258 pensioners per 1,000 population in 1996. However, several oblasts had more than 300 pensioners per 1,000 population. Such ratios seem likely to exert further strain on the revenues of already-overloaded local governments.

Marital Status

In most countries of the world, family members are the main source of emotional and economic support for the elderly. As such, one's marital status can strongly influence the quality of one's life. Studies[21] have shown that marriage has a positive impact on the survival and health behavior of older persons, particularly men. Marital status plays a major role in determining the living arrangements of older persons and directly influences the provision of care in cases of ill health and functional disability resulting from chronic disease.

There are substantial gender differences in the marital status of Russia's older population. In 1994, 80 percent of men aged 65 and older were married compared to 28 percent of women. Older women were much more likely than older men to be widowed (figure 12.4). Among persons aged 70 and older, women were three times as likely as men to be without their spouse. This gender disparity is the product of two primary factors: the aforementioned female/male difference in longevity, and the fact that women tend to marry men who are older than themselves. Also, remarriage rates for older men in most countries typically are higher than for older women.

The effects of World War II can be seen in data on widowhood. In 1979, 65 percent of women aged 60 and older were widowed compared to 50 percent in 1994. The percent widowed among women in 1979 was higher for every older age group than it was in 1994. The reason is that, in 1979, cohorts aged 60 and older were likely to be war widows. Women aged 60 in 1979 were around age 20 at the beginning of the war, and therefore likely to be married to men that were involved in the war. All female cohorts above age 60 in 1979 were likely to have a high proportion of war widows because, unlike in the United States, Russian men involved in combat were not concentrated in their 20s but rather spanned a wider age range. By 1994 the World War II widows were well over age 70; widowhood rates for cohorts younger than 70, which were not affected by the war, were lower.

World War II also affected the proportions of elderly who never married. In 1994, few men aged 65 and older (1.6 percent) had never married, whereas the proportion of elderly women who had never married was much higher (7.7 percent). The difference is due largely to the fact that many older women were of prime marriage age soon after the war, when there was a scarcity of potential spouses due to war deaths. At progressively younger ages, the share of never-married women and men begins to converge, with the proportion of never-married women decreasing and the proportion of never-married men increasing.

242

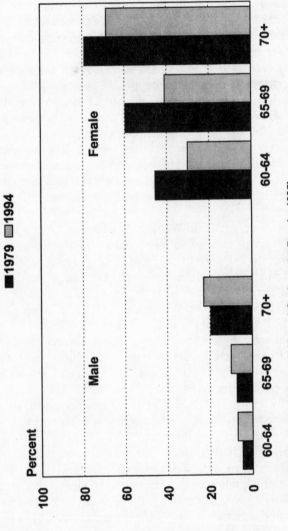

Figure 12.4 Percent Widowed, by Sex: 1979 and 1994

■ 1979 ▢ 1994

Source: Velkoff and Kinsella, 1993; and Goskomstat Russia, 1995b.

Data from the 1994 microcensus indicate that relatively few elderly—less than 4 percent—were divorced. This, however, is likely to change due to higher rates of divorce among younger cohorts. About 12 percent of women and 6 percent of men aged 55 to 59 in 1994 were divorced or separated, and proportions are higher among younger cohorts. As these cohorts reach age 65 and beyond, the growing number of elderly persons who potentially lack direct familial support may present special challenges to the nation's health care system.

Living Arrangements

Living arrangements are determined by a host of factors such as marital status, financial well-being, health status, and family size and structure, as well as cultural traditions including kinship patterns, the value placed upon living independently, the availability of social services and social support, and the physical features of housing stock and local communities. In turn, living arrangements affect life satisfaction, health, and most importantly for those living in the community, the chances of institutionalization.

Russian women aged 60 and older are nearly three times as likely to live alone as are men in this age group, which of course is related to gender differences in marital status. Over a third of women aged 70 and older were living alone in 1994, compared with just 12 percent of men. The propensity of the elderly to live alone in Russia is less than in many Western European countries; in Scandinavia and the Czech Republic, for example, between 45 and 50 percent of elderly women reside singly. Part of the reason for this difference is that in Russia, particularly in urban areas, there often is coresidence of adult children and their older parents. In 1994, 14 percent of married couples lived with one of their parents, and more than one-fourth of all single parents coresided with an older parent.[22] Many of the activities of these older family members are integral to family functioning. Older coresident parents often perform routine household tasks such as buying food, a daily chore that may involve a substantial amount of time.[23] In the past, because of the lack of day-care facilities in Russia, older coresident parents often cared for their grandchildren, thus enabling their adult children to work.[24] The recent decline in the number of day-care centers has inevitably made this aspect of grandparenting even more vital.

A closer look at available data on older women by urban/rural residence reveals little difference in the likelihood to live alone up to age 60. After age 60, however, rural women are considerably more likely to live alone than are their urban counterparts, and among women aged 70 and over, the proportion living alone in rural areas in 1994 was 45 percent versus 29 percent in cities. Comparable figures for men aged 70 and over were 15 and 11 percent, respectively.[25]

The rapid increase in Russia's oldest-old population might be expected to translate into a growing use of institutional health care and maintenance services. To date, however, available information indicates that institutionalization of older persons is not common. The capacity of (number of existing places in) old people's homes and nursing homes throughout the former USSR in the late 1980s has been estimated at between 320,000[26] and 380,000[27]; the higher estimate represents less than 1.5 percent of the USSR population aged 65 and over as of 1988. While the average Russian view of institutionalization may be extremely negative,[28] there does appear to be an unmet need for institutional services. Lengthy waiting lists for institutional admission have been the norm for many years, and time series data for Russia show a steady rise in the number of nursing/old people's homes, from around 700 in 1985 to more than 900 in 1996.[29] At the same time, the number of places in such institutions has remained fairly constant, suggesting a downsizing of the average facility. Older persons living alone, and especially never-married elderly men, are said to be at particularly high risk of institutionalization. In rural areas of the country, district hospitals frequently serve as long-term residences for the elderly, for social as well as health reasons.[30]

Educational Attainment

Educational attainment is an important determinant of an individual's living standard. High levels of education typically translate into better economic status, higher pensions, and better health status. Currently, the elderly in Russia have fairly low levels of educational attainment. In 1994, only 32 percent of men and 21 percent of women aged 65 and older had completed at least a secondary ed-ucation.[31] In contrast, 1996 data for the United States show that 65 percent of both elderly men and women had achieved this level. There are large gender differences in educational attainment at older ages in Russia; in 1994, more than one-quarter of elderly women had never finished primary school, compared with just 9 percent of elderly men.

One of the legacies of the Soviet regime was its improvement of educational opportunities and attainment throughout the former USSR. The main beneficiaries of this effort were the cohorts edu-cated after World War II. Data by age and sex from the mid-1990s show that the overall level of attainment increases for successively younger cohorts while the gender difference in attainment decreases with age. In fact, a greater proportion of women than men aged 50–54 have completed high school or a higher level of education. These patterns suggest that Russia's future elderly will have much higher levels of education than the current elderly and, theoretically, will enjoy the benefits that accompany these higher levels.

The Effects of Changing Economics

There is much interest in how the changing economic situation in Russia is affecting different subgroups of the population. Tradition-ally, Russia's elderly have been a group at risk. Elderly households during the Soviet period, particularly elderly women living alone, had higher-than-average poverty rates.[32] However, the latest studies of poverty suggest a relative improvement in the situation of the el-derly, to the extent that they now compare favorably with other sub-groups of the population. A recent World Bank study found that people past retirement age were less likely to be poor than were chil-dren or people in the working ages.[33] A profile of poverty produced by the Russian government corroborates this finding; in 1993, the poverty rates reported by Goskomstat for post-retirement-age men and women were lower than the national average. In addition to the research on poverty, studies that have utilized survey data to assess the impact of the changing economic situation on other spheres of life (e.g., nutritional status and access to health care) also have found that the majority of the elderly are not faring any worse than the rest of the population.[34] However, such aggregate findings may conceal the diversity of the pensioner population; the poverty studies indicate that certain subgroups of the elderly population (e.g., older women who are living alone) have a high likelihood of poverty.

Another change for older Russians involves participation in the formal labor force. The official retirement ages are 60 for men and 55 for women, but in the past many people continued to work beyond the official retirement age. The government encouraged this by increasing pensions for each year worked past the official retirement age.[35] Pensioners were also allowed to receive pension benefits while working. Approximately 22 percent of pensioners worked for wages while drawing pension benefits.[36] In 1992, 27 percent of men aged 60 to 72 were still active in the labor force. Women aged 60 to 72 had lower levels of economic participation, but a large proportion (39 percent) in the age group 55–59 were still active. One result of the changing Russian economy in the mid-1990s was a decline in labor force participation rates of older workers compared to those of younger workers (see table 12.1). Some of this decline may be attributed to early retirement, as older workers choose (or are forced) to leave the labor force rather than be laid off.[37]

Prospects for the Future

The issues associated with an aging population will create challenges for policy makers in Russia well into the next century. The sheer number of elderly, over 18 million in 1998, that the current government must provide services for has ramifications for health care services, pension outlays, and family life. To the extent that the recent mortality crisis also reflects increasingly poor health in the entire population, we may see a higher incidence and prevalence of disability in future cohorts of elderly. The existing social safety nets in Russia are not equipped to handle the present population of elderly, let alone the growing numbers in the near future. Further, the economic foundation needed to develop a comprehensive social security program will be lacking for years to come.[38] Russia's elderly will continue to rely heavily on their families for support, although the uncertain economic situation will affect the nature and adequacy of such support.

Table 12.1 Labor Force Participation Rates: 1992 and 1995 (percent economically active)

| | Male | | | Female | | |
Age	1992	1995	Change	1992	1995	Change
15–19	32.7	25.1	–7.6	29.2	22.1	–7.1
20–24	84.0	82.5	–1.5	74.4	71.0	–3.4
25–29	95.1	92.3	–2.8	85.4	80.7	–4.7
30–49	95.6	92.2	–3.4	91.6	87.6	–4.0
50–54	89.7	83.5	–6.2	81.0	73.1	–7.9
55–59	79.4	69.9	–9.5	39.4	30.0	–9.4
60–72	27.2	16.7	–10.5	12.7	7.7	–5.0

Source: Goskomstat Russia, 1996, Labor and Employment in Russia.

NOTES

This chapter reports the results of research and analysis undertaken by census bureau staff. It has undergone a more limited review than official census bureau publications. This report is released to inform interested parties of research and to encourage discussion. The use of data not generated by the U.S. Census Bureau precludes performing the same statistical reviews on those data that the census bureau does on its own data.

Unless otherwise indicated, the estimated and projected demographic figures in this chapter were prepared by the International Programs Center of the U.S. Census Bureau, based on data available through mid-1998.

1. There is a growing realization that the term "elderly" is an arbitrary concept, and that older individuals are generally as diverse in terms of socioeconomic characteristics as are younger persons. In this chapter, the term "elderly" is used primarily for referential and cross-national comparative purposes, and refers to persons aged 65 and older.

2. Sergei A. Vassin, "The Determinants and Implications of an Aging Population in Russia," in *Russia's Demographic Crisis,* eds. Julie Da Vanzo and Gwendolyn Farnsworth (Santa Monica: The RAND Corporation: 1996), 175–200.

3. Some analyses predict extremely low fertility rates in the early part of the twenty-first century that, if realized, would elevate the median age even faster (see, for example, Charles M. Becker and David D.

Hemley, "Demographic Change in the Former Soviet Union During the Transition Period," *World Development* 26, no. 11 (1998): 1957–1975.

4. Barbara A. Anderson and Brian D. Silver, "Demographic Consequences of World War II on the non-Russian Nationalities of the USSR," in *The Impact of World War II on the Soviet Union*, ed. Susan J. Linz (Totowa, NJ: 1985), 207–242; Alain Blum, "Uncovering the Hidden Demographic History of the USSR," *Population Today* 19, no. 7/8 (1991): 6–8.

5. Vassin, "The Determinants and Implications of an Aging Population."

6. The total fertility rate is the average number of children a woman could expect to bear over her reproductive life if the prevailing age-specific fertility rates remained constant.

7. Because of the lack of historical demographic data for the former Soviet Union, particularly referring to the period prior to World War II, it is impossible to accurately calculate the increase in the number of annual births. Instead, the relative size of cohorts (based on census data) must be compared. The results of this comparison suggest that the increase in births after World War II was not as substantial in Russia as it was in the United States.

8. Kevin Kinsella, "Changes in Life Expectancy 1900–1990," *American Journal of Clinical Nutrition* 55, Supplement, no. 6 (1992): 1196S-1202S.

9. One factor that may have affected the decrease in life expectancy in Russia is a change in the definition of infant mortality. In 1993, the World Health Organization's definition was introduced into the Russian health system. This definition is broader than the one previously used in Russia, and as a result, some infant deaths that previously were recorded as stillbirths are now considered to have occurred as live births. Applying this new definition would increase the reported infant mortality rate and thus lower life expectancy at birth, since the latter is a summary measure of mortality that includes infant deaths. Thus, even if the actual mortality level remained the same, such a statistical revision would create the impression of worsening mortality. However, the estimated decrease in life expectancy from this revision would be less than half a year (see Vladimir M. Shkolnikov, France Meslé, and Jacques Vallin, "Recent Trends in Life Expectancy and Cause of Death in Russia, 1970–1993," in *Premature Death in the New Independent States*, eds. José Luis Bobadilla, Christine A. Costello, and Faith Mitchell [Washington, D.C.: 1997], 34–65). A confounding factor in the analysis of mortality is that the dissemination of the new definition of a live birth has not necessarily been uniform across all areas of the country. It likely would take

months or years for the new definition to be widely and successfully implemented.

10. W. Ward Kingkade and Eduardo E. Arriaga, "Mortality in the New Independent States: Patterns and Impacts," in Bobadilla, et al., *Premature Death in the New Independent States,* 156–183.

11. Neil G. Bennett, David E. Bloom, and Sergey F. Ivanov, "Demographic Implications of the Russian Mortality Crisis," *World Development* 26, no. 11 (1998): 1921–1937.

12. U.S. Census Bureau, "International Data Base" (Washington, D.C.: International Programs Center, 1998).

13. Unpublished at the time of this writing.

14. U.S. Census Bureau, "International Data Base."

15. The administrative areas include oblasts, krays, republics, and autonomous regions, plus two cities. For ease we refer to them collectively as oblasts.

16. Although Russia is highly urbanized (over 70 percent of the population lives in urban areas), its rural population remains substantial, numbering approximately 40 million in 1996.

17. Russians define the working ages as 16–59 for men and 16–54 for women.

18. Goskomstat Russia, *Russian Statistical Yearbook* (Moscow, 1997).

19. Timothy Heleniak, "Internal Migration in Russia During the Economic Transition," *Post-Soviet Geography and Economics* 38, no. 2 (1997): 81–104.

20. Goskomstat Russia, *Russian Statistical Yearbook.*

21. Lee A. Lillard and Linda J. Waite, "Til Death Do Us Part: Marital Disruption and Mortality," *American Journal of Sociology* 100 (1995): 1131–1156; Barbara Steinberg Schone and Robin M. Weinick, "Health-Related Behaviors and the Benefits of Marriage for Elderly Persons," *The Gerontologist* 38, no. 5 (1998): 618–627.

22. Goskomstat Russia, *Type and Composition of Households in Russia: Data from the Microcensus of the Population, 1994* (Moscow, 1995).

23. Tracy Armstrong, *Access to Health Care Among the Elderly in Russia,* Ph.D. dissertation, University of Maryland, 1998; Jeanine D. Braithwaite, "The Old and New Poor in Russia," in *Poverty in Russia: Public Policy and Private Responses,* ed. Jeni Klugman (Washington, D.C.: 1997), 29–64.

24. David E. Powell, "Aging and the Elderly," in *Soviet Social Problems,* eds. Anthony Jones, Walter D. Connor, and David E. Powell (Boulder, CO: Westview Press, 1991), 172–193.

25. Goskomstat Russia, *Type and Composition.*

26. Rustam R. Muzafarov and Ernest M. Kurleutov, "The Provision of Primary Health Care to the Elderly in the USSR: Problems and Their

Solutions," in *Eldercare, Distributive Justice, and the Welfare State*, eds. Derek G. Gill and Stanley R. Ingman (Albany, NY: 1994), 175–202.

27. Vladislav V. Bezrukov, "Self-Care Ability and Institutional/Non-Institutional Care of the Elderly," *Journal of Cross-Cultural Gerontology* 8 (1993): 349–360.

28. Powell, "Aging and the Elderly."

29. Goskomstat Russia, *Russian Statistical Yearbook.*

30. Bezrukov, "Self-Care Ability."

31. Goskomstat Russia, *Education of the Population of Russia: Data from the Microcensus of the Population, 1994* (Moscow: 1995).

32. Monica S. Fong, *The Role of Women in Rebuilding the Russian Economy,* Studies of Economies in Transformation 10 (Washington, D.C.: The World Bank, 1993); Nataliya Rimashevskaya, "Poverty Trends in Russia: A Russian Perspective," in *Poverty in Russia,* 119–132.

33. Braithwaite, "The Old and New Poor in Russia."

34. Armstrong, *Access to Health Care;* and Barry M. Popkin, Namvar Zohoori, and Alexander Baturin, "The Nutritional Status of the Elderly in Russia, 1992 through 1994," *American Journal of Public Health* 86, no. 3 (1996): 355–360.

35. Powell, "Aging and the Elderly."

36. Mark C. Foley and Jeni Klugman, "The Impact of Social Support: Errors of Leakage and Exclusion," in *Poverty in Russia,* 189–210.

37. Simon Commander and Ruslan Yemtsov, "Russian Unemployment: Its Magnitude, Characteristics, and Regional Dimensions," in *Poverty in Russia,* 133–164.

38. Evgenii Andreev, Sergei Scherbov, and Frans Willekens, "Population of Russia: What Can We Expect in the Future," *World Development* 26, no. 11 (1998): 1939–1955.

CHAPTER 13

Promises to Keep: Pension Provision in the Russian Federation

Cynthia Buckley and Dennis Donahue

1. The Russian Federation shall be a social state, whose policies shall be aimed at creating conditions, which ensure a dignified life and free development of man. 2. The Russian Federation shall protect the work and health of its people, establish a guaranteed minimum wage, provide state support for family, motherhood, fatherhood and childhood, and also for the disabled and for elderly citizens, develop a system of social services and establish government pensions, benefits and other social security guarantees.

—Article 7 of the Constitution of the
Russian Federation, Ratified 1993

IN THIS CHAPTER WE EXAMINE THE WAYS IN WHICH the legacy of Soviet pension policies and post-1991 economic and social trends have constrained policy options concerning pension reform in the Russian Federation and have prevented serious reevaluation of pension provision or pension equity. While the Russian government inherited a pension system beset with difficulties and ill equipped for Russia's aging population, the Soviet pension system represented, in symbolic and financial terms, a widely valued social guarantee. We contend that the structural legacy and embedded expectations associated with the Soviet pension system thwart attempts to provide a unified and equitable pension system in the post-Soviet period.

While making numerous changes to the pension system in the post-Soviet period, the federation government remains severely constrained in either fulfilling the promises of the previous Soviet system, or instituting the type of large-scale structural reforms that might contribute to the long-term solvency of the system.

The Soviet Legacy: Inclusion and Ideology

Tracing its origins to the People's Commission on Social Provision of the 1920s, the Soviet pension system covered three specific categories of monthly transfers. First, transfers were made to families who had lost a breadwinner, a program initially oriented toward Red Army widows and their children.[1] Second, transfer payments were made to disabled individuals (invalidi), a policy that was ideologically oriented in a concern for those injured during the revolution and civil war. Lastly, a system of monthly payments to workers who had both reached retirement age (55 for women and 60 for men) and completed the required length of labor service (20 years for women and 25 years for men) was initiated. From its conception, the system of government pensions lacked adequate funding, often falling behind in benefit provision and scrambling for limited state resources.[2] However, with major expansions in coverage and increases in state revenue commitments, the Soviet pension system evolved from a limited system stressing self-help and work farms to an inclusive and extensive system of transfer payments.[3] In 1989 over 60 million citizens of the Soviet Union received monthly transfers from the central government in the form of a state pension, nearly triple the number of claimants in 1959 (only thirty years earlier).[4]

While the stability and coverage of the Soviet pension system grew, the rhetorical orientation toward pension provision also evolved. Soviet perspectives on state pensions originated in an initial concern for the poor and destitute (with both moral concerns and issues of public order at stake) focusing on the welfare of state employees, mothers, and children. Only later was there a move toward concerns regarding the social rights of individuals (particularly the aged) to state support and the role of pension provision in the overall contract between government and society.[5] No concerted reexamination of dependency on the state or re-calibration of boundaries of responsibility between the individual, families, and the state has appeared in the Russian Federation. Yet the administrative and financial difficulties of the pension system in the post-Soviet period have stimulated great debate.[6] The ideological legacy of the late Soviet period remains influential, and attitudes toward pensions formulated during the Soviet period make serious reform attempts difficult.

In the early Soviet period, several pension laws were established and many commissions created; however, direct resource transfers remained oriented toward mothers, small children, and veterans. Near central cities many "sanitoria" and residential cooperatives were created for the physically disabled *(invalidi)*, poor, and elderly, but they were structured to rely upon self-provision. Individuals were to be assisted by providing a context in which they could help themselves.[7] As the pension system became institutionalized in the early 1930s, soldiers, party workers, government officials, and strategic skilled workers were among the earliest occupational categories eligible for special resource transfers under the emerging pension system.[8] The poor, particularly invalids and the elderly, were portrayed as a social category in need of assistance and supervision, yet obligations toward them did not figure heavily in the rhetorical presentation of pension transfers, which tended to focus on old age or retirement pensions. Early calls for transfers did rely upon the vague idea of social obligation on the part of the state, but often linked such assistance to service (of the individual or family member) in the revolution and civil war. The strong emphasis on self-reliance is clear in reports of care for *invalidi* and the elderly on newly formed collective farms in the early 1930s. In the enthusiastic prose of the period, collective farm officials wrote progress reports to the journal *Sotsial'noe obespechenie,* detailing efforts to provide employment opportunities and resource transfers to *invalidi* and the elderly.[9] Far from an attitude of obligation from the central government, in numerous letters and articles rural officials and "pensioners" proudly stressed their self-reliance and independence from state transfers.

Article 120 of the 1936 constitution of the Soviet Union included the statement that all citizens deserved social provision, particularly in their old age. But no uniform statute assuring the provision of state pension coverage for most occupational categories existed until 1956. In that year legislation joined then disparate channels of old age pension provision (running through a combination of governmental agencies, firms, and trade unions) into a unified system with occupational coverage extending over most of the nonagrarian work force.[10] The pension requirements for age and years of service remained constant from their initial adoption in the 1920s through the expansion of the system in 1956 and the later inclusion of collective farmers in 1964. By 1960 over 20 million Soviet citizens received pensions through the central state, approximately 14 million for physical infirmity or loss of household head, and nearly 6 million for age and service. In time, the growth of the elderly population dramatically increased both the proportion and number of old-age pensions.[11] At the end of 1997, 75.9 percent of the over 38 million state pensions in the Russian Federation were old-age pensions, 12.6 percent were for physical infirmities, and 6.6 percent of all pensions went to recipients who had lost a head of household.[12]

The expansion in pension coverage coincided with a shift in rhetoric concerning the motivations behind pension provision, specifically old-age pension provision. Pensions to workers were viewed as delayed remuneration for labor provided to the state, a view reinforced through explicit taxes on enterprises and individuals supposedly intended for the pension fund. Far from a program to alleviate poverty among the elderly, or provide needs-based assistance, old-age pension payments were set in accordance with an individual's wage history. Pensions were provided without any needs testing to those who qualified by age and years of service to the state economy. In essence, old-age pensions became an implicit part of the labor contract, with workers accepting a wage rate in full expectation of a "delayed payment" during retirement. This attitude built upon the practice of higher pensions and earlier retirement ages for those in "strategic" professions, as they were due larger remuneration in their retirement years.

The first major standardization of the Soviet pension system in 1956 marked a shift from a complicated system of transfers organized through trade unions to a uniform governmental policy covering almost all occupations with the exception of collective farmers. Requirements for pension eligibility remained as they were set initially in the 1920s, with pension ages set at 55 for women and 60 for men, with labor requirements of 20 and 25 years respectively.[13] Dramatic improvements in public health during the period increased the effect of pension expansion. Decreases in infectious disease rates and improvements in infant mortality increased the number of individuals reaching pension age, while better adult mortality lengthened the average life expectancy after retirement age.[14] The presentation of pensions as delayed remuneration continued and was supported by the structure of the transfers, which enabled individuals to receive pension payments and wages if they elected to continue to work, an option that was actively encouraged as labor deficits emerged in the 1970s.[15] Pensions for individuals with physical infirmities, on the other hand, were reduced if wages were earned, indicating a different orientation toward the transfer. Similarly, *invalidi* payments were set much higher for individuals with at least some work experience in comparison to individuals without work experience (such as those with infirmities from childhood).[16] Pensions were primarily portrayed as an earned benefit for workers with long service records, not as a program focused on poverty eradication or morally motivated transfers to marginalized populations.

The 1956 pension laws maintained the lower retirement age and smaller tenure requirements for women that first emerged in some of the initial pension legislation of the 1920s. Lower retirement requirements for women were sometimes linked to women's allegedly weaker physical status, but most often they were associated with the heavier familial responsibilities that women bore under the Soviet regime in terms of child rearing, family provision, and in some cases care for elderly parents. The inclusion of reproduction as production (a long held Marxist belief) was made explicit by including mothers with a large number of children among those who qualified for early retirement due to especially strategic or difficult employment.[17] Explicitly gendered regulations rarely appeared in the legislative structure of the other two forms of government pensions, although most transfers for loss of household head went to families who lost a male breadwinner, a tendency that was doubtlessly linked to the higher income of men in the Soviet period and the focus on military losses in the original conceptualization of the transfer.

Nearly a decade later, the Soviet pension system experienced its last major legislative expansion when in 1964 plans were made to include collective farmers. Until their inclusion took effect in 1965, these farmers were dependent upon a combination of private plot income, wages, family transfers, and assistance from their collective

farms for support in their old age.[18] During debates on pension inclusion, the measurement of tenure was often raised. The seasonal
nature of agricultural labor and the persistence of wage payments
made by workday equivalent accounting made the calculation of
experience in years somewhat challenging. However, the focus on
years of experience also indicates a persistent orientation toward
old-age pension as an earned transfer that workers accumulated
through years of service. While collective farm pensions remained
administratively separate throughout the Soviet period, their orientation and structure were similar to the pension system for industrial
and service workers, although due to the process of wage and pension calculation pension payments for collective farmers were typically much lower than those of workers.

State pensions were widely perceived as earned, deserved, and
highly valued transfers. The orientation toward old-age pensions in
particular, that of delayed remuneration, differs from pension systems
primarily intended for poverty alleviation as a moral obligation to
provide for the needy, or to substitute for family caretaking. As a social guarantee, at least in the Russian Federation, pensions are viewed
differently from welfare payments or income transfers. They are seen
as delayed remuneration for services rendered. As part of a social
safety net, pensions are held as more important, as they are an earned
transfer. The Soviet orientation toward pension provision, that of delayed remuneration for services rendered, poses an especially difficult
barrier to pension reform. Individuals presently at or near pension age
have a historically embedded claim upon state pensions.

The actual administration of the Soviet pension fund differs dramatically from the historically developed expectations of Russian
citizens at or near pension age. While transfers to the pension fund
were made throughout the working life of present-day pensioners,
the financial pattern of the pension fund most resembled the "pay
as you go" approach, a system in which the pension contributions
of current workers pay the pensions of individuals currently on pension. Far from receiving delayed payment for their contribution to
the national economy, present pensioners are receiving clear transfers from workers presently contributing to the pension fund. The
monetary contributions of individuals presently on pensions were
transferred, long ago, to the pensioners of previous decades.

Even though pensions were loosely calibrated to wage levels
(and therein pension contributions), pay-as-you-go pension systems

do not truly link individual contributions paid to the amount of transfer received over the retirement lifetime. In essence, workers support the older generation and will rely upon the younger generation to support them when they attain old age. Workers do potentially benefit during their laboring years from reduced familial obligations (as they are not responsible for the financial support of elderly relatives), but their direct remuneration from the program is delayed. Pay-as-you-go pension systems are widespread, and nearly universal among the countries of the former Soviet bloc.[19] During prolonged periods of economic growth and high fertility, such plans may provide stable financing for state pensions, as economic and demographic growth yield increasing contributors. However, economic development is typically linked with public health improvements, which extends the required person-years of pension support for each individual pensioner. Across the globe, pay-as-you-go systems are currently in crisis, as they struggle to come to grips with economic and demographic developments that severely threaten the solvency of pension funds. The experience of the Russian Federation in this regard is especially instructive.

Demographic Challenges

Population aging is one of the most dramatic demographic trends in the Russian Federation. As of 1997, 30.5 million permanent residents of the Russian Federation were past pension age (60 for men and 55 for women) and over 29 million citizens were registered to receive state pensions for old age. As seen in table 13.1, the number and proportion of residents past pension age has risen dramatically. In 1959, slightly over 11 percent of the total population was past pension age, and there were nearly five people of working age for every one pensioner. A mere 40 years later the proportion past pension age has almost doubled, to 20.7 percent, and Russia contains only 2.77 individuals in the working ages for every one pensioner. The proportion of the population past pension age differs dramatically by region. Within Russia, the elderly population continues to be concentrated in rural areas, where infrastructure development is challenged and service provision relatively low in comparison with urban areas. While urban areas have 3.01 working-aged residents for each individual of pension age, rural regions have only 2.21. Long-term trends related to fertility decline and mortality improvement, not only in Russia but also across the industrialized world, have placed severe strains on the state pension system, strains that are heightened in Russia by the expansive nature of pension legislation there. While estimates indicate that less than half of all individuals past pension age were covered by the old-age pension system in 1959, coverage by 1997 was nearly universal.

As table 13.1 clearly indicates, the demographic context in which the Russian pension system operates has changed dramatically since the initial standardization of the system in 1956, or the expansion to cover collective farmers in 1965. Under a pay-as-you-go system, decreasing numbers of contributors and increasing numbers of claimants in the long term demand either increases in contribution levels, decreases in coverage, declining pension value, or a combination of all of the above. Longevity improvements also strongly influence the demographic context for pension provision. A tremendous amount of attention has been paid to the declining life expectancy of Russian males, and it is a very serious demographic development. However, when seen in the long term and viewed in terms of life expectancy at retirement age, the improvements in mortality experienced for men (although marginal at present) and especially women has extended the relative cost of each individual reaching pension age by increasing the average number of years they live to receive pension.[20]

Table 13.2 illustrates that the pay-as-you-go pension system, inherited from the Soviet Union, presents a differential burden to the successor states in the CIS. The Slavic countries have the highest proportion of their population past pension age. Ukraine and Russia face the highest relative burden, with fewer than three potential workers per pensioner. Under a unified system, the larger working populations of Central Asia may have assisted in making the Soviet old-age pension system viable for a longer period of time. With the breakup of the union, the Russian Federation is left with a particularly acute demographic dilemma.

Relatedly, international migration between Russia and the near abroad has increased, in absolute numbers, the pension-aged population of the Russian Federation. According to legislation adopted shortly after the fall of the Soviet empire, citizens of the Soviet Union are technically eligible for both citizenship and access to the Russian pension system. While migration into the Russian Federation has been at levels far lower than expected, net migration figures

Table 13.1 Pension-Aged Population* in the Russian Federation, 1959–1997

	1959	1970	1979	1989	1997
% of population pension-aged	11.76%	15.38%	16.33%	18.50%	20.73%
Pension-aged population	13,827,000	19,987,000	22,436,000	27,196,000	30,500,000
Working age/pension age	4.96	3.64	3.70	3.08	2.77
Estimated coverage**	43.34	57.03	81.57	92.66	96.95
Of which:					
Urban population	10.17%	13.78%	14.70%	17.21%	19.73%
Urban pension-aged	6,264,335	11,118,658	13,958,648	18,578,111	21,175,000
Urban working/pension age	6.17	4.02	4.31	3.42	3.01
Rural population	13.52%	17.98%	19.96%	22.06%	23.44%
Rural pension-aged	7,562,464	8,868,342	8,477,897	8,617,440	9,325,000
Rural working/pension age	3.96	2.67	2.69	2.34	2.21

Sources: Rossiiskii Statisticheskii Ezhegodnik (Russian Statistical Yearbook) (Moscow, 1995); *Demograficheskii Ezhegodnik* (Demographic Yearbook) (Moscow, 1990); *Demograficheskii Ezhegodnik Rossii* (Demographic Yearbook of Russia) (Moscow, 1997).
*Pension ages are 55 years for women and 60 for men. Working age/pension age refers to the ratio of workers to pensioners.
**Estimated coverages are based on the reported number of old-age pensions received and the total population past pension age.

Table 13.2 Population Past Pension Age in the Commonwealth of Independent States, 1999

Country	Total Population	Population Past Pension Age	Percent of Population	Ratio of Working Aged to Pension Aged*
Ukraine	49,811,000	11,641,000	23.4	2.49
Belarus	10,402,000	2,231,000	21.4	2.76
Russia	146,394,000	30,270,000	20.7	2.91
Georgia	5,422,000	978,000	18.0	3.10
Moldova	4,461,000	735,000	16.5	3.59
Armenia	3,409,000	504,000	14.8	4.05
Kazakstan	16,825,000	2,174,000	12.9	4.54
Azerbaijan	7,908,000	919,000	11.6	4.85
Kirghizia	4,546,000	471,000	10.4	5.27
Tadjikistan	6,103,000	475,000	7.8	6.64
Uzbekistan	24,102,000	1,936,000	8.0	6.82
Turkmenistan	4,366,000	321,000	7.4	7.44

Sources: U.S. Census International Database, Table 094. Midyear population estimates for CIS countries. http://www.census.gov/cgi-bin/ipc/idbagg.

*Working age in this table begins at age 15 rather than age 16 due to census five-year age groupings. Pensions begin at 55 for women and 60 for men.

indicate that the population past pension age in the Russian Federation increased by 326,025 between 1993 and 1996. While the net increase for migrants past pension age (and for all migrants) into the Russian Federation has declined from the peak seen in 1994, migrant elders may present special challenges to pension provision and social support. First, migrant streams are far from homogeneous in terms of nationality composition.[21] Increased diversity among the pension-aged population brings cultural specificity and perhaps linguistic differentials into play. At worst, the interaction of nationality and demographic changes can fuel nationalistic and exclusionary concerns.[22] Additionally, the very nature of migration often separates individuals from long-standing social networks, which are especially important as individuals transit into retirement, raising the possibility that pension-aged migrants will require additional assistance to adjust to their new surroundings.

The demographic trends discussed above, with the possible exception of recent in-migration, reflect long-term developments in fertility and mortality within the Russian Federation. The pay-as-you-go structure of the Russian pension system is particularly ill suited to the rapidly aging population of the federation. Regardless of political or economic change, the Soviet pension system would by now have been faced with solvency problems. Considering the rapid and dramatic changes in economic structure and political activity, the Russian Federation faces even more serious challenges to the long-term stability of its pension system.

Economic Stability? Lacking a Strong Foundation

Since its emergence in January 1992, the Russian Federation has faced catastrophic economic conditions. Low productivity, aging infrastructure, and outdated technology, while inherited from the Soviet period, have vexed the industrial and agricultural performance of the federation. These structural factors, along with persistent difficulties relating to privatization, ownership, and accountability, stand as barriers to marketization and thwart attempts to revitalize the Russian economy.[23] Since the fall of the Soviet Union in 1991, economic and socio-demographic trends have accentuated the difficulties associated with pension provision in rural and urban areas.[24] Space here precludes a detailed discussion of the effects of the economic crisis on the pension system. This section will focus upon four specific symptoms associated with the economic transition that strongly influence the context in which the pension system operates and in which discussion of reform options takes place: unemployment, the rise in poverty, payment arrears, and the government budget crisis.

Unemployment, relatively unknown (or at least hidden) during the Soviet period, is an often-cited negative consequence of privatization and marketization in Russia. Symbolically, the existence of unemployment represents a break with previous guarantees of full employment for all. In relation to the pension system, unemployment negatively affects the absolute and relative number of contributors to the pension fund in the short term, and makes it potentially difficult for individuals to gain adequate working tenure to qualify for all but minimal pensions in the long term. Official unemployment remains relatively low, considering the high level of economic difficulties in the federation, a trend most analysts attribute to underregistration (as benefits are extremely small) and to hidden unemployment. Many individuals are in essence unemployed, but maintain ties to their enterprises in hopes of receiving past wages, believing that once they sever ties with an enterprise they are even less likely to receive back wages.[25] As such individuals are not making monthly contributions to the federal tax system (including pension transfers), it is unclear as yet how this will affect the calculation of their years of labor service.

Related to difficulties associated with unemployment, both hidden and registered, is the rising level of poverty documented in the federation in the post-Soviet period. In some regions pensioners represent as many as 80 percent of those in poverty.[26] While the calculation of the poverty line is fraught with difficulties, especially in light of high reliance on private plot production and barter, estimates show between 30 and 45 percent of the total population living on incomes below the recommended minimum standard of living. In 27 regions, according to 1995 data, the official average pension was set at a value lower than the minimum living standard for pensioners, and in Ingushetia, Tuva, Chitinskaya, Sakha, and Magadan, average pension payments were 75 percent or less of the minimum standard.[27] Pensioners suffer not only due to low pension transfers, but also as a result of overall economic difficulties that often yield family support networks incapable of assisting elders. In most cases, research indicates that pensioners, although close to or below the poverty line, often provide wealth transfers in cash and kind to impoverished adult children and their families.[28]

High poverty levels, unemployment, and inflation—chronic problems in the Russian Federation—increase the negative effect of delays in pension payments. While delays in pension provision vary by region due to increased reliance on oblast-level officials, the system as a whole was over 30.1 billion rubles behind in payments as of October 1998.[29] Both the World Bank and the International Monetary Fund have been active in recent years in attempts to clear the pension payment arrears through the use of long-term loans and credits, but arrears continue, and both pension and wage arrears appear staggering.[30] Most importantly, such outside support not only decreases the autonomy of the Russian Federation in seeking avenues of pension reform, it also delays an even larger pension crisis when loans and credits come due. On the micro-level, delays in the payment of pension transfers act to decrease the real value of pension transfers due to high inflation. While the pension fund has actively sought to index pension payments to changes in price levels (indexing every three months), it has been neither entirely successful nor popular.[31] There is also no evidence that arrears are indexed to the time of payment. Typically, they are held on account, and paid without indexation.

Unemployment, poverty, and wage and pension arrears are all symptoms of the overarching budget crisis faced by the Russian Federation, a situation that provides challenges to the pension system at many levels.[32] Budget deficits at the regional level encourage regional officials to use pension funds for maintaining other social programs, according to accusations made by President Yeltsin.[33] Regional officials charge the central government with delays in fund transfers and insufficient support.[34] At the root of the budgetary crisis is the seeming inability of the central government to collect taxes generally, and enforce contributions to the pension fund specifically. Tax collection is stymied by the persistence of wage arrears, high reliance on barter, and the inability or unwillingness to hold functioning enterprises accountable for tax payments. In July 1997, pension fund chairman Vasilii Barchuk vowed to get tough with debtor enterprises, as the pension fund was owed a total of 70 trillion rubles (approximately U.S. $12 million), but pension fund contributions from both firms and individual workers remain woefully delinquent.[35]

Separate and Unequal:
Regional Issues in Pension Provision

The process of governmental decentralization in the federation and the uneven nature of the pension burden significantly affect the collection of pension taxes in the Russian Federation when viewed from the perspective of the regions. Pension burdens are highest for the European regions of the federation, with Siberia and the Far East experiencing relatively low pension burdens. This pattern of differentiation is primarily driven by the distribution of old-age pensions. Recipients of old-age pensions are strongly concentrated in central European Russia, where in some cases they comprise over 30 percent of the total population and represent a formidable potential voting block. Related to the older population, recipients of pensions for the physically disabled are also concentrated within the central European regions of the federation. While this may be linked in part to better medical provision (and thus increased likelihood of identification and registration), this pattern is most likely driven by the age structure of the population. In highly concentrated regions, between 4 and 6 percent of the population receive some sort of *invalidi* transfers, which are divided into three levels on the basis of infirmity. By contrast, the regional distribution of pensions due to the loss of household head differs significantly from old-age and infirmity pensions. Like infirmity pensions, the proportion of the population covered is small (under 6 percent even in highly concentrated regions). These pension transfers, however, are concentrated in the regions of Siberia and the Far East, where old-age pensions and pensions for physical infirmities are relatively rare.

The picture of pension burdens is therefore highly regionalized, which in the current context of decentralization in the federation raises serious administrative difficulties. Regional (oblast) centers for the Russian pension fund exist in each oblast or republic center. Here tax receipts are balanced with tax estimates, with excesses sent to Moscow and shortfalls resulting in a request for funds from the center. The redistributive role of the central pension fund is significant. While the Far East and Siberia have few pensioners, over one-fourth of the populations in several European oblasts are pension-ers. Not surprisingly, many regions that should supposedly be donor regions are seen as reluctant to contribute pension funds to the center by pension officials in recipient oblasts.[36] This leads not only to interregional infighting, but to significant variation in the average value of pension transfers, as noted above.

Marked regional inequity and ongoing difficulties with the specific nature of federalism within Russia further complicate the context for pension reform. The emerging difficulties with tax collection, regional cooperation, pension distribution, and payment lags add to the problems inherited from the Soviet pension system. Nonetheless, the population past pension age remains reliant upon state pensions. Evidence from the 1994 micro-census indicates that government pensions are the major income source for persons past pension age, with over 80 percent of those past pension age reporting income in the form of a government old-age or service pension. Despite payment lags and declines in real value, pensions remain the cornerstone of income for the population past pension age and a valued aspect of the social contract. The extreme difficulties associated with pension provision in the federation have motivated several administrative changes to the pension system, but they have yet to significantly curtail benefits or coverage.

Pension Changes in the Russian Federation

The Russian Federation has generally maintained the social assurances set forth by the Soviet pension system, albeit at lower values and with sometimes sporadically provided transfers. Pension responsibilities of oblast-level administrators have increased, and the administrative system for collective farmers and industrial workers has merged in order to increase efficiency.[37] Even though the Russian Federation inherited a system fraught with payment difficulties, several programs have been adopted over the past eight years to expand pension system coverage and programs. First, as mentioned above, pension rights were granted to all citizens of the former Soviet Union after the breakup of the union in 1991. Second, efforts have been made to increase in-kind transfers through the development of cadres of social workers who make home visits to the elderly and physically infirm in order to provide physical assistance.

By 1995 there were 142,506 regional social-service centers in the federation, and nearly one million (904,066) Russian residents received in-home visits by social workers.[38] Third, a fourth pension category, social pensions, began to grow. The number of recipients of social pensions, intended as a minimum safety net for the very poor, grew from 990,000 in 1993 to 1,269,000 in 1997.[39] While social pensions are typically set at 25 percent of the minimum living standard, and aimed only at those at the very margins of survival, it is quite likely that they will increase in the future. Social pension recipients are concentrated along the southern tier of the federation and in the Far East, where the cost of living is highest and the economic crisis particularly sharp.

There also have been some legislative attempts to trim pension costs and increase the financial stability of the pension system. Several attempts to curb pension access, particularly for individuals still actively engaged in the labor market, have been made, although final adoption of a ban on wage income has yet to be adopted. These attempts have been reinforced by policies that correlate pension level with years of service, in an attempt to encourage pensioners to delay retirement.[40] Attempts to limit pension increases have faced strong opposition and as yet have not been codified. In spite of recent protests, pension taxes have also been raised, from one percent of individual wages to three percent, and enterprise responsibilities have also risen.[41] Such tax *increases* were met with opposition and claims from some sectors that the IMF and World Bank were at fault for the rise. No concerted attempt to increase pension ages, change the basic elements of the pay-as-you-go system of finance, or curtail pension coverage has been openly discussed.

Constrained Choices

The Russian Federation, like many Western countries, presently supports a pension system (specifically an old-age pension system) that is not financially viable in the long term. Demographic shifts have dramatically increased the number of claimants and diminished the number of contributors. While the problems associated with pension provision in the Russian Federation have a great deal in common with those of other aging countries, the economic and political crisis within Russia intensifies pension difficulties. In this chapter we have presented an overview of the demographic and economic forces challenging the stability of the pension system. At present, although thus far able to maintain wide-scale social transfers, the Russian pension system is in serious crisis. It is dependent upon resource infusions from abroad, unable to consistently disburse payments, and unable to collect pension taxes. The potential political power of old-age pensioners as a voting block and the importance of transfers from elderly parents to their adult children only intensify the risks associated with pension instability. Clearly the situation cannot continue. Yet attempts to modify the pension system in order to improve its stability have met with strong resistance.

One specific element in the strong resistance to serious pension reform in the Russian Federation can be found in the embedded ideological approach of the Soviet state toward old-age pensions. Individuals past or nearing retirement in the Russian Federation labored under a social contract guaranteeing future returns to labor in the form of old-age pensions. Not only were state pensions anticipated, but alternative investment options for retirement provision were unavailable. For workers who created savings accounts for retirement, the early financial crisis of the Russian state (monetary reform, bank failures, inflation) erased the most of the value of such holdings. Historicized expectations and an absence of alternatives increase both the symbolic role of pension transfers and their financial importance. While present programs to encourage individual retirement accounts in Russia may benefit the young, for individuals at or approaching retirement, state pension transfers remain critically important, and therefore very difficult to renegotiate.

NOTES

1. See A. Vinokurov, *Narodnoe komissia sotsialnogo obespecheniia* (Moscow: 1919).
2. Narodnoe Kommisariat Truda, *Ob ulychshenii penionnogo obespecheniia invalidnosti po sluchaiu poterikormel'tsa o po starosti,* 179 Statute 76, 23 May 1929.
3. For details on the growth of coverage patterns during the development of the pension system see Cynthia Buckley, "Obligations and Expectations: Renegotiating Pensions in the Russian Federation," *Continuity and Change* 13, no. 3 (1998): 317–338.
4. *Narodnoe khoziastvo SSR* (Moscow: 1990).

5. Linda Evans and John Williamson, "Old Age Dependency in Historical Perspective," *International Journal of Aging and Human Development* 27, no. 2 (1988): 75–80; and also Jill Quadagno, *Aging in Industrial Society* (New York: Academic Press, 1972).

6. See N. N. Simonova, ed., *Netrudosposobnoe naselenie v perekhodnii period* (Moscow: Russian Academy of Sciences, 1998), 18.

7. *Narodnoe komissia sotsialnogo obespecheniia, sotsialnoe obespechenie za 5 let* (Moscow, 1923).

8. *Pensii po gosudarstvennomy sotsialnomy strakhovaniiu* (Moscow, 1948), 28–42.

9. See, for example, "V Stalinskii podkhod za uluchshenie sotsobespecheniia," *Sotsial'noe obespechenie*, no. 12 (1932): 3–5. In nearly every issue of the journal between 1932 and 1974, a story of the efforts made on a specific collective farm to provide opportunities and assistance to individuals in the three pension categories appears.

10. The 14 July 1956 statute can be found in *Sotsialnoe obespechenie v Sovetskoi Rossii: sbornik ofitsial'nikh materialov* (Moscow: 1962), 7–12.

11. Buckley, "Obligations and Expectations," 319.

12. See *Sotsial'noe polozhenie i uroven' zhizni naseleniia Rossii: ofitsial'noe izdanie* (Moscow: Goskomstat Rossii, 1998), 228. Other pension categories include social pensions devoted to the very poor, and service pensions (a form of old-age pension with lower age and tenure requirements often associated with dangerous or strategically important work).

13. *Sotsialnoe obespechenie v Sovetskoi Rossii: sbornik ofitsial'nikh materialov* (Moscow: 1962), 7–12.

14. E. M. Andreev, L. E. Darskii and T. L. Khar'kova, *Demograficheskaya istoriia Rossii: 1927–1959* (Moscow: Informatika, 1998).

15. See V. Shapiro, *Sotsial'naia aktivnost' pozhilykh liudei v SSSR* (Moscow: Izdatel'stvo, 1983); and M. Sonin and A. Dyskin, *Pozhuliiu chelovek v semi i obshchestve* (Moscow: Finansi i statistiki, 1984).

16. See P. M. Margieva, *Sotsial'naya zashita invalidov: normativnie aky i dokumenty* (Moscow: 1994). Pensions for individuals with physical infirmities were oriented toward financial assistance and compensation for family members providing care. Few programs, either historically or presently, focused on the integration of the physically challenged into society generally or the work force specifically. For more information, see the chapter by Ethel Dunn in this volume.

17. For example, see the discussion on women pensioners in V. E. Gordon, *Chem starost' obespechim* (Moscow: Mysl', 1988); and Shapiro, *Sotsial'naia aktivnost'*.

18. V. D. Arkhipov, *Pensii kolkhoznikam* (Moscow: 1996), 3–16.
19. An exception is found in Latvia, which has begun a shift to individual retirement accounts in response to encouragement from the World Bank and IMF. Michael Wyzan, "Latvia leads way on pension reform," RFE/RL report, 30 September 1997, available at *http://search.rferl.org/newsline/1997/09/300997.html*
20. Buckley, "Obligations and Expectations." See also the chapter by Velkoff and Kinsella in this volume.
21. Cynthia Buckley, "Exodus?: Out-Migration From the Central Asian Successor States to the Russian Federation," *Central Asian Monitor,* no. 3 (1996): 16–22.
22. A. G. Vishnevskii, "Demograficheskie izmeneniia i natsionalizm," *Sotsiologicheskii zhurnal,* no. 1 (1994): 22–34.
23. Clifford G. Gaddy and Barry W. Ickes, "A Simple Four-Sector Model of Russia's 'Virtual Economy,'" Center for Social and Economic Dynamics, The Brookings Institution, May 1998.
24. C. Buckley and W. Hickenbottom, "Taxation Possibilities for Elderly Support in Rural Russia," *Comparative Economic Studies* 37, no. 1 (Spring 1995): 19–37.
25. *Izvestiya,* 26 May 1999, 3, states that only 10 of Russia's 89 administrative regions did *not* report wage arrears (meaning 79 were behind in payment). Summary reported in RFE/RL report, 14 June 1999.
26. N. M. Pavlova, "Dinamika urov'nia bednosti v sem'iakh pensionerov," in Simonova, *Netrudosposobnoe naselenie,* 66–77.
27. *Uroven' zhizni naseleniia Rossii* (Moscow: Goskomstat, 1996): 68–73.
28. See Thomas A. Mroz and Barry Popkin, "Poverty and the Economic Transition in the Russian Federation," *Economic Development and Cultural Change* 44, no. 1 (1995): 1–31; and Buckley, "Obligations and Expectations." During the Soviet period, pension transfers were relatively generous, and downward wealth transfers (from elders to adult children) were the norm, a pattern that appears resistant to short-term change.
29. See RFE/RL reports 2, vol.1, no. 14, June 1999. Deputy Prime Minister Matvienko claimed that by May of 1998 arrears had fallen by half, to 16.5 billion rubles. As did many of her predecessors, she vowed to eradicate the payment debt.
30. Robert Lyle, "Russia, IMF, World Bank Financing to Clear Pension Arrears," RFE/RL report 30, April 1997.
31. See RFE/RL report, 10 July 1998. In addition to raising individual contributions to the pension fund, Deputy Prime Minister Oleg Sysuev called for the end of pension indexation. While not adopted at that time, it remains a potential policy option.

32. See N. Shemlev, "Kriszis vnyutri kriszisa," *Voprosy ekonomiki,* no. 10 (1998): 4–17.

33. See RFE/RL report, 27 June 1997, available at http://search.rferl.org/newsline/1997/06/270697.html. In a radio address to pensioners, Yeltsin vowed to pursue ruthlessly regional officials who had misused pension funds, in a clear attempt to shift blame away from the central government concerning pension arrears.

34. Buckley, "Obligations and Expectations."

35. See RFE/RL report, 27 June 1997.

36. L. H. Zhukova, manager of the Vladimir Oblast Pension Fund, interview by author, November 1995, Vladimir, Russia; and V. N. Babaev, manager of the Nizhni Novgorod Pension Fund, interview by author, Nizhni Novgorod, January 1996.

37. See Buckley, "Obligations and Expectations."

38. *Sotsial'noe obespechenie,* no 7 (1995): 9.

39. *Sotsial'noe polozhenie,* 1998, 212. See also E. N. Yakovleva, ed., *Rossiia–1997: Sotsial'no-demograficheskiia situatsiia* (Moscow: 1998).

40. See RFE/RL report, available at http://search.rferl.org/newsline/1997/12/221297.html.

41. See RFE/RL newsline, 22 July 1998, available at http://search.rferl.org/newsline/1998/07/1-RUS/rus percent2D220798.html.

CHAPTER 14

The Social Crisis of
the Russian Military

Deborah Yarsike Ball

Introduction

THE RUSSIAN MILITARY, LIKE RUSSIA AS A WHOLE, is experiencing a
systemic crisis. Historically, the military was a favored institution
that was given tremendous resources and enjoyed a position of
high status in society. It was used as an instrument of youth socialization and uplift. Today it is no longer favored and has few
resources at its disposal, but the need to socialize youth is greater
than ever before. The military, because of institutional inertia, still
sees the task of socializing youth as its mission, but it is incapable
of handling even its own social problems, let alone addressing and
ameliorating those of society's younger generation. In fact, the
military exacerbates the very social problems it believes it should
address.

This chapter will first examine the many social ills prevalent in
the Russian military as well as the extent to which the military's status in society has plummeted. The military's role as a socializing
agent in Soviet times will then be reviewed in order to understand
how the Russian military views its socialization role today. A spiritual crisis has enveloped Russian society, and the military believes
that it is the best institution to address this crisis. The military, however, needs to undergo thorough reform itself and reestablish its re-
spectability in society before it can contemplate having a positive
role in socializing Russian youth.

The Social Ills of the Russian Military

One of the major problems confronting the Russian military is that it is subject to the same social ills that afflict the rest of society, including poor health care, drug abuse, sexually transmitted diseases, housing shortages, poorly educated youth, crime, and wage arrears.

Health Issues

The health problems prevalent in Russia obviously affect the military as well. Although many young people are dodging the draft, those who do serve are largely unfit for military service. In fact, recent statistics reveal that almost half of those drafted are not fit for military service for health reasons.[1] Civilian and military physicians alike must work with limited resources. The military recognizes that healthy personnel are a key component of combat readiness, but it is operating in a larger environment that lacks the basic requirements for good health: quality water is not available in all the regions of the Russian Federation, food is frequently contaminated, and heat and electricity are often turned off because of insufficient funds. The defense ministry is attempting to address these problems and has issued a Military Order to improve the level of preventive health care in order to stop problems before they become serious. The Order directs officers to ensure that servicemen are provided with clean living conditions, healthy and noncontaminated meals, baths and basic laundry services, and other basic household amenities.[2] The military claims that "the medical service has stepped up its information analysis, tightened monitoring functions, and started to work even more closely with offices of the procuracy in light of [the Order's] requirements." The evidence indicates that the military has a long way to go to improve conditions for Russian servicemen, and given its budget constraints, it is difficult to envision improvements in the foreseeable future.

The military has seen a dramatic increase in the number of its personnel requiring serious treatment for ailments such as cardiovascular disease and malignant tumors. The number of oncological illnesses has risen at military medical institutions to 23,000 patients/year. But the military is a mirror of the larger society in which it resides: "One out of five Russian inhabitants suffer from cancer in one form or another."[3]

The number of cases of tuberculosis (TB) has doubled in the armed forces from only a few years back. In response, the Main Military Medical Directorate (GVMU) has developed a six-year program to combat TB in the army. The goal of this program is to reduce the rate of illness by 10 percent annually. The goal of reducing TB by 10 percent suggests that the military is using the same type of vaccine that is otherwise used only in underdeveloped countries. Given limited resources, in particular the availability of needles, it is questionable whether the military will be able to achieve its objective of reducing the rate of illness in servicemen by even 10 percent.[4]

Psychiatric disorders have also increased among servicemen. In the last two years alone there has been a 30 percent increase in such disorders among soldiers and noncommissioned officers, and a 19 percent increase among officers. Among the central causes given for such problems are the stressful state of conditions for families trying to make ends meet in Russia as well as alcohol and drug addiction. Most astounding is the report that suicides accounted for 27 percent of all military fatalities in 1998.[5] Conscripts commit more suicides (60 percent) than officers and warrant officers (40 percent),[6] but the number is quite large for both groups. These are astonishing statistics that would never be tolerated in a developed nation.

Despite the enormity of this problem, the recommended response is typical of the old Soviet approach. The chief of the Main Military Medical Directorate of the Russian Ministry of Defense, Colonel-General Ivan Chizh, suggests supplementing "assistance to those suffering from psychiatric disorders" with more comprehensive measures, such as having the military press publish articles that will "instill [vospitanie] moral and psychological stability in the servicemen."[7] Chizh apparently does not comprehend the enormity nor the cause of the problem. Needless to say, less exhortation and more attention to solving the underlying causes of the problem would be a more effective means of ameliorating the servicemen's plight. For instance, improving the economic condition of military personnel and their families, eliminating hazing in the barracks, and providing proper clothing and food would go a long way toward improving the mental health of military personnel.

Drug Abuse

Drug abuse is an enormous problem in Russia. The number of drug users has increased roughly 250 percent between 1993 and 1998. In the past ten years, there has been a twelve-fold increase in the number of deaths attributed to drug abuse, and the number of drug-related deaths among children "increased by a factor of 42."[8] Young people between the ages of 18 and 25 years comprise 80 percent of the drug addicts, and it is precisely this age group from which people are called to serve in the military. Drugs appear to have replaced alcohol as the first-choice substance of abuse. According a recent report, "the number of children who are addicted to narcotics is six times more than the number of the persons in the same age group who drink alcoholic beverages."[9]

The rate and scale of the spread of narcotics in Russia point to an epidemic, and the military has not been able to shield itself from this nefarious activity. Statistics about criminal activities indicate that more than half of the soldiers apprehended with drugs in their possession began to use them for the first time during their military service.[10] The Russian defense ministry's main newspaper notes that drug use in the military reflects the drug problem throughout Russian society. "Despite the tightening of measures to keep 'pot lovers' out of the draft, their penetration into the army ranks continues."[11] The military's claim that it has tried to keep drug addicts out of the army is disingenuous. First, it admits to not having a system to identify the addicts and root them out.[12] At the same time, the military acknowledges that it conscripts teenagers even if there are many needle marks on their arms: "if a person has pricked veins, that still is not a reason to reject him or her for military service." Unless it can prove that the youth in question is an addict rather than a casual drug user, the military conscripts him.[13]

The problem of drug use in the military is of great concern. Entrusting weapons to possible addicts places at risk the safety of society at large. Of even greater concern is whether drug addicts have penetrated the ranks of the Strategic Missile Troops, the branch that contains the nation's nuclear weapons, or the 12th GUOMO, the directorate that controls the nuclear weapons' launch codes.

AIDS and Other Sexually Transmitted Diseases

The number of servicemen believed to be HIV positive has increased in the Russian Armed Forces. Until recently the military has been reluctant to discuss the issue, asserting that there were no cases of AIDS in the military. But a recent article on drug use acknowledges that the prevalence of AIDS has increased in the past three to four years because the increase in drug addiction has aggravated the spread of AIDS through the use of shared needles. Thus far, the army has admitted only to having servicemen who have tested positive for the HIV infection rather than AIDS itself, because military policy is to discharge personnel from service once they start manifesting the symptoms of AIDS.[14]

The military has been reluctant to talk about other sexually transmitted diseases (STDs), but given the rapid increase in STDs in Russia, the military cannot be immune to this problem. One reason for the increase in STDs is the prevalence of prostitution, which was prohibited in the Soviet era and thus was not as widespread as at present. Venereal disease has become so threatening that the Ministry of Health recently announced that it would not object to the legalization of prostitution so that it could work with a trade union in the industry to develop health standards. The military's reluctance to address this issue directly is unfortunate, because this is one area where, if given the resources, it could positively impact Russian youth. In a recent interview, the chief public health physician of the Ministry of Defense provided no statistics but only said that there has been a notable growth in syphilis as well as a number of other diseases.[15] Similarly, the head of the military medical directorate would only say that syphilis and AIDS became a problem in Russia not too long ago and that "it is hard for the army to construct an 'iron curtain' around them."[16] The military is currently providing a sanctuary for young people rather than taking a more aggressive stance and directly confronting the problem of AIDS and STDs.

Hazing

The Russian military leadership at times seems baffled over the large number of youths who avoid military service as well as the large number of deserters. They claim that "Russian citizens have lost their sense of responsibility for the country's safety" and that rather than encouraging youths to join the military, "it has become fashionable 'to save the boys from the horrors of the barracks.'"[17] The practices that take place in the barracks are indeed horrific. The practice of *dedovshchina,* or bullying and hazing, is routine in the Russian military. *Dedovshchina* encompasses much more brutality than the usual fraternal practice of humiliating the incoming class by having them clean toilet stalls, run outside without clothes, consume great quantities of alcohol, and possibly even endure some paddling. Boys are beaten up with fists and shovels and often require hospitalization. Rape is not an uncommon occurrence. The treatment is so ignominious that many cannot cope and commit suicide. Having heard intimate details of the practice of *dedovshchina,* other youths undertake extreme measures, including self-mutilation, to avoid military service.

The practice of *dedovshchina* began in 1967 with the introduction of a new law on military service.[18] Conscripts were to serve three years instead of four in the navy, and two years rather than three in the other branches of the military. In addition, annual induction into the military was replaced by a semiannual call-up that made available a fresh batch of raw recruits every six months. The reduction in service time undermined the training and development of a strong professional noncommissioned officer corps that oversaw order in the barracks. What emerged was a system whereby senior conscripts established control of the barracks through the process of physical brutality. Ironically, when the fresh recruits became the *stariki* (seniors) in the barracks, they adopted precisely the same brutal tactics as their predecessors. In the end, the senior Russian officer corps bears the blame for allowing this method of control to be adopted in the military. When junior officers complained, they received a demerit in their files for being unable to control the troops under their command. Needless to say, reporting on the brutality quickly stopped.

What appears to be a new phenomenon in the post-Soviet era is that the practice of *dedovshchina* is being conducted not merely by the conscripts but by officers. In one instance, lieutenants' "brains, inflamed by alcohol, suggested the only option for solving all their problems—it was necessary to beat up their subordinates. . . . As a result, six men were severely beaten up." In another instance, an officer serving in the Caucasus "slammed [a private's] neck so hard that he fractured the kid's laryngeal cartilage."[19]

Housing and Salary

A social contract that guaranteed officers housing, wages, and medical care for their families, as well as a pension, existed between the Soviet military and the state. These benefits were expected to continue for Russian officers in the post-Soviet era. Russian officers have inherited the legal right to these same benefits, but unfortunately, this right exists primarily on paper. Officers go for months without receiving their wages, and often the money they do receive is inadequate to support their families. One reason the money is insufficient is that there is not enough housing for the officers' families, and an officer has to pay rent if he is even sufficiently lucky to find an apartment. A survey I conducted in the summer of 1995 of 600 Russian field-grade officers in 12 regions of Russia revealed that the majority of officers (67 percent) were dissatisfied with military service. When asked how they viewed the overall economic situation in Russia at the time, 93 percent viewed it as very bad or fairly bad. Perhaps more significantly, when the officers were asked whether their material well-being—a phrase that encompasses salary, health care, housing, and other benefits discussed above—would have been better if the Soviet Union still existed, three-fourths of the officers said they would indeed have been better off in the old system. One-fifth of the officers believed their material well-being would have been the same. Unfortunately, four years later, these figures probably remain dismal, because many officers today are destitute, with little hope for improvement, whereas in 1995 there was still some hope of economic progress in the not-too-distant future.[20]

The result is an enormous shortage of young officers in the military, as many of the best young officers have left: "They are tired of roaming from one place of service to another, and of bad housing conditions, and are lured by good prospects and better payment in commercial and other civilian structures."[21] For those officers who remain, the impact on the military is equally dire. As a result of their economic plight, these officers are compelled to seek additional work outside the military (in addition to engaging in illegal activities, which will be discussed below). The ramifications of this pattern cannot be underestimated. There can be no order in a military where situations prevail in which an officer, moonlighting as a taxi driver, picks up one of his sergeants who can afford the ride as a result of illegal activities in which he is engaged. Combat effectiveness and morale are diminished when the officer spends his time thinking about how to raise money to feed his family rather than focusing on military matters. Chaos reigns in the barracks because there is no one present to hold the troops accountable. Accordingly, the professionalism of the armed forces is thoroughly undermined.

The standard of living for conscripts has also declined precipi-
tously. Soldiers frequently live in old, condemned buildings that are
on the verge of collapse. For example, in one building there was one
toilet available for 94 men, whereas military regulations require that
one be available for every 12 servicemen.[22] As the men waited in
line, fights would erupt. The dietary situation is also pathetic. The
soldiers' diet often consists of little more than broth and bread.

Education Level of Military Conscripts

The general education level of the military manpower pool "has no-
ticeably declined," according to Lieutenant-Colonel Vladimir
Skubayev, chief of the professional-psychological selection group of
the Serpukhov Military Institute of Missile Troops. Skubayev further laments that Russian youth have in-depth knowledge of "cheap
literature" and popular Western films, but are disappointingly igno-
rant of great Russian writers: "The heroes of Yumatov and Lanov
from 'Officers' have been replaced by the American 'Rambo.'"
Skubayev attributes this fact to the weakness of the military-patriotic indoctrination program that was pervasive in the Soviet Union.
"We stopped popularizing military service, lost the halo of roman-
ticism around our officers, with a single mark of a pen destroyed the
organized systems of initial [beginning] military training tested
through the years in schools."[23] According to general staff data,
only 3 percent of the spring 1998 conscripts had completed any
higher education. More significant (and astonishing), only 3.6 percent had completed primary education.[24] A military with such a low
level of education among its conscripts will never constitute an effective fighting force nor be a school of upbringing.

Crime

Crime is an enormous problem in the military, and it is not bounded
by rank. From the top generals to the conscripts, crime is rampant.
Embezzlement is common, and includes the sale of weapons, muni-
tions, and any other property. Military personnel sell stinger-type
weapons, air-to-ground missiles, tanks, planes—basically anything
that can be moved. Even honest officers condone the behavior because they often have no other means to pay their staffs. Organized
crime has penetrated the armed forces, and former army officers are

apparently prominent in various mafia organizations as well.[25] The minister of defense, Igor Sergeev, admitted that in 1997 roughly 18,000 officers were charged with criminal activity. The activities and behavior of senior officers have been particularly bad. They not only inappropriately use conscripts to build dachas for themselves, but have developed businesses where they profit by using conscripts to build dachas for others. In the early half of the 1990s, 300 generals built dachas in the suburbs of Moscow using military conscripts and stolen material.[26] Prior to becoming defense minister, General Lev Rokhlin publicized corruption among his fellow flag officers. Among the many cases he discussed was the disappearance of $23 million received by the defense ministry's budget chief, Vasili Vorobev, from the sale of ammunition to Bulgaria.[27] To date, no charges have been brought against Vorobev.

Much of the increase in the crime rate can be attributed to the new culture of drug use. The number of crimes that were committed by soldiers who were using drugs increased three-fold between 1996 and 1998.[28] In addition, once soldiers are hooked on drugs, they need to steal to support their habit.

Wage Arrears

One of the military's most lamentable practices has been its failure to pay its people. The problem of wage arrears has resulted not so much from insufficient funds coming from Moscow. Rather, upon receiving the troops' salaries, senior officers take the cash fund and invest it to make a quick profit. They then turn around six months after having "borrowed" the money, and pay military personnel their long-awaited wages. In some cases, of course, the profit has been lost and along with it the soldier's wages. Needless to say, such practices have led to a severe decline in the prestige of the Russian military.

Loss of Prestige in the Military

In the Soviet era, the high prestige of the military in society contributed to its ability to serve as the moral educator of youth. But the military is no longer a hallowed and respected institution. The glory of saving the country from the Nazis in World War II is no longer enough to sustain its honored place in society. Gone are the days when the military commanded the lion's share of the state budget, when its accomplishments—real and contrived—were ritualistically lionized by an adoring state-controlled press, and when it enjoyed official status as a key socializing agent for society's youth. Today, Russia's military has its power shut off because it cannot pay its bills. It is portrayed as weak and ineffective by the press. And, while it claims an important role in combating various social ills and educating youth, it is in fact exacerbating these very problems.

As if this were not enough, the military's international prestige has declined as well. The mighty superpower that competed with the United States is no longer considered even a great power by many in Russian society. Even the vast majority of Russian field-grade officers (80 percent) do not view the military as a superpower equal to the United States.[29] Yet restoration of that superpower status is extremely important to most (83 percent) of the officer corps.

The decline in the military's status in recent times has undermined its ability to serve as a role model and educator of youth. Unfortunately, unless change is imposed from the outside, institutions rarely have sufficient insight or desire to change their methods of operation. As a result, the Russian military is still pursuing the Soviet approach to addressing its problems.

To fully understand the military's role today in educating youth and combating social problems, it is important first to understand what was meant by education in the Soviet context. The Russian political and military leadership, like its Soviet predecessor, views education as a means of imbuing youth with a sense of moral responsibility. But more than education is required to deal with the many social ills afflicting Russian youth and by extension the military.

The Soviet Era

The primary purpose of education in the Soviet Union was to inculcate the citizenry with the values of the regime and to mobilize it to work toward the goals delineated by the leadership. Lenin maintained that "the old schools provided purely book knowledge," whereas "the entire purpose of training, educating and teaching the youth of today should be to imbue them with communist ethics."[30]

In other words, education in the Soviet Union was first and fore-most a process of socialization, or *vospitanie,* to use the Russian term. The Soviet Union placed great emphasis on *vospitanie,* and the military was a key institution responsible for instilling the nation's youth with proper values.[31]

In fact, in creating an effective fighting force, the Soviet military, in contrast to western militaries, accorded comparatively greater im-portance to socializing soldiers than to training them. Soviet mili-tary thought maintained that moral and political superiority would be the ultimate factors determining success on the battlefield. To be sure, training was important, but proper upbringing [*vospitanie*] would give the Soviet military an important edge vis-à-vis its adver-saries. At the same time, the military emphasized the importance of upbringing not only to ensure its combat superiority, but because as an institution through which the vast majority of young Soviet men passed, it was a means of achieving political indoctrination. Officers were "not only commanders . . . but teachers participating in edu-cational and upbringing work in the full sense of the word."[32] Offi-cers were given the task of being moral educators and transmitting good social values to youth, for this was the last opportunity for the leadership to reach out to youth and indoctrinate them with the regime's values.

At the end of the Soviet era, when communism was being dis-credited under glasnost—Gorbachev's policy of openness that per-mitted greater freedom of the press and personal expression—the military was one of the few remaining organizations with enough le-gitimacy to reach out to youth and provide them with moral guid-ance. During the waning days of the Soviet Union, there was much discussion about the lack of spirituality (*dukhovnost'*) in society, and the leadership was grappling for something to replace commu-nist ideology and its utopic promises of a glorious future. In two speeches alone, Gorbachev referred to "spiritual renewal," "spiri-tual potential," "spiritual life," "spiritual enrichment," "spiritual values," "spiritual sphere," "spiritual culture," "spiritual immobil-ity," "spiritual richness," "spiritual progress of society," "spiritual development," "spiritual experience," and "spiritual deadend."[33] As these many references indicate, spirituality was a complex term with varied meanings that depended on the context in which it was used. It was not, however, intended to convey the ecclesiastical sense of the word as it is usually used in the West, but rather to convey a sense of morality and the need for a higher level of guidance to be good citizens.

Russia Today

Given the present state of Russian society, it is hardly surprising that the notion of a spiritual crisis has gained wide currency. And although the Russian educational establishment, of course, no longer focuses on imbuing youth with communist ethics, the notion of teaching youth how to be better citizens and instilling them with a sense of morality and spirituality, of giving them more than "book knowledge," remains a strong component in Russian thinking today.

Promoting the military as an educational institution is contrary to Western liberal practices. The West historically has been suspicious of its military, viewing it not only as a defender against outside aggression, but also as a potential internal threat to democratic rule. To be sure, in the West the military is viewed by some as capable of "making men out of boys," or having a positive impact on race relations. These successes, however, are viewed more as a byproduct than as the goal of the organization. This is not the case in Russia.

In fact, the Russian leadership's policy is similar to the old Soviet approach of relying heavily on the military to provide youth with a moral upbringing, albeit with a different content. As the new Russian state struggles to adopt democratic modes of operation, it does not have many tools at hand to cope with inevitable challenges and tends to rely on the Soviet approach to dealing with social issues. Just as people tend to operate according to the procedures to which they are accustomed, the Russian system is still very much Soviet from a social perspective.

In 1993, the Russian government approved the *Basic Provision of the Military Doctrine of the Russian Federation,* the first reformulation of military doctrine since the demise of the Soviet Union.[34] The document assessed vital military issues such as whence the major threat would most likely emanate. But, as in Soviet times, the *Basic Provision* outlined an unrealistically expansive view of the role of the military in society. A document focusing on military doctrine repeatedly stressed the importance of military-patriotic education and predraft training for high school–age youth, and measures to raise the military's prestige in society, improve the education of servicemen, and ensure cooperation between the high command on the one hand and state, public, and religious organizations on the other. The Russian political leadership, just like its Soviet predecessor, views the military as an important mechanism for educating youth and instilling in them a moral code.

Interestingly, the *Basic Provision* does not use the term "spirituality" in its analysis. In the early days of the Russian regime the future looked bright, and the notion of an emerging spiritual crisis did not appear on the horizon. However, by the time Russia published its *National Security Concept of the Russian Federation* in 1997, it was clear that a spiritual crisis was in the making and that overcoming it was vital to the nation's security. The *National Security Concept* draws numerous links between the nation's security and preservation of "spiritual traditions and norms of social life."[35] The military correctly picked up on this theme in its analysis of the document and noted that the "absence of a spiritual basis capable of uniting society is strongly felt."[36]

A recent round-table discussion on training-indoctrination (*vospitanie*) work in the military academies noted its importance for the training of a young officer.[37] Examples of such upbringing work include having military students conduct military assemblies with local school children and work with disadvantaged families in a sports camp. According to the military, what is important is not the number of events, but that they be conducted "with spirit" rather than in a formal, mechanistic manner. The argument is made that spiritual work is as important to one's well-being as food. If people go to the event "with pleasure," then the military "is involved in a business that is no less important than sowing or harvesting."

The commander in chief of the Strategic Missile Forces, Colonel-General Vladimir Yakovlev, noted that the military educational institutes had to prepare students for the twenty-first century by providing them with specialties in nuclear weapons, electronics, cybernetics, and the use of missiles, including weapons of the next century such as the modern "Topol." But equally important, he said, was "to strive to instill [*vospitat'*] in the students patriotism and high moral qualities, and to raise their intellect and culture."[38] "Our graduates are entrusted with the nuclear missile shield of the nation, and only a person with a firm moral foundation and ethical principles is able to understand the whole depth of responsibility lying on his shoulders." Yakovlev goes on to say that "it is possible to teach a student to work on equipment and prepare good specialists. But, without a special spiritual temperament, if you like, a 'missile character,' a true officer will not turn out from him."

In fact, the military has begun a general campaign to convince the media and cultural figures to portray the military in a positive light because "the minds of young people are being filled with notions wherein the people's spiritual values have been eroded."[39] An article in *Krasnaia zvezda* noted that "the state is not in a position to fully withstand the destruction of cultural traditions, and many of the mass media, primarily television and radio, are forming a negative image of the country's present and past and the life of servicemen."[40] An assessment of the situation in the barracks reveals that the media's portrayal of the military is largely correct. The Russian military, in an era of limited finances, is relying on the old Soviet technique of using propaganda and education [*vospitanie*] to lift morale and convince youth to work more diligently and to care about themselves and their country. Given the dismal state of the Russian military, much more will be needed.

Conclusion

Nothing less than a complete transformation will enable the military to command the respect it once held in Soviet society. The military exacerbates numerous social problems and is driving youth away from this previously revered institution. Some in the military are working to adopt rules so that officers are not punished if they report hazing in the barracks. This move could be a first step toward eliminating *dedovshchina* as a priority for the military. It would not require a large infusion of money into the system. Until the military accepts that it must institute fundamental reforms, and begins to carry them out, it will not only fail to win the hearts and minds of the nation's youth but also contribute to the further deterioration of their social condition.

NOTES

This work was performed under the auspices of the U.S. Department of Energy by Lawrence Livermore National Laboratory under contract no. W-7405-Eng–48. The views expressed herein are those of the author and not those of LLNL of the U.S. government.

1. Roy Medvedev, "Will the 'Military Opposition' Enter the Kremlin Uninvited?" *Rabochaia Tribuna* (Moscow), 21 March 1998, translated in *Foreign Broadcast Information Service (FBIS)*, 26 March 1998. For an excellent overview of the health problems afflicting Russia's youth, see Murray Feshbach, "What a Tangled Web We Weave: Child Health in Russia and its Future," written for SAIC, Inc., July 1998.

2. The Russian Federation Minister of Defense Order (1996) on "Sanitary and Epidemiological Oversight in the Armed Forces of the Russian Federation" is discussed in Petr Altunin and Ivan Ivaniuk, "Voennaia meditsina obsluzhivaet bolee 6 millionov patsientov, no ee glavnyi prioritet—meditsina voiskovaia," *Krasnaia zvezda,* 4 June 1999, 1.

3. Petr Altunin and Ivan Ivaniuk, "Voennaia meditsina obsluzhivaet bolee 6 millionov patsientov, no ee glavnyi prioritet—meditsina voiskovaia," *Krasnaia zvezda,* 4 June 1999, 1.

4. Altunin and Ivaniuk, "Voennaia meditsina," 1.

5. Altunin and Ivaniuk, "Voennaia meditsina," 1.

6. Aleksandr Ovchinnikov, "Statistics and Basic Trends of Suicide in the Russian Armed Forces," *Noviye Izvestia,* 12 March 1998, translated in *Current Digest of the Post-Soviet Press (CDPSP)* 50, no. 13 (1998): 13.

7. Altunin and Ivaniuk, "Voennaia meditsina," 1.

8. All the figures in this paragraph are taken from "Drug Abuse in Russia: A Threat to the Nation," *Rossiiskaia gazeta,* 3 March 1998, 3, translated in *CDPSP* 50, no. 10 (1998): 1.

9. Irina Zhirnova, "U opasnoi cherty," *Krasnaia zvezda,* 8 July 1999, 1.

10. Zhirnova, 1.

11. Altunin and Ivaniuk, 1.

12. Altunin and Ivaniuk, 1.

13. Zhirnova, 1.

14. Zhirnova, 2.

15. Dmitrii Iurov, "Predupredit' bolezni legche . . . ," *Krasnaia zvezda,* 25 May 1999, 4.

16. Altunin and Ivaniuk, 1.

17. V. M. Zakharov, "Military Education in Russia: How to Reform It?" *Military Thought* 6 (April 1997): 48.

18. I am grateful to Lieutenant-Colonel Dmitri Trenin, deputy director of the Carnegie Moscow Center, for explaining the origins of *dedovshchina* to me. Lt.-Col. Trenin served in the Soviet and Russian military from 1972 to 1993.

19. "Boys Beaten Up By Seniors and Fathers Too. By Their Commanders," *Komsomolskaia Pravda*, 5 March 1998, translated in *FBIS*, 6 March 1998.

20. For a more complete discussion of the Ball survey, see Deborah Yarsike Ball, "The Unreliability of the Russian Officer Corps: Reluctant Domestic Warriors," *Jane's Intelligence Review* 8 (May 1996); and Deborah Yarsike Ball and Theodore Gerber, "The Political Views of Russian Field-Grade Officers," *Post-Soviet Affairs* 12 (April-June 1996).

21. Zakharov, "Military Education in Russia," 48.

22. Pavel Anokhin, "A 'Division of Deserters' Is on the Run," *Rossiiskie vesti*, 26 December 1997, translated in *CDPSP* 50, no. 1 (1998): 15.

23. "Raketchik XXI veka: kakim emu byt'?" *Krasnaia zvezda*, 8 June 1999, 2.

24. Ilya Bulavinov, "Draft Contingent Is Limited—Intellectually," *Kommersant-Daily*, 7 October 1998, translated in *Current Digest of the Post-Soviet Press* 50, no. 40 (1998): 19.

25. Chris Donnelly, "Prospects for Reform of the Russian Armed Forces," 30 July 1999, unpublished manuscript.

26. John M. Kramer, "The Politics of Corruption," *Current History* 97 (October 1998): 331.

27. Richard F. Staar, "Russia's Military: Corruption in the Higher Ranks," *Perspective* 9 (November-December 1998).

28. Zhirnova, 2.

29. This is taken from the Ball survey, May-July 1995.

30. V. I. Lenin, "The Tasks of the Youth Leagues," 2 October 1920, in *V. I. Lenin Selected Works* (New York: International Publishers, 1971), 609, 613 respectively.

31. For a more complete discussion of the military's role as a socializing agent, see Deborah Yarsike Ball, "The High Politics of Soviet Socialization Policy: A Comparison of Civil-Military Relations Under Khrushchev and Gorbachev" (Ph.D. diss., University of Michigan, 1994), 61–83.

32. A. V. Barabanshchikov, *Pedagogicheskie osnovy obucheniia sovetskikh voinov* (Moscow: Voenizdat, 1962), 5.

33. M. S. Gorbachev, "O khode realizatsii reshenii XXVII s'ezda KPSS i zadachakh po uglubleniiu perestroiki," 28 June 1988, in *Izbrannye rechi i stat'i*, (Moscow: Politizdat, 1988); "Revoliutsionnoi perestroike—ideologiiu obnovleniia," 18 February 1988, also in *Izbrannye rechi i stat'I*, 6:70–72.

34. "Voennaia doktrina Rossii," *Rossiiskie vesti*, 18 November 1993, 1–2.

35. "Kontseptsiia natsional'noi bezopasnosti Rossiiskoi Federatsii," *Krasnaia zvezda* 27 December 1997, 4.

36. "Rossiia gotova otstaivat' svoi interesy," *Krasnaia zvezda* 27 December 1997, 1.
37. "Raketchikh XXI veka: Kakim emu byt'?" *Krasnaia zvezda*, 8 June 1999, 2.
38. "Kommentarii glavnokomanduiushchego RVSN general-polkovnika Vladimira Iakovleva," *Krasnaia zvezda*, 8 June 1999, 2.
39. Vladimir Kaushanskii, "Otzovites', deiateli kul'tury! 'Kul'tura i bezopasnost' otechestva'," *Krasnaia zvezda*, 6 March 1998, 3.
40. Kaushanskii, 3.

PART III

Replacing the Safety Net?

CHAPTER 15

U.S. Foreign Assistance to the Russian Federation for Medicine and Health

Edward J. Burger, Jr.

TECHNICAL ASSISTANCE FOR HEALTH AND SOCIAL WELFARE for Russia—indeed, for all of the former Soviet republics—has been a much less well-conceived and -supported effort than was characteristic of earlier counterparts. Political support has been inconsistent. Its several parts cannot be said to adhere to an overall set of goals and strategies. What follows is a brief review of the major components of U.S. technical assistance for the Russian federation for health and medicine since 1991. Two examples of earlier, highly successful health-related foreign assistance programs are described for the purpose of extracting some principles. Following this is a summary of the debate that ensued in 1991–1994 over the proper size and character of our foreign policy (including health) for the Russian Federation.

USAID-Funded Health Assistance to the Russian Federation

U.S. foreign assistance on behalf of health for what were termed the New Independent States (NIS) began with a flourish. In 1991, the

U.S. foreign policy community suddenly faced a series of challenges (and opportunities) triggered by the dissolution of the Soviet empire. At the same time, international financial institutions such as the World Bank were handed a new set of members—the former constituent nations of the Soviet bloc. The principal focus initially was serving humanitarian goals in the face of the threat of a severe economic crisis in 1991.

Some of the earliest health and social assistance programs for Russia following the dissolution of the Soviet system were humanitarian and food assistance projects in 1992 and 1993. In January 1992, the U.S. Department of Defense, under the title Operation Provide Hope, delivered excess food, medicine, and medical supplies to Russia. The same year, the U.S. Department of Agriculture supported food assistance to Russia. Additionally, the U.S. government, in 1992 and 1993, purchased commodities for distribution by nine U.S. private volunteer organizations as charitable donations, and the Department of Defense transported hospital equipment and supplies from a decommissioned U.S. military hospital to Moscow and Vladivostok.

The most significant initiative began in 1992, with the convening of the Washington Coordinating Conference on Assistance to the New Independent States, headed by Secretary of State James Baker. The goal was to determine appropriate humanitarian assistance for the former Soviet states. Health and medicine were represented at that conference in the form of a medical working group, which in 1992 dispatched a delegation of 30 health care professionals from 13 countries to visit medical institutions in ten of the former Soviet republics. This delegation divided its numbers and tasks into three areas—public health, pharmaceutical materials, and hospitals and clinical medicine. The delegates were impressed by the extensiveness of the former Soviet system ("one that provided what every government attempts: access for care to the greatest number of people at reasonable cost"). The Russian hosts strongly admonished the delegation to limit humanitarian assistance. ("Humanitarian assistance can have an anesthetizing effect on the recipients, numbing them to the responsibility of blending their own good will with expressed determination to work hard and prioritize in the national interest.") A common plea from the Russian quarter was "help us to help ourselves."[1] The delegates foresaw a loosening of the authority of the centralized federal Ministry of Health, a further decline in the financial resources available to the health care system, and a resultant disenfranchisement of citizens from access to care.

A second series of reports on the worsening health situation was developed in late 1992. These reports focused on a breadth of public health issues and recommended a series of targeted humanitarian types of assistance.[2]

One of the principal outcomes of the medical working group's report was the most notable and productive of all of the health initiatives in the former Soviet republics supported by the U.S. Agency for International Development, commonly known as AID. This program, known as the Hospital Partnership Program, consisted of a series of partnership linkages between pairs of hospitals in the United States and in the former Soviet republics. Twenty-six partnerships were ultimately created, generally built around educational activities and professional exchanges concentrating on disease categories corresponding to the major burden of disease and contributors to excess mortality in the former Soviet realm. Principal examples were cardiovascular disease, diabetes, and infectious disease.

The Hospital Partnership Program was a perfect example of one of the things academic and practicing physicians can do best—impart a body of knowledge and experience to their professional counterparts. The program mobilized an eager segment of American medicine to devote voluntarily its time and expert knowledge. The program promised to confirm that professional exchanges bring with them the highest level of leverage. Those trained, in time, train others. Further, unlike most other AID-sponsored programs, which have been managed by outside AID contractors, the Hospital Partnership Program's architects established *de novo* a new, not-for-profit intermediary organization, the American International Health Alliance, devoted solely to this project, and awarded that privilege on a noncompetitive basis. Finally, on the scale of foreign assistance programs generally, it was relatively inexpensive. An initial budgetary allocation of $2.5 million for ten initial partnerships in the former Soviet republics was to be spent over a period of three years. In spite of this, the AID bureaucracy gave the Hospital Partnership Program very ambivalent support at best, and at times outright hostile opposition. The program had not been invented within the AID structure but rather brought to it from the outside. Its management arrangement bypassed the classic AID-contractor apparatus, and it was concerned with matters of clinical medicine—a subject generally alien to AID's interest or experience.

By far the most ambitious (and most expensive) AID-sponsored health program for the New Independent States was the Health Care Finance and Service Delivery Reform Project—ultimately known as the Health Reform Project. This project aspired to reshape the organization and financing of medical care in as many as five regions of the former Soviet Union. The reshaping was to hew to the fashions currently of interest in the United States—competition, market forces, and privatization. The orientation was entirely an economic and organizational one. Clinical medicine and its practitioners were actively excluded. As the original request for proposal stated, "The specific purpose of the Health Reform Project is to help increase economic efficiencies, quality of care, access, and provider choices in the NIS through market-oriented reforms in the health finance and delivery system."[3]

The AID contract for the Health Reform Project was awarded to an AID contractor who, in turn, enlisted a series of additional subcontractors. The principal contractor, Abt Associates, proceeded to "reform" the organization and financing of health care as commissioned in five regions of the NIS with an initial budget of $44 million and a proposed ultimate expenditure of $75 million. The strong orientation of this program toward reliance on current American principles—market forces and competition—was clearly out of phase with the political and economic realities of the time in Russia, whose health expenditures reached, at most, 3 percent of a declining GDP and whose employers were not paying employees' wages. Further, the Russians realized that the Americans' own experiment with these principles was a questionable pattern to follow. Finally, the imposition of institutions designed to increase efficiency threatened a large number of traditional Russian arrangements and personnel. Ultimately, the entire Health Reform Project was truncated—partly at the insistence of the Russian hosts, with no little embarrassment to the American operatives.[4]

The USAID health assistance program for Russia has included additional, less ambitious components. One of these, the Rational Pharmaceutical Management Project, administered by two AID contractors, had as its nominal goals the strengthening and automating of drug registration procedures, rationalizing of drug procurement and management of drug inventories, and promotion of the "rational" use of therapeutic drugs.[5] A more recent cooperative arrangement between USAID and the American Medical Association is aimed at "improving the re-professionalization of the physician community in Russia through the strengthening of professional organizations and the institution of a process of certification and accreditation of physicians' educational achievements."[6]

Lessons from the Past

It is useful to look at earlier examples of health-related foreign assistance deemed highly successful by later reviewers, to determine the ingredients of that success. Two examples are offered from a period prior to the establishment of AID in 1961. One is a health program in Latin America beginning in 1940. The other is a health-related foreign assistance effort in Greece that was part of the Truman Point Four program, beginning in 1947.

The Institute for Inter-American Affairs

Nelson Rockefeller assumed the post of coordinator for inter-American affairs in 1940. This position reflected Rockefeller's strong interest in Latin America and his and the president's desire to build economic and cultural linkages with the southern hemisphere.[7]

The impending European war brought a new urgency to the task of strengthening relationships with Latin American neighbors. Several southern hemisphere countries were sympathetic with German ambitions. As the probability of war approached, many believed that the stationing of U.S. troops and equipment at strategic locations in Latin America would become necessary. Information was needed. Removal of threats of malaria and other hazards of the endemic diseases of the tropics was a necessity. The goodwill of the nations and avoidance of political opposition were believed vital. Rockefeller saw the advantages of a specific health-related initiative to serve both humanitarian and strategic objectives.

In November 1941, Rockefeller approached the War Department with a proposal for a massive "Public Works Improvement" program in Latin America to be centered in locations likely to be chosen as U.S. bases. At the same time, in concert with cabinet members, Rockefeller developed a "Preparedness Program" that was to engage sanitary engineers and medical personnel.

This effort enjoyed the consistently strong support of President Roosevelt, who approved an initial request of $25 million on January 1, 1942 for a program whose primary objectives included the assurance of a safe and healthful environment for U.S. troops and for workers producing materials vital to the war effort. On March 24 of that year, Roosevelt authorized the coordinator to assume responsibility for an even broader series of projects in health, sanitation, nutrition, housing, transportation, and public works.[8] With the advice of the Rockefeller Foundation, the Institute for Inter-American Affairs was established as a quasi-governmental corporation in order to assure flexibility and freedom from the restrictions of general governmental operations.

Physicians and sanitary engineers were seconded from the Public Health Service and the military—many of whom remained in residence in Latin America for years. Steps were taken to engage close cooperation with the host governments through the establishment in each country of a *servicio* (Servicio Cooperativo Interamericano de Salud Publica, or SCISP) as the operational element—usually located within the ministry of health. The entire operation was directed by a distinguished tropical disease expert, Dr. George Dunham. The United States committed itself to a long-term project and a specific funding level—usually above 50 percent of the initial expense. The understanding in all cases was that the host Latin American country would eventually assume 100 percent of the cost. The institute eventually expanded its activities to 18 Latin American countries.

By 1944, the tide of war had turned against Germany, and the probability of its coming to the Americas had diminished. Rockefeller modified the list of goals from military to societal and commercial. In congressional hearings that year he argued that health measures in Latin America were important "not only from the point of view of immediate production of military support, but also from the point of view of laying foundations for the expansion of markets based on a rising standard of living."[9] By 1945, the coordinator reported that the "principal objective of the operations of the Institute [was] to promote economic development and economic stability by raising the standard in the other American republics."[10]

Looking backward, the Institute for Inter-American Affairs and its health and medical program were extremely successful. The program, from the beginning, was a closely collaborative one with the host governments—principally through the *servicios* within the governmental structures. It enjoyed substantial continuity and longevity, coming to an end only in 1958. The program, in collaboration with the Rockefeller Foundation, built hospitals, nursing schools, and health clinics, and supported training programs for visiting nurses and health education programs for the general public. It provided service, expert advice, and training to over 1,500 physicians in 18 Latin American countries. By 1945, 300 Latin Americans had received scholarships and travel grants to the United States.

The program had the personal attention and support of the president. Equally important, its constant promoter and defender, Nelson Rockefeller (the program incurred numerous jealousies and detractors), carefully linked its narrow health and medical goals to other prominent and overarching foreign policy and strategic goals.

Greece

On February 2, 1946, a little-known diplomat in Moscow, George Kennan, sent a now famous "long telegram" describing the threat of an expansionist Soviet Union. He proposed the "containment" of Soviet ambitions by encouraging the establishment of a barrier of stable and democratic states. This barrier of containment became the basis of the Truman Doctrine, announced in the president's speech in March 1947. Following World War II, Greece, by agreement, became a British protectorate. However, in February 1947 the British government secretly informed the United States that it would no longer supply assistance to Greece and Turkey. Within three weeks, on March 12, President Truman spoke before a joint session of Congress to request a major program for those two countries, at a cost of $400 million. The rationale was prevention of Greece's falling under the influence of Soviet communism, with the possible subsequent "collapse of free institutions and loss of independence." Truman pointed to the particular leadership role of the United States in maintaining peace.

This strong and unequivocal articulation of the Truman Doctrine led in July to the dispatching of a combined military and civilian mission—the American Mission for Aid to Greece. A civil war raged in that country. It had barely begun to rebuild after the ravages of World War II. The balance of payments was strongly in the direction of net indebtedness, threatening economic collapse and possible famine. By November, the American Mission had developed a strategy that included a combination of physical security, improving economic conditions, and a series of thrusts designed to improve health and social welfare.

The program lasted seven years and reached a peak in spending by 1950–1951. At that point, there were 181 American specialists and advisers in Greece—experts in agriculture, electric power, road building, civil aviation, health, labor union organization, income tax, and social security. The total expenditures for the seven years were $609 million.[11]

Once again, health was one of the instruments used to further larger foreign policy goals. Specialists developed rural potable water supplies, put in place programs to reduce malaria, and modernized hospitals and clinics. Once again, too, physicians and others were seconded from the U.S. Public Health Service to serve a variety of functions in Greece. In the course of this program, President Truman, in 1949, proposed his now famous fourth point of the foreign policy Point Four program, influenced interestingly by the success of the earlier Institute for Inter-American Affairs:

> ... to embark on a bold new program for making the benefits of our scientific advances and industrial progress available for the improvement and growth of underdeveloped areas. More than half the people of the world are living in conditions approaching misery. Their food is inadequate. They are victims of disease. Their economic life is primitive and stagnating. Their poverty is a handicap and a threat both to them and to more prosperous areas. For the first time in history, humanity possesses the knowledge and skill to relieve the suffering of these people. ... The material resources which we can afford to use for assistance of other peoples are limited. But our imponderable resources in technical knowledge are constantly growing and are inexhaustible.[12]

The Context: Broader Foreign Policy Goals

It is the observation of this author that our health-related foreign assistance to mature nations and transition economies works best not only for its humanitarian purposes, but as an instrument for the achievement of broader foreign policy goals. It is useful at this point to look back at the brief history of our general strategy for the Russian Federation following the breakup of the Soviet Union, to consider where health-related assistance might have played a more forthright role.

Beginning in 1992, a group of American economists, advisory to the Russian government, urged the devotion of a large fund of money, to be contributed by several Western governments, for the purpose of stabilizing the Russian economy and easing its transition from a centrally financed system to a market economy. Failure to persuade the governments of the G-7 countries on the first try led the advisers to craft a proposal for a $27 billion foreign assistance fund—partly from national governments, and partly from the international financial community. The rationale included assistance to the Russians in meeting a deepening financial crisis from both foreign debt and domestic credits, the urgent need for assistance to Russian industries both to produce for a market and to convert from defense-related activity, the need to help forestall a looming high inflationary crisis, and the need to assist the Russian citizenry through support of the social safety net and its components during the difficult period of economic and political transition.[13] Nearly one-third of the total financial assistance program was to be devoted to the "social fund," of which a substantial portion was earmarked for health.

The American advisers noted that, while Russian leaders had dedicated themselves to economic and political reform, the absence of Western financial assistance during the reform period had already begun to lead to a number of serious consequences—fiscal and social—for Russia. Economic hardships were increasing. The budget depended on inflationary financing, threatening to lead to hyperinflation. Social unrest was a possibility, and the reformers' own credibility was becoming undermined. Independently, others also saw the importance of attending to social safety net challenges during the economic and political transition.[14] Parallels were raised with the goals and achievements of the earlier Marshall Plan. Those who drew the comparisons characteristically noted the importance of health and a decent standard of living in assuring political stability.[15]

Once again, the advisers' position was not persuasive. Much discussion ensued then and more recently over the appropriateness of another "Marshall Plan–type" initiative for Russia.[16] Typically, arguments against the Marshall Plan formula for Russia rested on the historical absence of key economic and legal institutions in Russia. Critics emphasized that these institutions had never existed in Russia, in contrast with Western Europe, where they had simply been temporarily suspended because of the war.[17]

Absence of support for the general underlying idea of a stabilizing fund led the economic advisers, in 1994, to bring to the attention of the World Bank in stark terms the adverse consequences of temporizing further or, worse, of failing to craft a coherent strategy.[18] These consequences were described as the possible collapse of a nascent democracy in the face of highly unstable economic and political conditions. The advisers predicted possible serious instability, either through hyperinflation or catastrophic unemployment not cushioned by an adequate social safety net. The results, devastating not only for Russia but for the whole world, might include a "contagion of anti-social behavior"—tax evasion, flight from domestic currency, further inflation, and criminality. While late in the day, the proponents of assistance to Russia continued to urge a "well-designed combination of internal reforms and large-scale international assistance" for the purpose of social and economic stability.[19]

The larger, "Marshall Plan–type" of assistance and coherent strategy were not realized. There was no overarching program of economic stabilization to accompany political reform, and there was no corresponding social safety net component. Assistance in the social safety net sector, including health, has been piecemeal and without the type of coherence and long-term political support needed for a truly successful effort. The bilateral assistance from the U.S. government and that from the World Bank have been accompanied by a wide variety of individual efforts of varying character and motivation, sponsored by religious groups, individual initiatives, and nongovernmental organizations. These efforts have also not reflected an overall, coherent strategy.

Finally, it is perhaps instructive to look at the experience of another sector—rule of law—where the leadership of the legal profession in the United States assumed early on the direction of legal assistance to Russia and the NIS following the dissolution of the Soviet Union. Shortly after that event, the then leadership of the American Bar Association concluded that bringing the rule of law to the former Soviet republics and to Eastern and Central Europe was in the interest of both those nations and our own. With some anxiousness on the part of the bar membership, the leadership put in place a new institution, the Central and East European Law Initiative, designed to bring the voluntary contribution and experience of American attorneys and judges to bear on reforming legal systems abroad. The American Bar Association and the U.S. Congress have consistently supported AID funding over a period of a decade for this program. Approximately 5,000 American lawyers and judges have shared their expert knowledge and skills with their counterparts in Russia. The program has enjoyed continuity. It has been highly productive. Perhaps most important, the U.S. professional legal community early on seized the role of setting the character and dimensions of our rule-of-law foreign assistance to the NIS and Eastern Europe.

Conclusions and Lessons from This Experience

Success in the past in U.S. foreign assistance in the health field appears to have been due to a very clear articulation of goals. Perhaps most important, health and medicine have been considered not only in their humanitarian sense, but as instruments of a larger, overarching foreign policy objective. For the transition economies and Russia in particular, these two conditions—clear goal articulation and the presence of consistent larger foreign policy objectives—have not been unequivocally met. The U.S. government (as indeed, the community of Western governments) has exhibited a very unclear overarching foreign policy toward the Russian Federation since 1991, focusing varyingly on military-strategic issues, the economic and political transition, trade and commerce, and humanitarian needs. In the absence of clear resolve and, correspondingly, an already declining constituency favorably disposed toward appropriate foreign assistance generally, there has been little appetite for a bounded, clearly articulated set of foreign policy goals toward the former Soviet republics. Health could not be an instrument to further broader goals, as these broader goals were unclear. Assistance for health and medicine, purely as a humanitarian matter, has been given varying support since 1991, beginning with an initial flurry of enthusiasm followed by grudging support by the administering AID bureaucracy.

Concurrent with this ambivalent support and continuing debate over the United States' proper role, the philanthropic community of foundations backed away almost entirely from support of endeavors and institutions in Russia. Apart from the Fund for Open Society, the independent sector absented itself in wholesale fashion from concerns about health in the former Soviet republics, arguing that the dimensions of the challenge were so daunting as to claim all of their resources without measurable effect.

The West failed to agree on an overarching and coherent strategy for the transition economies. Opposition to any "Marshall Plan–type" activity prevailed—relying on the argument that the Russian Federation did not possess the traditions and institutions necessary to utilize assistance of that scale.[20] Political support for the concept was overwhelmed by political opposition.

Some of the predictions ventured by the proponents of a coherent strategy and financial assistance program have materialized, and some are still emerging: hyperinflation became a serious problem; central government control has been weakened; there has occurred a portfolio of anti-social behaviors including tax evasion, criminality, and flight from the domestic currency; and impacts on the social structure have been extremely harsh. In the words of one commentator, "the costs of societal transformation have proven to be more formidable than was originally anticipated and have fallen disproportionately on the shoulders of those who are the least able to bear them."[21]

What lessons can be taken from this narrative for foreign assistance in the health and social welfare sector? What are the key elements that have assured successful and productive programs in the past, and whose absence has limited the effectiveness of the recent health-related assistance to Russia?

The most successful health initiatives appear to have been not isolated elements of foreign aid but explicitly components of a larger foreign assistance strategy. Health assistance in Greece and in Latin America in the 1940s and 1950s was an instrument of an explicit, overarching foreign policy framework. With the end of the Cold War, the West and the United States were not able or politically willing to mount that larger effort. Consequently, the components of our technical assistance effort, including health, were treated with less than the threshold support required to assure fully effective results.

The outstanding health and social assistance programs of the past enjoyed the strong and unequivocal support of leaders who understood the strategic importance of supporting health assistance as a security issue as well as a humanitarian gesture. Those leaders defended health programs against detractors and critics, not uncommonly crafting the political rationale so as to blunt opponents' criticisms, but always couching those messages in language understandable to the electorate at large. Indeed, the organized effort by the administration to educate the American public and work with Congress toward acceptance of the Marshall Plan was extraordinarily impressive. A special citizens' Committee for the Marshall Plan, comprising a breadth of economic and social interests, was organized to inform the American people of the plan and to enlist their support. In Congress, the foreign affairs committees of both houses and a newly created select committee prepared the members thoroughly and systematically, with extensive consultation with the executive branch.[22] Interestingly, as one commentator has noted, assistance to the republics of the former Soviet Union early on enjoyed broad bipartisan support in Congress, but this support was eventually supplanted by a crescendo of concerns for the form and details of implementation of that assistance.[23]

Important features of past efforts included the promise of continuity over a sufficient period of time to realize intended goals, administrative arrangements that assured flexibility and relief from some of the constraints of governmental management, and the strong and consistent support of the president himself. Cooperative administrative and professional linkages with host governments are clearly important. Finally, past technical assistance efforts for health relied at times heavily on the advice of outside, seasoned experts. These kinds of collaborations assure the technical quality of health-related assistance programs and add an important political constituency to the programs' support that a government bureaucracy by itself cannot furnish.

NOTES

1. Medical Working Group, Experts Delegation to the New Independent States, "Country Reports" (for presentation to the Coordinating Conference on Assistance to the New Independent States, Lisbon, 23–24 May 1992).

2. International Federation of Red Cross and Red Crescent Societies, "Medical Assessments and Public Health Reports from the Former Soviet Union," a collection of reports written, compiled, or translated by Lawrence M. Probes, M.D., Public Health Delegate, Moscow Regional Delegation, February-October 1992.

3. U.S. Agency for International Development, Request for Proposal (RFP) Number OP/CC/N-93–16, "Health Care Finance and Service Delivery Reform Project No. 110–0004," 4 August 4 1993.

4. P. J. Stavrakis, "Bull in a China Shop: USAID's Post-Soviet Mission," *Demokratizatsiya* 4, no. 21 (1996): 247–270.

5. A. Savelli, J.-P. Sallet, A. Zagorski, O. Duzey, and H. Haak, "Ryazan Oblast Rational Pharmaceutical Management Project: Russian Pharmaceutical Sector" (Management Sciences for Health, Arlington, VA, November 1994).

6. Program Description, "Cooperative Agreement between USAID and the American Medical Association for a Program," 1997.

7. C. Reich, *The Life of Nelson A. Rockefeller* (New York: Doubleday, 1996); C. Erb., *Nelson Rockefeller and U.S.-Latin American Relations, 1940–1945,* Ph.D. thesis, Clark University, Worcester, MA.

8. Erb, *Nelson Rockefeller.*

9. U.S. House of Representatives, Hearings on the National War Agencies Appropriations Bill, 1994: 140–141.

10. Coordinator for Inter-American Affairs, "Annual Report of the Institute of Inter-American Affairs for the fiscal year ending June 30, 1945."

11. J. C. Warren, "Origins of the 'Greek Economic Miracle': The Truman Doctrine and Marshall Plan Development and Stabilization Programs," in *The Truman Doctrine of Aid to Greece: A Fifty-Year Retrospective,* ed. E. T. Rossides (New York: The Academy of Political Science, and Washington, D.C.: The American Hellenic Institution Foundation, 1998).

12. Public Papers of the Presidents, Harry S Truman, Washington, D.C., 1964, 114; and B. Kondis, "The United States' Role in the Greek Civil War," in Rossides, *The Truman Doctrine.*

13. J. Sachs and P. Boone, "Strengthening Western Support for Russia's Economic Reforms," unpublished memorandum, 28 December 1992.

14. P. Ackerman and E. Balls, "Financing the Russian Safety Net" (Center for the Study of Financial Innovation, London, September 1993).

15. J. M. Silberman and C. Weiss, "Restructuring for Productivity: The Technical Assistance Program of the Marshall Plan as a Precedent for the Former Soviet Union," paper written for the Industry Development Division, Operations and Sector Policy, Vice Presidency, The

World Bank, Washington, D.C., November 1992; and C. Dahlman, unpublished memorandum to Russell Cheetham, The World Bank, 10 November 1992.

16. C. Tarnoff, "The Marshall Plan: Design, Accomplishments, and Relevance to the Present," Report #97–62F, Congressional Research Service, The Library of Congress, Washington, D.C., 6 January 1997; W. W. Rostow, "Lessons of the Plan: Looking Forward to the Next Century," in *The Marshall Plan and Its Legacy: A Foreign Affairs Reader,* P. Grouse, ed. (New York: Foreign Affairs, 1997); L. Gordon, "The Marshall Plan and the Former Soviet Union," remarks presented at the symposium "Lessons from the Era of the Marshall Plan," Harvard University, 4 June 1997.

17. Gordon, "The Marshall Plan."

18. Dahlman, unpublished memorandum.

19. J. D. Sachs, "Russia's Struggle with Stabilization: Conceptual Issues and Evidence" (paper prepared for Annual Bank Conference on Development Economies, The World Bank, Washington, D.C., 28–29 April 1994).

20. Sachs and Boone, "Strengthening Western Support."

21. Z. Ferge, "Social Policy Challenges and Dilemmas in Ex-Socialist Systems," in *Transforming Post-Communist Political Economies,* ed. National Academy of Sciences (Washington, D.C.: National Academy Press, 1997).

22. H. B. Price, *The Marshall Plan and Its Meaning* (Ithaca, NY: Cornell University Press, 1995).

23. C. Tarnoff, "The Former Soviet Union and U.S. Foreign Aid: Implementing the Assistance Program," Report #95–170F, Congressional Research Service, The Library of Congress, Washington, D.C., 18 January 1995.

CONTRIBUTORS

MARK G. FIELD is an associate of the Davis Center for Russian Studies and an adjunct professor, School of Public Health at Harvard University. He is also emeritus professor at Boston University and a senior sociologist at the Department of Psychiatry at the Massachusetts General Hospital. He holds the A.B., A.M., and Ph.D. degrees from Harvard University. His major professional interests are health conditions and health care in the former Soviet Union and comparative health care systems.

JUDYTH L. TWIGG is an assistant professor of political science at Virginia Commonwealth University. She holds a B.S. in physics from Carnegie Mellon University, an M.A. in political science from the University of Pittsburgh, and a Ph.D. in political science from the Massachusetts Institute of Technology. Her research interests center on the reform of health care structure and financing in Russia. She has published articles on this topic in *Europe-Asia Studies, Social Science and Medicine, The American Journal of Public Health, Transition,* and *Health and Place,* among other journals. Her work in this area has been funded by the Social Science Research Council, the National Council on Eurasian and East European Research, and the International Research and Exchanges Board.

DEBORAH YARSIKE BALL is a political-military analyst specializing in Russian affairs in the Nonproliferation, Arms Control, and International Security Directorate at Lawrence Livermore National Laboratory. She has been a fellow at Harvard University's Center for Science and International Affairs, as well as Stanford's Center for International Security and Arms Control. Her current work focuses on preventing the theft of weapons-usable nuclear material from the former Soviet Union. Her other interests include the safety and security of nuclear weapons in the former Soviet Union, Russian military and political affairs, and civil-military relations. Her articles have appeared in journals such as *Jane's Intelligence Review, Post-Soviet Affairs,* and *Armed Forces and Society.*

JULIE V. BROWN is associate professor of sociology at the University of North Carolina at Greensboro. She is the author of a number of articles on socio-cultural aspects of health and illness, responses to mental disabilities, the medical care system, and medical professionals in Russia and the Soviet Union.

CYNTHIA BUCKLEY is associate professor of sociology and the Associate Director of the Center for Russian, East European and Eurasian Studies at the University of Texas. She is the author of several articles on the social demography of the former Soviet Union. Her work presently focuses upon intergenerational wealth transfers and pension reform across the region.

EDWARD J. BURGER, JR., M.D., SC.D., is director of the Institute for Health Policy Analysis, Washington, D.C. He is a former member of the faculty of the Harvard School of Public Health and was a professor at Georgetown University Medical School. As a member of the staff of the White House Office of the President's Science Advisor in the 1970s, Dr. Burger was responsible for fostering a series of cooperative medical, scientific, and environmental agreements with the Soviet Union during the period of détente. Over the past several years, he has been deeply involved in U.S.-Russian health and medical policy issues. He currently directs a program of the American College of Physicians for continuing medical education for Russian physicians.

JUSTIN BURKE received a B.A. in Soviet and Eastern European Studies from Boston University. He worked as a Moscow correspondent for the *Christian Science Monitor* from June 1990 until November 1993. Among the events that he covered were the Moscow coup attempts of August 1991 and October 1993, the conflicts in Moldova, Tajikistan, and the Nagorno-Karabakh region of Azerbaijan, and the fall of Najibullah's regime in Afghanistan. During the 1995–1996 academic year, he was a visiting scholar at the Davis Center for Russian Studies at Harvard University. From 1996 to 1999, he was the associate director/editorial manager of the Forced Migration Projects of the Open Society Institute.

WALTER D. CONNOR is professor of political science, sociology, and international relations at Boston University, and a fellow of the Davis Center for Russian Studies at Harvard University. Before coming to Boston University, he was a member of the faculty at the University of Michigan (1968–76), and served in the U.S. Department of State (1976–84). Most recent among his several books is *Tattered Banners: Labor, Conflict, and Corporatism in Post-Communist Russia.*

DENNIS DONAHUE is a graduate student in the department of sociology and a research trainee at the Population Research Center at the University of Texas. His research interests are poverty, stratification, and global demographic trends. His M.A. research focuses on occupational changes and structural inequalities in the Russian Federation.

ETHEL DUNN is executive secretary of Highgate Road Social Science Research Station. She has an M.A. in history and a certificate from the Russian Institute at Columbia University. She and Stephen P. Dunn are the authors of *The Peasants of Central Russia* (1967, reissued in 1988 with a new introduction). The disabled in Russia represent her major research interest, but she has also written on sectarians in Russia, the Small Peoples of the far north, on women and the family, on Central Asia and Kazakstan, and on current developments in rural Russia.

KEVIN KINSELLA is a study director with the Committee on Population of the National Research Council in Washington, D.C. He presently directs projects involving the development of an international research agenda on aging, and the collection of bioindicators in population-based surveys. Prior to his assignment to the National Research Council, Kinsella was chief of the Aging Studies Branch, International Programs Center, U.S. Census Bureau, where he had been employed since 1979. His professional activities have focused on the role of women in development, population projections for developing countries (particularly in Latin America), and the demography of aging internationally.

JOHN M. KRAMER is Distinguished Professor of Political Science, Mary Washington College, Fredericksburg, Virginia, and concurrently serves as professor, department of strategy and policy, United States Naval War College, Newport, Rhode Island. He is a former research associate of the Russian Research Center at Harvard University, and a Fulbright-Hays fellow in Czechoslovakia and Yugoslavia. He has authored *The Energy Gap in Eastern Europe* (DC Heath, 1990) and numerous articles on political and social issues in post-communist polities.

DAVID E. POWELL is the Shelby Cullom Davis Professor of Russian Studies at Wheaton College (Norton, MA) and an associate of the Davis Center for Russian Studies, Harvard University. He is the author or editor of four books as well as dozens of articles on various social, economic, and political issues in the Soviet Union and post-Soviet Russia.

NINA L. RUSINOVA is senior researcher at the St. Petersburg Branch of the Institute of Sociology of the Russian Academy of Sciences. She has written numerous articles on social aspects of health care, health policy, and health reform in Russia and the USSR.

KATE SCHECTER has worked as a consultant for the World Bank for the last two years, specializing in health care reform and child welfare issues in the former Soviet Union and Eastern and Central Europe. She taught political science at the University of Michigan from 1993 to 1997. In 1997, she received a grant from the National Council for Soviet and East European Research to do research on the politics of health care reform in Russia. She has written extensively about the Soviet socialized health care system and recently published three chapters in *Physicians in New Worlds: Immigration of Physicians from the Former Soviet Union to Israel, Canada, and the United States* (Praeger Press, 1998). She received her M.A. in Soviet studies from Harvard University, and Ph.D. in political science from Columbia University. In addition, she has made three documentary films for PBS about the former Soviet Union, and is the co-author of *Back in the USSR* (Scribner's, 1988) and *An American Family in Moscow* (Little, Brown, 1975), two journalistic accounts of living in the USSR.

VALERIE SPERLING received her Ph.D. in political science from the University of California, Berkeley, in 1997. She spent the following year on a postdoctoral fellowship at Harvard University's Davis Center for Russian Studies. She is currently a visiting assistant professor at Clark University. Her book on the emergence and development of the Russian women's movement, *Organizing Women in Contemporary Russia: Engendering Transition,* was published by Cambridge University Press in October 1999.

VICTORIA VELKOFF is acting chief of the Aging Studies Branch, International Programs Center, U.S. Bureau of the Census, where she has been employed since 1991. She has a B.A. in economics and an M.A. in Russian and East European Studies from the University of Michigan. She has a Ph.D. in sociology and demography from Princeton University. While at the census bureau, Dr. Velkoff's professional activities have been concentrated in two areas: aging and women in development. Her latest research has focused on gender and aging throughout the world, centenarians, and caregiving.

INDEX